AF566467

Gastroesophageal Reflux Disease

Gastroenterology and Hepatology

Executive Editor

J. Thomas LaMont, M.D.

Chief, Division of Gastroenterology
Beth Israel Hospital
Boston, Massachusetts
and
Charlotte F. and Irving W. Rabb Professor of Medicine
Harvard Medical School
Boston, Massachusetts

1. *Crohn's Disease*, edited by Cosimo Prantera and Burton I. Korelitz
2. *Clinical Gastroenterology in the Elderly*, edited by Alvin M. Gelb
3. *Biliary and Pancreatic Ductal Epithelia: Pathobiology and Pathophysiology,* edited by Alphonse E. Sirica and Daniel S. Longnecker
4. *Viral Hepatitis: Diagnosis • Treatment • Prevention*, edited by Richard A. Willson
5. *Gastrointestinal Infections: Diagnosis and Management*, edited by J. Thomas LaMont
6. *Gastroesophageal Reflux Disease*, edited by Roy C. Orlando

ADDITIONAL VOLUMES IN PREPARATION

Gastroesophageal Reflux Disease

edited by

Roy C. Orlando
Tulane University Medical School
New Orleans, Louisiana

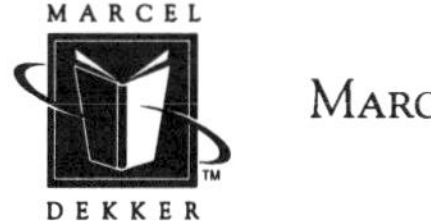

Marcel Dekker, Inc. New York • Basel

ISBN: 0-8247-0389-8

This book is printed on acid-free paper.

Headquarters
Marcel Dekker, Inc.
270 Madison Avenue, New York, NY 10016
tel: 212-696-9000; fax: 212-685-4540

Eastern Hemisphere Distribution
Marcel Dekker AG
Hutgasse 4, Postfach 812, CH-4001 Basel, Switzerland
tel: 41-61-261-8482; fax: 41-61-261-8896

World Wide Web
http://www.dekker.com

The publisher offers discounts on this book when ordered in bulk quantities. For more information, write to Special Sales/Professional Marketing at the headquarters address above.

Current printing (last digit):
10 9 8 7 6 5 4 3 2 1

PRINTED IN THE UNITED STATES OF AMERICA

To My Mother, Father, Sister, Wife, and Children

Preface

Common and complex, gastroesophageal reflux disease (GERD) has seen an explosion in interest from both lay and scientific communities. As a result, information has been pouring in. And no wonder—symptoms and signs of GERD seem to be everywhere, affecting millions of people on every continent and in a variety of ways. On one hand, they masquerade innocently enough as heartburn, yet, on the other, they represent an insidious disorder that can lead to esophageal epithelial destruction, Barrett's esophagus, and esophageal adenocarcinoma—a deadly cancer whose frequency has increased dramatically in the past half-century. GERD, however, is not confined to the esophagus; it represents one of the known causes for such commonplace diseases of the oropharynx and airways as laryngitis, pharyngitis, pneumonia, and asthma. Not surprisingly, then, given the breadth of pathology, physicians and other healthcare providers are confronted with a wide range of important questions about its cause, natural history, and risks, in addition to the appropriate application of diagnostic tests and therapeutic medical and surgical approaches. Indeed, the therapeutic landscape for GERD and its complications has changed materially—with antacids, the old standard bearer, giving way to increasingly more powerful acid-suppressant and prokinetic medications, and surgically with traditional open fundoplication competing effectively with laparoscopic fundoplication. Moreover, endoscopic laser-based photodynamic therapy has emerged as a novel method of ablating dysplastic and superficial neoplastic tissue in Barrett's esophagus, and endoscopic treatment of esophageal strictures has improved as a result of refinements in stent technology.

Given the explosion of interest, information, and technology in GERD, this represents an ideal time to take stock and assess where we are and what gaps remain to be filled. Toward this end, we have assembled an international group of recognized experts to produce this state-of-the-art volume covering all aspects of GERD: epidemiology (Chap. 3), risk factors (Chap. 2), pathophysiology (Chaps. 5 and 6), clinical course and manifestations (Chap. 1), diagnostic testing (Chap. 4), medical treatment (Chap. 10), surgical treatment (Chap. 11), esophageal complications such as stricture and Barrett's esophagus (Chaps. 7 and 8), and extraesophageal complications such as laryngitis and asthma (Chap. 9). In addition, Chapter 12 provides in-depth coverage of GERD in infants and children. Readers of this book should also take note that there are two chapters on the pathophysiology of GERD: Chapter 5 covers the esophageal antireflux and acid clearance mechanisms and Chapter 6 covers the noxious elements in the gastric refluxate and factors comprising tissue resistance. This division was not arbitrary but a means to explore two divergent views on the pathophysiology of GERD. Chapter 5 reflects the current view that GERD is a motor disorder and Chapter 6 reflects a contrary view, that GERD is in part, if not completely, an epithelial disorder (shades of *H. pylori* and peptic ulcer disease). In summary, based on the effort expended by the authors in creation of this work on GERD, we expect readers in the field of healthcare to come away with a better appreciation of our current knowledge about this intriguing disorder.

Roy C. Orlando

Contents

Contributors

Eugene M. Bozymski, M.D., F.A.C.P., F.A.C.G. Professor of Medicine and Chief of Endoscopy, Department of Medicine, University of North Carolina, Chapel Hill, North Carolina

W. Keith Fackler, M.D. Center for Swallowing and Esophageal Disorders, Department of Gastroenterology, Cleveland Clinic Foundation, Cleveland, Ohio

Walter J. Hogan, M.D. Professor of Medicine and Radiology, Division of Gastroenterology and Hepatology, Department of Medicine, Medical College of Wisconsin, Milwaukee, Wisconsin

John David Horwhat, M.D. Walter Reed Army Medical Center, Washington, D.C., and Uniformed Services University of the Health Sciences, Bethesda, Maryland

Peter J. Kahrilas, M.D. Marquardt Professor of Medicine, Division of Gastroenterology and Hepatology, Department of Medicine, Northwestern University Medical School, Chicago, Illinois

Lars R. Lundell, M.D., Ph.D. Professor, Department of Surgery, Sahlgren's University Hospital, Gothenburg, Sweden

Peter R. McNally, D.O. Gastrointestinal Section, Department of Medicine, Dwight D. Eisenhower Army Medical Center, Fort Gordon, Georgia

Susan R. Orenstein, M.D. Professor and Chief, Department of Pediatric Gastroenterology, University of Pittsburgh School of Medicine and Children's Hospital of Pittsburgh, Pittsburgh, Pennsylvania

Roy C. Orlando, M.D. Chief, Section of Gastroenterology and Hepatology and Professor, Department of Medicine, Tulane University Medical School, New Orleans, Louisiana

Dawn Provenzale, M.D., M.S. Director, GI Outcomes Research, Department of Gastroenterology, Duke University Medical Center, Durham, North Carolina

Joel E. Richter, M.D. Chairman and Professor, Department of Gastroenterology, and Director, Center for Swallowing and Esophageal Disorders, Cleveland Clinic Foundation, Cleveland, Ohio

Nicholas J. Shaheen, M.D., M.P.H. Assistant Professor, Department of Medicine, University of North Carolina, Chapel Hill, North Carolina

Reza Shaker, M.D. Professor and Chief, Division of Gastroenterology and Hepatology, and Director, MCW Dysphagia Institute, Department of Medicine, Medical College of Wisconsin, Milwaukee, Wisconsin

Guoxiang Shi, M.D., Ph.D. Research Assistant, Division of Gastroenterology and Hepatology, Northwestern University Medical School, Chicago, Illinois

Stuart John Spechler, M.D. Chief, Division of Gastroenterology, Department of Medicine, Dallas Veterans Affairs Medical Center, Dallas, Texas

Guido N. J. Tytgat, M.D., Ph.D., F.R.C.P. Professor, Department of Gastroenterology and Hepatology, Academic Medical Center, Amsterdam, The Netherlands

Roy K. H. Wong, M.D. Chief, Gastroenterology Service, Walter Reed Army Medical Center, Washington, D.C., and Director, Division of Digestive Diseases, Uniformed Services University of the Health Sciences, Bethesda, Maryland

Gastroesophageal Reflux Disease

1

Clinical Manifestations, Natural History, and Differential Diagnosis of Reflux Esophagitis

Peter R. McNally
Dwight D. Eisenhower Army Medical Center, Fort Gordon, Georgia

INTRODUCTION

Gastroesophageal reflux disease (GERD) is an extremely common disorder, but it has many "faces," in terms of symptoms and signs of *esophageal* damage produced by gastroesophageal reflux. The material in this chapter will review the clinical manifestations, natural history, and differential diagnosis of GERD. The extraesophageal symptoms and signs of GERD are covered in another chapter.

CLINICAL MANIFESTATIONS

Symptoms

Heartburn

The most common manifestation of GERD is heartburn (1,2). Usually, heartburn is described as a burning sensation located behind the sternum. Patients often place an open hand over the sternum and wave it from the xiphoid to the neck to relate a sensation of discomfort moving to and fro. These symptoms occur typically after meals (3), especially when reclining after a large meal high in fat

---

The opinions and assertions contained herein are the private views of the author and are not to be construed as reflecting the view of the Department of the Army or the Department of Defense.

content (4). The initial symptoms of heartburn for women frequently manifest during pregnancy (5). The heartburn experienced during pregnancy usually remits postpartum, but offers a sound historical reference to compare with digestive complaints later in life. Mild heartburn usually improves with consumption of buffering substances such as antacids, baking soda, or milk, which act to both neutralize acidic reflux and stimulate esophageal peristalsis, which clears the esophagus of any gastric refluxate (6). The presence of heartburn symptoms is helpful in establishing the diagnosis of GERD; however, the frequency and the severity of the symptoms are not helpful in establishing the degree of mucosal damage seen endoscopically (7).

A cause-and-effect relationship between the exposure to a known precipitant of gastroesophageal reflux and the symptoms of heartburn are often present and helpful in making the diagnosis of GERD. Numerous foods, lifestyles, drugs, and medical conditions are associated with heartburn; see Table 1.

A consistent relationship between the onset of heartburn symptoms and meal composition is common (8,9). The acidity and/or hyperosmolarity of cola beverages, tomato juice, and citrus juices can directly irritate esophageal mucosa and precipitate symptoms (10). After-dinner liqueurs containing carminatives and

Table 1 Common Causes of Heartburn

Food	Lifestyle and activities	Drugs and medications	Medical conditions
Alcohol	Bending, stooping	Alcohol (distilled spirits, wine, beer)	CREST
Carminatives (spearmint, peppermint)	Cycling	Alpha-adrenergic antagonists (phentolamine)	Diabetes mellitus
Chocolate	Reclining or horizontal position after eating	Anticholinergics	Pregnancy
Citrus fruit juices	Tight-fitting garments	Beta-adrenergic agonists (isoproterenol)	Prolonged NG tube
Coffee (caffeinated and decaffeinated)		Calcium channel antagonists	Raynaud's syndrome
Cola beverages		Diazepam	Scleroderma
Fat		Nitrates	Sjögren's and sicca syndrome
Tomato juice/food		Progesterone	Xerostomia (head and neck irradiation)
		Smooth muscle relaxants	Zollinger-Ellison syndrome
		Tobacco or nicotine (smoked, chewed, or patches)	

chocolate or fatty foods can either directly or indirectly promote relaxation of the lower esophageal sphincter (LES) and predispose to gastroesophageal reflux. Coffee (caffeinated and decaffeinated) and tea have also been reported to cause heartburn (11). Finally, alcohol can promote esophageal injury by penetration of the cytoprotective esophageal mucus layer, disruption of tight junctions between squamous epithelium, and inhibition of the LES (12).

Certain lifestyles and activities of daily living can precipitate heartburn. Assuming a reclining or horizontal position after eating is notorious for precipitating heartburn in those predisposed (13). Loss of the gravitational effect on gastroesophageal emptying and the truncation of the distance from the ruminant meniscus to the LES are thought to be responsible. Exercise promoting abdominal Valsalva and bending or stooping, especially after eating, can predispose to gastroesophageal reflux and heartburn as well (14).

Many medical conditions predispose to symptoms of heartburn. Rheumatological disorders such as Raynaud's syndrome, scleroderma, and CREST (calcinosis, Raynaud's phenomenon, esophageal dysmotility, sclerodactyly, telangiectasias) are associated with esophageal dysmotility characterized by impaired esophageal clearance, hypotonic LES pressure, and delayed gastric emptying (15–17). Progressive systemic sclerosis (PSS) with diffuse scleroderma is the most virulent form. It is seen predominantly in white women, aged 40–50 years (18). Esophageal disease is reported in 70–90% of PSS cases and usually correlates with the presence of Raynaud's phenomenon (19). The reflux disease associated with these rheumatological disorders is much more virulent than seen in idiopathic GERD. In idiopathic GERD the incidence of peptic stricture and Barrett's esophagus is 5–7% and 10%, respectively, while in PSS 40.6% of patients have strictures and 37% have been reported to have Barrett's esophagus (20–23).

Patients with long-standing diabetes mellitus can have significant symptoms of heartburn (24). The severity of GERD associated with diabetes mellitus correlates with duration of disease and the presence of gastropathy and retinopathy. Neurological and myopathic damage to the stomach and esophagus can impair gastroesophageal clearance and basal LES sphincter pressure leading to GERD (25).

Women often experience their first symptoms of heartburn during pregnancy (26–29). Two physiological factors are responsible for pregnancy-related heartburn. First, the higher gestational levels of estrogen and progesterone inhibit LES pressure, and second, the mechanical pressure of the gravid uterus against the stomach promotes gastroesophageal reflux. While the inhibitory effects of estrogen and progesterone are maximal on the LES during the first trimester and resolve postpartum, the mechanical effects of the gravid uterus on the stomach and LES may lead to the most severe symptoms during the last trimester (30).

Heartburn symptoms in the presence of diarrhea or duodenal ulcers unrelated to *Helicobacter pylori* infection should always alert the clinician to the possibility of Zollinger-Ellison syndrome (ZES). Miller and others have reported 40–60% of patients with ZES will have severe GERD (31,32).

Indwelling nasogastric tubes can act like a wick that promotes gastroesophageal reflux (33). Injury can be profound with long esophageal erosions and strictures. Injury usually requires 5–7 days, but more rapid onset can occur when gastric acid suppression is inadequate or when gastric outlet obstruction is present (34).

Saliva is vital to the natural defense of the esophagus against reflux injury (35). The act of swallowing bicarbonate-rich saliva acts to both buffer refluxed gastric acid and promote peristaltic clearance (36). The mucopurulent saliva is also an important component to the cytoprotective layer of the esophagus (35). Xerostomia due to head and neck irradiation, Sjögren's and sicca syndromes are predisposing factors for the development of GERD (37,38).

Regurgitation

Regurgitation is the effortless retropulsion of gastric contents through the esophagus into the oral cavity without nausea, retching, or abdominal contractions. Frequently it occurs with a belch, bending, or other maneuver that increases intra-abdominal pressure (39,40). The regurgitated gastric contents often have a bitter or acidic taste. A history of bilious stains on the pillowcase may suggest nocturnal regurgitation.

Water Brash

Water brash refers to a foaming at the mouth caused by hyperproduction of salivary juice. In contrast to regurgitation, water brash is not bitter; it has a salty or a bland water-like taste. The sialorrhea seen in water brash is mediated by the presence of acid in the esophagus that stimulates a vagal, esophagosalivary reflex (41,42). Increased saliva production promotes swallowing and peristaltic clearance of the esophagus. The saliva itself is a bicarbonate-rich slime important in restoring local esophageal cytoprotection and buffering residual esophageal acid film (43,44).

Dysphagia

Dysphagia is the symptom of impaired transit of a swallowed bolus (45). These symptoms are seen in up to 40% of patients with long-standing GERD and may herald the presence of an esophageal stricture, esophageal dysmotility, Schatzki ring, or even esophageal carcinoma (46,47). The occurrence of dysphagia to solid foods is characteristic of obstructive etiologies, while dysphagia to liquids suggests esophageal dysmotility. When the dysphagia occurs primarily with solids, and is rapidly progressive with significant associated weight loss, esophageal carcinoma should be suspected.

Odynophagia

Odynophagia is the symptom of painful swallowing. This symptom is usually described as a sharp or lancinating pain located behind the sternum. Although severe erosive esophagitis or esophageal ulceration from reflux can cause painful swallowing, both are uncommon causes of odynophagia. Symptoms of odynophagia should always suggest the possibility of infectious or pill-induced esophagitis; see Table 2.

The most common esophageal infections reported to cause odynophagia are *Candida* sp., herpes simplex virus (HSV), cytomegalovirus (CMV), and human immunodeficiency virus (HIV) (48). Esophageal infections are usually preceded by immune suppression, such as AIDS, chemotherapy, diabetes mellitus, and corticosteroids (49–53). In the setting of AIDS, esophageal infections are often multiple and more complicated.

Table 2 Causes of Odynophagia

Infectious esophagitis	Pill-induced esophagitis
Common	Most common drugs listed
Candida sp.	Alendronate (Fosamax)
Cytomegalovirus (CMV)	Antibiotics (doxy-tetracycline, clindamycin, trimethoprim-sulfa)
Herpes simplex virus (HSV)	Ascorbic acid
Human immunodeficiency virus (HIV)	Empromium bromide (not available in the U.S.)
Uncommon	Ferrous sulfate
Actinomycosis	Nifedipine (procardia XL, slow release)
Aspergillosis	NSAIDs (ASA, indomethacin, ibuprofen, naprosyn)
Bacterial esophagitis	Potassium chloride (slow-release preparations)
Human papilloma virus	Quinidine gluconate (Quiniglute)
Tuberculosis	Theophylline
Varicella	Zidovudine (AZT)
Risk factors: immune suppression: HIV, diabetes mellitus, chemotherapeutic drugs, broad-spectrum antibiotics, corticosteroids (inhaled, oral, or parenteral)	Risk factors: anatomical: strictures, extrinsic compression from aorta, left atrium; pill characteristics: large size, slow release, acidic coat; how consumed: prior to sleep with little or no water

Over 70 drugs are said to cause pill-induced esophagitis (54,55). Odynophagia and retrosternal chest pain are the most common symptoms of pill esophagitis. The mucosal injury caused by pills can be profound; reports of inflammatory esophageal mass with stricture formation and even esophageal perforation have been reported (56,57). Esophageal anatomy, pill composition, and the manner in which pills are taken can predispose to pill esophagitis. Points of esophageal stasis from the aortic arch, left atrium, or strictures may offer a nidus for pills to stick and slowly leach mucosal irritants. Taking pills with little or no water and retiring to bed shortly thereafter promotes slow pill transit through the esophagus and increased contact time with the mucosa (58). Several medications are commonly associated with pill esophagitis in the elderly, i.e., Alendronate, ASA, NSAIDs, potassium chloride, and quinidine gluconate (59–61).

Noncardiac (Atypical) Chest Pain (NCCP)

The esophagus and heart have similar embryonic evolution. Hence many afferent sensory pathways are shared, rendering some similarities between esophageal and cardiac pain (62). Although, the pain from heartburn is usually mild to moderate in severity, some patients may experience severe chest pain descriptively identical to classic angina: crushing retrosternal pressure sensation with radiation over the precordium to the neck, jaw, or left upper extremity, associated with diaphoresis, shortness of breath, and a sense of impending doom (63). Symptoms of heartburn usually occur after meals, while symptoms of angina usually occur with exertion or activity that accelerates heart rate and systolic pressure (double product) beyond the capacity of coronary arterial flow (64). When angina occurs at rest it is considered unstable or due to coronary vasospasm—Prinzmetal or variant angina (65). Research on patients with known coronary artery disease has suggested that the pain from severe heartburn can lead to a sympathetic reflex increase in double product and precipitate reversible ischemic chest pain (66,67). Although the symptoms of chest pain caused by esophageal disease may be severe, they never lead to death. It is imperative to always prioritize the cardiac evaluation and management of all patients with severe chest pain.

The difficulty in discriminating between chest pain caused by coronary versus esophageal disease was emphasized by a recent study by Voskuil et al. (68). They studied 28 patients referred to a cardiologist for evaluation of ''anginal'' chest pain. All patients underwent independent history and examination by a specialist in cardiology and gastroenterology, followed by comprehensive cardiac and gastrointestinal evaluations. History taken by a cardiologist correctly predicted angina in only 40% of cases, while history by a gastroenterologist was accurate in predicting esophageal origin in only 30% of cases.

The esophageal causes of NCCP are rooted in multiple origins, including both acid-reflux-mediated pain and acid-reflux-precipitated esophageal dysmotility (69,70). Other nonacid-reflux causes of NCCP include primary esophageal dysmotility (nutcracker, diffuse esophageal spasm, nonspecific esophageal dysmotility syndrome), the newly characterized NCCP syndrome of ''hypersensitive, hyperactive, and poorly compliant esophagus,'' altered nociception, and a variety of psychiatric disorders including panic attacks (71–74). Overall, most authorities suggest that GERD accounts for 50% of unexplained NCCP, about one-third of cases are due to esophageal dysmotility or esophageal noncompliance, and the remainder are due to musculoskeletal, psychiatric, or other causes (62).

Clinical Signs

Gastrointestinal Bleeding

Heme-Occult-Positive Stool. Occult bleeding from esophagitis is common. Some reports describe positive fecal occult tests in over a quarter of patients with Barrett's esophagus (75,76). However, the esophagus is not the sole source of occult bleeding in many of these cases.

Hematemesis. It has been estimated that esophagitis is the source of bleeding in 2–6% of patients presenting with upper gastrointestinal hemorrhage (77,78). Four factors appear to predispose to esophageal bleeding: Barrett's esophagus, ingestion of ASA and NSAIDs, rheumatological conditions (CREST), and diabetes mellitus.

Murphy et al. have shown that discrete esophageal ulcers in patients with Barrett's esophagus are a unique risk factor for esophageal bleeding (79). They studied 78 patients with histologically confirmed Barrett's esophagus by serial endoscopies for 1–11 years (mean 3.3 years). Discrete ulcers were identified in 36 of 78 patients (46%) at some time during the follow-up period. Nineteen of these patients (24%) had active gastrointestinal bleeding during follow-up.

There are now several reports of life-threatening upper gastrointestinal hemorrhage from esophageal ulcers caused by ASA and NSAIDs (80). These ulcers have a characteristic appearance: namely, they are usually solitary, large, ulcers with normal surrounding mucosa. Most are located in the midesophagus near the aortic arch or left atrium; see Figure 1 (61).

In a large retrospective review of over 140 patients with PSS or CREST, Duchini and Sessoms found that 15% of their patients had at least one episode of gastrointestinal hemorrhage (81). Of the 22 patients with gastrointestinal hemorrhage 36% had multiple episodes and 18% required chronic transfusions. The most common cause of the bleeding was either telangiectasias (41%) or GERD (32%).

Faigel and Metz studied records of all patients hospitalized at their center with diabetic ketoacidosis over a 30-month period and found that 25 of 193 (13%) of these patients had significant upper gastrointestinal hemorrhage (25). Each of

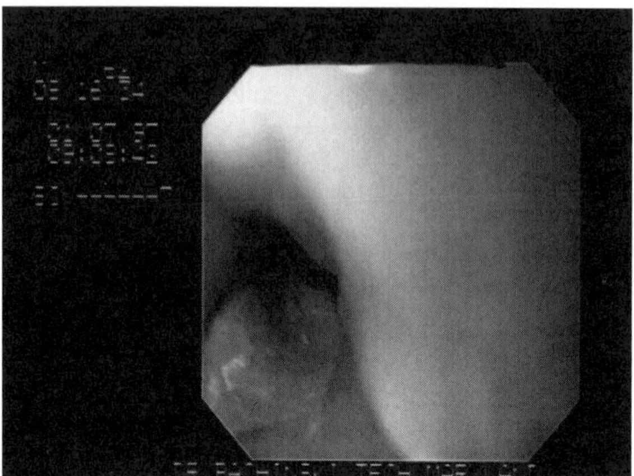

Figure 1 Endophotograph of pill esophagitis, showing a large midesophageal ulcer (top) and a pill resting in an esophageal ulcer (bottom). (Courtesy of Matthew B. Z. Bachinski, M.D.)

the patients evaluated with endoscopy was found to have esophagitis. Other sources of upper gastrointestinal bleeding included Mallory-Weiss tear, gastritis, duodenitis, and duodenal ulcer. Gastrointestinal hemorrhage was more common among those patients with a longer duration of diabetes and complications of retinopathy and gastroparesis (25).

Iron Deficiency

Iron deficiency anemia has been reported with riding erosions of the esophagus, so called ''Cameron lesions''; see Figure 2 (82). Their presence seems to be associated with the size of the hiatal hernia sac, with an increase in prevalence the larger the hernia sac. The cause of these riding erosions is thought to include ischemia, mechanical trauma, and acid mucosal injury. Cameron lesions are seen in 5.2% of patients with hiatal hernia who undergo EGD examinations. In two-thirds of the cases multiple, not solitary, lesions are seen. Cameron lesions can clinically present with silent chronic gastrointestinal bleeding and iron-deficiency anemia or as acute upper gastrointestinal bleeding, which is life threatening, in up to one-third of cases (82). Both medical and surgical antireflux therapy have successfully prevented recurrent iron deficiency (83).

Weight and GERD

Although obesity is often thought to cause GERD, it has been shown that acid reflux is not more common among the obese (84). However, a diet rich in fat

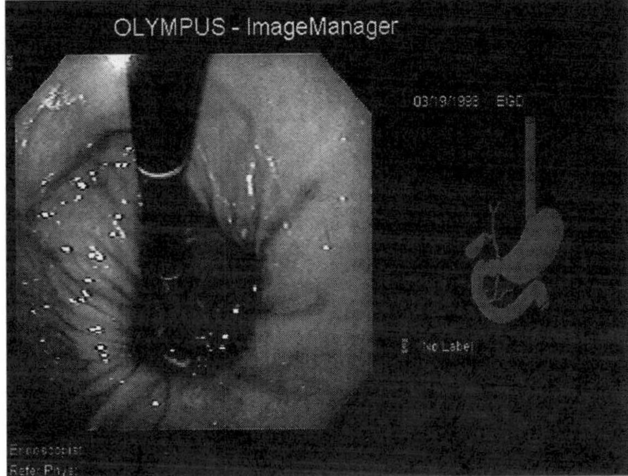

Figure 2 Endophotograph of a Cameron lesion: retroflex view of the stomach showing a large hiatal hernia with four linear erosions, Cameron lesions. (Courtesy of Leonard Little, M.D.)

content promotes gastroesophageal reflux by neurohumoral delay of gastric emptying and inhibition of the LES (85). When rapid weight loss occurs in the face of symptoms of solid food dysphagia, esophageal carcinoma must be excluded (40,45).

CLINICAL COURSE

General

In Western countries, reflux esophagitis is the most common disease of the upper gastrointestinal tract (86,87). A survey of the prevalence of heartburn in the United States found that 7% of persons suffer daily heartburn, 14% notice heartburn weekly, and 44% experience it once a month (1,88). The frequency of heartburn symptoms is much more common among persons with comorbid illness. Pregnant women frequently have daily heartburn, 25 to 48% reported in studies from Europe (27–29). Gastroesophageal reflux disease may present at any age, but is more common among adults with a mean age at onset of 50–56 years (89). Except for the period of pregnancy, women tend to present with esophagitis later in life than men (90). The course of esophagitis is more severe among the elderly (91).

Most patients endure symptoms of heartburn for 1–3 years before seeking medical care (92). Overall, the prognosis of GERD is excellent with over 80%

of patients with noninflammatory GERD showing improvement or resolution of symptoms with medical treatment (93). However, when erosive esophagitis is identified, most cases (70%) become chronic (93). The major complications of GERD are peptic stricture, Barrett's esophagus, and gastrointestinal bleeding. In patients with erosive esophagitis, the prevalence of peptic stricture ranges from 10 to 20% and that of ulceration is 5% (92,94). Barrett's epithelium has been observed in 8–20% of patients with erosive esophagitis and 44% of those with peptic stricture (95–97). Between 2 and 6% of patients with GERD will develop significant gastrointestinal bleeding.

What Is the Likelihood of Esophagitis and Barrett's Esophagus Among the General Population Self-Medicating Symptoms of Heartburn?

Corder et al. conducted a postal survey of adults with chronic symptoms of heartburn (more than once per week for over 3 months), who had never been evaluated by a physician (98). Of the 177 subjects interviewed, most were taking alginates for symptom relief (68%) and only 6% were taking over-the-counter H_2-receptor antagonists. Of the 106 subjects who agreed to undergo endoscopy, 46 (44%) were identified to have macroscopic esophagitis. Most of the esophagitis was grade I or II, but three patients (3%) had mild strictures and six (6%) subjects had Barrett's esophagus. The authors concluded that the prevalence of premalignant conditions and stricture complications of GERD among persons self-medicating symptoms of heartburn is low, but the finding of macroscopic esophagitis is quite high (44%).

Who Seeks Medical Attention for Heartburn Symptoms?

Johnston et al. have objectively compared the psychosocial characteristics and social support patterns of patients with heartburn who do and do not seek medical help with healthy persons without heartburn (99). In general, the heartburn sufferers seeking medical care were older and the heartburn was more severe. However, when these variables were controlled for, patients who sought medical help experienced greater phobia, obsessionality, somatization, life hassles, and had less adequate close social support than those who did not seek medical attention.

Symptom Relationship to Endoscopic Findings

Heartburn may be the leading symptom of and eructation may be the most common complaint of erosive esophagitis, but symptoms are not helpful in differentiating between gastroesophageal reflux without inflammation and reflux esophagitis. Interestingly, among patients with typical symptoms of gastroesophageal reflux, prolonged esophageal pH monitoring was found to be normal in 27%. In some cases, the disease is asymptomatic or the symptoms are atypical. Many patients regard mild symptoms of heartburn to be "normal" and do not seek medical assistance. Tew et al. conducted an illness behavior questionnaire on 140 subjects referred for investigation of heartburn (100). When the subjects with and without endoscopic evidence of esophagitis were compared, no difference in the response to the illness questionnaire was evident. This suggests that the severity of esophageal mucosal damage does not correlate with the severity of illness behavior.

Collen et al. have shown that mucosal injury of GERD increases significantly for each decade of life (91). Also, among persons presenting with symptoms of pyrosis, mucosal disease (erosive esophagitis and Barrett's) is much more common in those over 60 years of age (81% vs. 47%); however, there were no significant differences in severity of symptoms.

Frequency of Evolution from Symptomatic Nonerosive to Erosive Disease

Pace et al. retrospectively studied the clinical outcome for 33 outpatients with nonerosive symptomatic heartburn treated with conservative medical therapy (101). Abnormal esophageal pH measurements were used as the gold standard to establish the diagnosis of GERD. Therapy consisted of antacids, alginate, and/or domperidone. Their study population was middle aged (45.9 years), predomi-

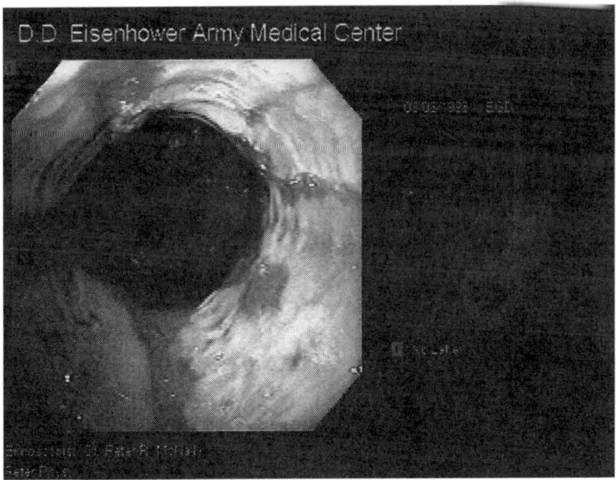

Figure 3 Endophotograph of GERD: typical erosive esophagitis with apparent proximal extension of the squamocolumnar junction.

nantly male (2:1 ratio), and 27% smoked and/or drank alcohol. The mean duration of symptoms was 3.7 years, range 0.4–20 years. They found that after 6 months of conservative therapy for nonerosive GERD, roughly 40% (14 of 33) became symptom free and only five of 33 (15%) showed endoscopic progression to erosive esophagitis (Fig. 3). When esophageal pH data were analyzed, total pH score and percent duration of pH < 4 during daytime and nighttime were not predictive of which patients would exhibit endoscopic progression. Unfortunately, the authors did not evaluate whether age, gender, presence of hiatal hernia, or consumption of alcohol or tobacco predisposed to the development of erosive esophagitis.

Frequency of Progression from Erosive Disease to a Complication

Isolauri et al. studied 87 consecutive patients initially evaluated for symptoms of gastroesophageal reflux from 1973 to 1976 to determine the natural history of GERD (102). Their standard of practice was to offer conservative therapy including lifestyle modifications, antacids, alginates, and/or metoclopramide, or surgery. None were offered H_2-receptor antagonist or proton pump inhibitor therapy. All patients underwent extensive baseline evaluation with provocative upper gastrointestinal radiography, endoscopy, esophageal pH monitoring, and Bernstein-Baker test.

Of the 60 patients available for follow-up (mean 19.5 years, range 17.1–22 years), 50 received only medical treatment. Most of the patients in the medical treatment group had no esophagitis ($n = 30$) or only mild esophagitis, five with grade 1 at baseline endoscopy. Upon follow-up, nine of 50 (18%) patients showed endoscopic progression: grade 0 to grade 1 (five), grade 1 to grade 2 (two), and grade 2 to Barrett's esophagus (two). Symptoms improved in 36 of 50 (72%) patients and most (68%) were not on medical therapy at follow-up.

Of the 10 patients treated with a surgical antireflux procedure, symptoms improved in all and follow-up endoscopy showed the prevalence of erosive esophagitis decreased from 60% to 10%. Surprisingly, four of the 10 patients treated with surgery developed Barrett's esophagus.

The authors concluded that in the long term, symptoms of gastroesophageal reflux tend to decrease, but the pathological process persists in most and the disease is not self-limiting. The most disturbing finding of their study was that six of 60 (10%) patients progressed to Barrett's esophagus. Although these findings are important and interesting, one should be cautious in generalizing the results of this retrospective study. The suggestion by Isolauri that the pathological process of GERD is progressive and leads to the development of Barrett's esophagus in 10% of cases is contrary to most previous published experience. For instance, Cameron et al. have shown that the segment of Barrett's esophagus did not increase in length over 7 years of careful follow-up (103). Also, numerous studies of erosive esophagitis followed after successful fundoplication or therapy with proton pump inhibitors have rarely documented evolution of Barrett's esophagus or elongation of the metaplastic segment (104).

DIFFERENTIAL DIAGNOSIS: CLINICAL, ENDOSCOPIC, HISTOLOGICAL

Clinical Features

Often it is clinically important to distinguish symptoms of GERD from other causes of chest and esophageal pain including caustic ingestion, pill-induced injury, and infection. A thorough history including inquiry about the duration and time of onset of symptoms, risk factors, associated medications, and medical conditions can often be helpful in determining the cause.

Caustic alkaline or acid ingestion is usually accompanied by immediate profound symptoms. In children caustic ingestion is often accidental, while in teens and adults suicide gesture is the common motive. Usually there is no confusion with acute caustic ingestion; however, the clinician must be vigilant and mindful of this possibility as a cause of acute, severe esophageal symptoms especially among those with emotional and/or psychiatric instability. Later in life, caustic injury to the stomach and esophagus may predispose to GERD and esophageal cancer.

The clinical history for pill esophagitis is in striking contrast to that of patients with symptomatic GERD; see Table 3. With pill-induced esophagitis the onset of symptoms is usually acute, while with GERD the symptoms are often present for 1–3 years before clinical presentation. Symptoms of GERD are usually responsive to antacids, while symptoms of pill esophagitis are resistant. Odynophagia is a common symptom with pill or infectious esophagitis, but rare among patients with GERD. Risk factors for pill esophagitis include conditions that may cause sites for esophageal stasis, while GERD is more prevalent among those with medical conditions predisposing to esophageal dysmotility; see Table 3.

Patients with infectious esophagitis usually offer a clinical history very dissimilar to those with symptomatic GERD. Like pill esophagitis, odynophagia is the cardinal symptom of infectious esophagitis, while it is an uncommon symptom among those with GERD. The presence of impaired immunity should suggest the possibility of infectious esophagitis. It is important to emphasize that immune impairment may be subtle, i.e., due to chronic alcoholism, diabetes mellitus, or inhaled corticosteroids. With advanced AIDS, the esophageal infections tend to

Table 3 Comparison of Pill Esophagitis and GERD

	Pill esophagitis	GERD
History	Acute onset, temporal ingestion of a pill	Long history of symptoms (1–3 years)
Onset	Nocturnal common	Any time, especially postcibal
Symptom relief with antacids	Often transient or none	Often prompt relief
Risk factors	Sites for potential esophageal stasis: aortic arch, left atrium, mediastinal adenopathy, and stricture	Esophageal dysmotility (LES hypotonia, impaired esophageal clearance, aperistalsis)
Commonly associated medications	Alendronate, antibiotics, ascorbic acid, iron, NSAIDs, potassium, quinidine, zidovudine (AZT)	Anticholinergics, beta-agonists, calcium channel antagonists, diazepam, nitrates, progesterone, muscle relaxants, nicotine
Associated medical conditions	Atrial fibrillation, congestive heart failure, hilar adenopathy, aortic aneurysm	Scleroderma, Raynaud's syndrome, diabetes mellitus, prolonged nasogastric tube, pregnancy

be multiple, causing severe odynophagia, often resulting in profound weight loss and nutritional impairment.

Endoscopic Features

Unique endoscopic features distinguish GERD from other causes of esophagitis; see Table 4 (105,106). Esophageal injury from acid reflux disease occurs predominantly in the distal esophagus. Although the esophageal injury seen with GERD may extend proximally, a pattern of distal-to-proximal extension is always evident.

Powder-based-caustic ingestions tend to cause more oropharyngeal damage, while liquid-based preparations tend to affect the entire esophagus. The degree of caustic injury varies according to the pH and volume of the caustic agent consumed. A black discoloration of the esophagus signifies third-degree injury and risk for perforation.

A solitary, midesophageal ulcer with normal surrounding mucosa is the typical endoscopic finding of pill esophagitis. Pill ulcers often occur where the aortic arch or the left atrium indents on the esophagus.

Infectious esophagitis is usually extensive, with proximal-to-distal esopha-

Table 4 Comparison of Endoscopic Findings

Condition	Findings
GERD	Usually starts distally at the squamocolumnar junction and progresses proximally. New Savary-Miller classification: Grade 1: Single or multiple erosions, on a single fold: erosions may be erythematous or erythemato-exudate Grade 2: Multiple erosions affecting multiple folds: erosions may be confluent Grade 3: Multiple, circumferential erosions Grade 4: Ulcer, stenosis, or esophageal shortening (brachy esophagus) Grade 5: Barrett's epithelium: cylindrical reepithelialization in the form of a small island, or tongue
Lye ingestion	Powder preparations of lye cause more oropharyngeal damage, while liquid preparations tend to affect the entire esophagus. Degree of injury varies according to pH and volume consumed: First degree: erythema and edema Second degree: ulceration and membranous exudate Third degree: penetrating ulceration, black discoloration
Pill esophagitis	Usually a focal ulcer, variable size from pinpoint to several centimeters. Most common in the midesophagus, at sites of stasis: left atrium, aortic arch, left mainstem bronchus, etc. May be associated with stricture formation.
Infectious esophagitis	*Candida*: multiple gray-white to yellow plaques, may be small to confluent with luminal narrowing. Adherent to mucosa; underlying mucosa is friable and often bleeds with removal of exudate. May see oral thrush. HSV: early lesion: 1–3-mm vesicles, mid- to distal esophagus; later lesion: central slough making discrete ''volcano'' ulcers with raised edges. Can involve entire esophagus. May see companion oral lesions. CMV: may see single or multiple ulcers, initially superficial, later characteristically the ulcers are deep, large, and solitary. Coincident involvement of the stomach is common. HIV: initially see multiple small, aphthoid-like lesions during transient fever and body rash; later may become giant ulcers.

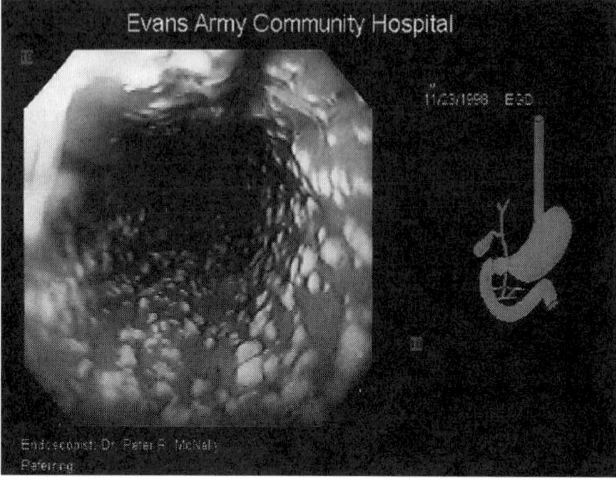

Figure 4 Endophotograph of *Candida* esophagitis: multiple white plaques.

geal involvement commonly seen. *Candida* esophagitis is characterized by raised white plaques, which can become confluent; see Figure 4. Esophageal ulceration is seen with both herpes simplex virus (HSV) and cytomegalovirus (CMV) infection. The esophageal ulcers seen with the HSV are referred to as ''volcano ulcers,'' because of the common feature of a raised edge; see Figure 5, while the esophageal ulcers seen with CMV tend to be more superficial, but may become confluent and very large; see Figure 6.

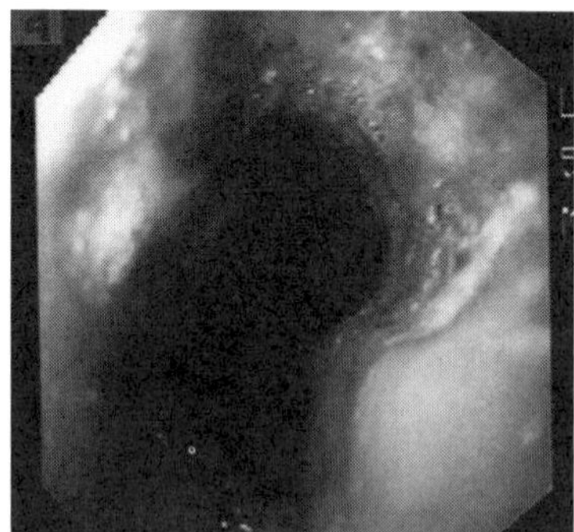

Figure 5 Endophotograph of HSV esophageal ulcer: deep esophageal ulcer with raised edge—''volcano ulcer.'' (Courtesy of Matthew B. Z. Bachinski, M.D.)

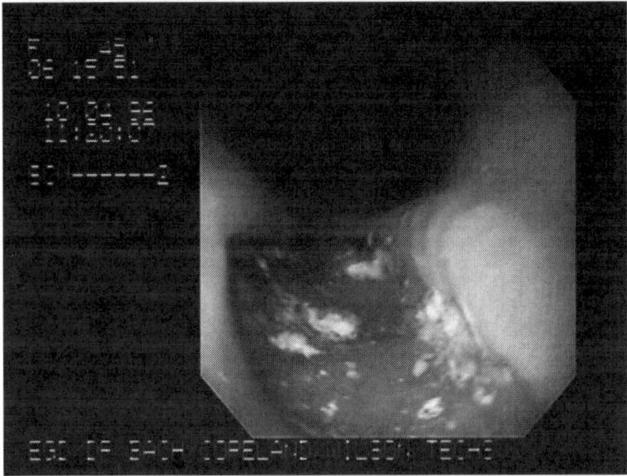

Figure 6 Endophotograph of CMV esophageal ulcer: very large confluent ulcer. (Courtesy of Matthew B. Z. Bachinski, M.D.)

Radiographic Features

Radiographic examination of the esophagus for evaluation of GERD, caustic ingestion, pill, and infectious esophagitis may provide some unique and diagnostic findings, but it has been supplanted by endoscopy as the preferred first test. The diagnostic radiographic features seen with each of these entities are listed in Table 5 (107,108).

The single most important misconception about radiographic findings from the barium esophagram is that the presence of hiatal hernia signifies GERD. Hiatal hernia is a common radiographic finding among Western populations, seen in 40% of person's 50 years of age and 60% of person's 70 years of age (109). However, in a very large, long-term, follow-up study by Palmer, it was discovered that only 9% of individuals with radiological confirmation of hiatus hernia experienced reflux symptoms and only one-third of those with symptoms had endoscopic findings of esophagitis (110). Although the presence of a hiatal hernia alone does not cause GERD, it appears to be an important contributor to the pathophysiology of disease among those with a defective LES barrier and/or esophageal clearance, being present in over one-third of patients with esophageal erosions, ulcers, or strictures (111,112).

Histological Features

Severe esophagitis from any cause may be endoscopically indistinguishable. Endoscopic biopsies with appropriate histological staining are helpful in distinguish-

Table 5 Comparison of Radiographic Findings

Condition	Findings
GERD	Usually starts distal at the squamocolumnar junction, may identify erosions, ulcers, or strictures. Barrett's esophagus is reported to have a unique mosaic appearance. Hiatal hernia is a common finding, but when identified only 9% of individuals have reflux symptoms and only 1/3 of patients with symptoms have endoscopic findings of esophagitis. Conversely, 63–84% of patients with reflux esophagitis were found to have hiatal hernia.
Lye ingestion	Contrast radiography usually not done due to risk of barium mediastinitis or aspiration of gastrograffin. Early examination may underestimate injury. EGD is the preferred test.
Pill esophagitis	Nonspecific findings of single or multiple esophageal ulcers, usually in the midesophagus and occasionally associated with stricture formation. EGD is the preferred diagnostic test.
Infectious esophagitis	*Candida*: nonspecific, cobblestone, serpiginous ulcers with raised edges, shaggy appearance. HSV: nonspecific, small erosions to large deep ulcers in the midesophagus. CMV: nonspecific, discrete, superficial lesions to large, flat elongated ulcer(s). HIV: nonspecific, solitary ulcer.

ing these forms of esophageal injury; see Table 6. Characteristic histological findings of reflux esophagitis include hypertrophy of the basal zone and elongation of the papillae such that they extend more than two-thirds of the way to the mucosal surface (113,114). With low grades of esophagitis, only reactive epithelial changes will be seen. The presence of intraepithelial polymorphonuclear cells or eosinophils suggests high-grade changes of GERD (113,114). Caustic ingestion causes a series of time-related histological changes: first liquefaction necrosis, then sloughing casts, and finally fibroblastic proliferation and collagenous repair. Pill esophagitis causes focal mucosal desiccation, with absence of surrounding involvement and/or infectious causes by appropriate stains. *Candida* esophagitis is characterized by mycelia invasion and budding yeast forms, best seen with periodic acid Shiff or Gormethamine silver stain. Herpes esophagitis is histologically characterized by the presence of multinucleated giant cells and infection of epithelial cells with intranuclear inclusion bodies (Cowdry A bodies). Sampling the *edge* of the ulcer to obtain squamous epithelium provides the highest yield for HSV esophagitis. CMV esophagitis is identified by infection of fibroblasts with both intranuclear and intracytoplasmic inclusion bodies. Sam-

Table 6 Comparison of Histological Findings

Condition	Findings
GERD	Papillae elongation and the presence of lymphocytes, eosinophils, and neutrophils. Mucosal erosions or ulcers. Barrett's esophagus characterized by presence of metaplastic columnar epithelium with presence of goblet cells by periodic acid Schiff or Alcian Blue stain.
Lye ingestion	Acute phase (1–4 days): liquefaction necrosis, vascular thrombosis. Subacute phase (5–14 days): sloughing of casts, granulation tissue, extensive fibroblastic activity, and collagenous repair.
	Cicatrization (15 days–3 months): further fibroblastic proliferation and collagenous repair.
Pill esophagitis	Variable: mucosal desiccation, acute and chronic inflammation, absence of viral and fungal infection.
Infectious esophagitis	*Candida*: invasion with mycelia elements and copious budding yeast forms. Periodic acid Shiff or Gormethamine stain best for diagnosis.
	HSV: Biopsies from the *edge* of ulcers show multinucleated giant cells, infection of epithelial cells intranuclear inclusion bodies (Cowdry A bodies). Immunoperoxidase stains and culture are helpful.
	CMV: biopsies from the *base* of ulcers show infection of fibroblasts with evidence of both intranuclear and intracytoplasmic inclusion bodies. Immunoperoxidase stains and culture are helpful. Stomach lesions should be biopsied, because coincident gastric infection is common.

pling the *base* of the ulcer to obtain fibroblasts provides the best yield for CMV esophagitis.

REFERENCES

1. Nebel OT, Fornes MF, Castell DO. Symptomatic gastroesophageal reflux: incidence and precipitating factors. Am J Dig Dis 1976; 21:953–956.
2. Klauser AG, Schindlbeck NE, Muller-Lissner SA. Symptomatic gastro-oesophageal disease. Lancet 1990; 335:205–208.
3. Price SF, Smithson KW, Castell DO. Food sensitivity in reflux esophagitis. Gastroenterology 1978; 75:240–243.
4. Iwakiri K, Kobayashi M, Kotoyori M, Yamada H, Sugiura T, Nakagawa Y. Relationship between postprandial esophageal acid exposure and meal volume and fat content. Dig Dis Sci 1996; 41:926–930.

5. Borum ML. Gastrointestinal diseases in women. Med Clin North Am 1998; 82: 21–50.
6. Homan CS, Maitra SR, Lane BP, Thode HC Jr, Finkelsteyn J, Davidson C. Histopathologic evaluation of the therapeutic efficacy of milk and water dilution for acid injury. Acad Emerg Med 1995; 2:952–958.
7. Berstad A, Hatlebakk JJ. The predictive value of symptoms in gastro-oesophageal reflux disease. Scand J Gastroenterol 1995; 211:1–4.
8. Rodriguez S, Miner P, Robinson M, Greenwood B, Maton PN, Pappa K. Meal type affects heartburn severity. Dig Dis Sci 1998; 43:485–490.
9. Grande L, Manterola C, Ros E, Lacima G, Pera C. Effects of red wine on 24-hour esophageal pH and pressures in healthy volunteers. Dig Dis Sci 1997; 42:1189–1193.
10. Feldman M, Barnett C. Relationship between the acidity and osmolarity of popular beverages and reported postprandial heartburn. Gastroenterology 1995; 108:125–131.
11. Brazer SR, Onken JE, Dalton CB, Smith JW, Schiffman SS. Effects of different coffees on esophageal acid contact time and symptoms in coffee-sensitive subjects. Physiol Behav 1995; 57:563–567.
12. Pehl C, Wendl B, Pfeiffer A, Schmidt J, Kaess H. Low-proof alcoholic beverages and gastroesophageal reflux. Dig Dis Sci 1993; 38:93–96.
13. Katz LC, Just R, Castell DO. Body position affects recumbent postprandial reflux. J Clin Gastroenterol 1994; 18:280–283.
14. Moses FM. The effect of exercise on the gastrointestinal tract. Sports Med 1990; 9:159–172.
15. Sjogren RW. Gastrointestinal features of scleroderma. Curr Opin Rheumatol 1996; 8:569–575.
16. Bassotti G, Battaglia E, Debernardi V, Germani U, Quiriconi F, Dughera L, Buonafede G, Puiatti P, Morelli A, Spinozzi, Mioli PR, Emanuelli G. Esophageal dysfunction in scleroderma: relationship with disease subsets. Arthritis Rheum 1997; 40:2252–2259.
17. Weston S, Thumshirn M, Wiste J, Camilleri M. Clinical and upper gastrointestinal motility features in systemic sclerosis and related disorders. Am J Gastroenterol 1998; 93:1085–1089.
18. Medgser TA, Masi AT. Epidemiology of systemic sclerosis (scleroderma). Ann Intern Med 1971; 74:714–721.
19. Poirier TJ, Rankin GB. Gastrointestinal manifestations of progressive system scleroderma based on a review of 364 cases. Am J Gastroenterol 1972; 58:30–44.
20. Recht MP, Levine MS, Katzka DA, Reynolds JC, Saul SH. Barrett's esophagus in scleroderma: increased prevalence and radiographic findings. Gastrointest Radiol 1988; 13:1–5.
21. Zamost BJ, Hirschberg J, Ippoliti AF, Furst DE, Clements PJ, Weinstein WM. Esophagitis in scleroderma: prevalence and risk factors. Gastroenterology 1987; 92:421–428.
22. Katzka DA, Reynolds JC, Saul SM, Plotkin A, Lang CA, Ouyang A, Jimenez S, Cohen S. Barrett's metaplasia and adenocarcinoma of the esophagus in scleroderma. Am J Med 1987; 82:46–52.

23. Anselmino M, Zaninotto G, Constantini M, Ostuni P, Ianniello A, Boccu C, Doria A, Todesco S, Ancona E. Esophageal motor function in primary Sjögren's syndrome: correlation with dysphagia and xerostomia. Dig Dis Sci 1997; 42:113–118.
24. Camilleri M. Gastrointestinal problems in diabetes. Endocrinol Metab Clin North Am 1996; 25:361–378.
25. Faigel DO, Metz DC. Prevalence, etiology, and prognostic significance of upper gastrointestinal hemorrhage in diabetic ketoacidosis. Dig Dis Sci 1996; 41:1–8.
26. Katz PO, Castell DO. Gastroesophageal reflux disease during pregnancy. Gastroenterol Clin North Am 1998; 27:153–167.
27. Bainbridge ET, Temple JG, Nicholas SP, Newton JR, Boriah V. Symptomatic gastro-oesophageal reflux in pregnancy. A comparative study of white Europeans and Asians in Birmingham. Br J Clin Pract 1983; 37:53–57.
28. Bassey OO. Pregnancy heartburn in Nigerians and Caucasians with theories about etiology based on manometric recordings for the oesophagus and stomach. Br J Obstet Gynaecol 1977; 84:439–443.
29. Nagler R, Spiro HM. Heartburn in pregnancy. Am J Dig Dis 1962; 7:648–655.
30. Larson JD, Patatanian E, Miner PB Jr, Rayburn WF, Robinson MG. Double-blind, placebo-controlled study of ranitidine for gastroesophageal reflux symptoms during pregnancy. Obstet Gynecol 1997; 90:83–87.
31. Miller LS, Vinayek R, Frucht H, Gardner JD, Jensen RT, Maton PN. Reflux esophagitis in patients with Zollinger-Ellison syndrome. Gastroenterology 1990; 98:341–346.
32. Bondeson AG, Bondeson L, Thompson NW. Stricture and perforation of the esophagus: overlooked threats in Zollinger-Ellison syndrome. World J Surg 1990; 14:361–363.
33. Miyoshi H, Yata M, Matsuo N, Sameshima Y, Harima T. Nasogastric tube feeding and esophageal disorders. Intern Med 1998; 37:102.
34. Buchman AL, Waring JP. Mucosal bridge formation in the esophagus caused by injury from a nasoenteric feeding tube. J Parenteral Enteral Nutr 1994; 18:278–279.
35. Helm JF, Dodds WJ, Hogan WJ. Salivary response to esophageal acid in normal subjects and patients with reflux esophagitis. Gastroenterology 1987; 93:1393–1397.
36. Helm JF, Dodds WJ, Pelc LR, Palmer DW, Hogan WJ, Teeter BC. Effect of esophageal emptying and saliva on clearance of acid from the esophagus. N Engl J Med 1984; 310:284–288.
37. Korsten MA, Rosman AS, Fishbein S, Shlein RD, Goldberg HE, Bieher A. Chronic xerostomia increases esophageal acid exposure and is associated with esophageal injury. Am J Med 1991; 90:701–706.
38. Sheikh SH, Shaw-Stiffel TA. The gastrointestinal manifestations of Sjögren's syndrome. Am J Gastroenterol 1995; 90:9–14.
39. Axelrad AM, Fleischer DC. Esophageal tumors. In: Feldman M, Scharschmidt BF, Sleisenger MH, eds. Sleisenger and Fordtran's Gastrointestinal and Liver Disease, 6th ed. Philadelphia: WB Saunders, 1998:540–554.
40. Parkman HP, Cohen S. Heartburn, regurgitation, odynophagia, chest pain and dysphagia. In: Haubrich WS, Schaffner F, Berk JE, eds. Bockus Gastroenterology, 5th ed. Philadelphia: WB Saunders, 1995:30–40.

41. Brown CM, Snowdon CF, Slee B, Sandle LN, Rees WD. Effects of topical oesophageal acidification on human salivary and esophageal alkali secretion. Gut 1995; 36: 649–653.
42. Mandel L, Tamari K. Sialorrhea and gastroesophageal reflux. J Am Dent Assoc 1995; 126:1537–1541.
43. Brown CM, Rees WD. Review article: factors protecting the oesophagus against acid-mediated injury. Aliment Pharmacol Ther 1995; 9:251–262.
44. Goldin GF, Marcinkiewicz M, Zbroch T, Bityutskiy LP, McCallum RW, Sarosiek J. Esophagoprotective potential of cisapride. An additional benefit for gastroesophageal reflux. Dig Dis Sci 1997; 42:1362–1369.
45. Decktor DL, Allen ML, Robinson M. Esophageal motility, heartburn, and gastroesophageal reflux: variations in clinical presentation of esophageal dysphagia. Dysphagia 1990; 5:211–215.
46. Singh S, Stein HJ, DeMeester TR, Hinder RA. Nonobstructive dysphagia in gastroesophageal reflux disease: a study with combined ambulatory pH and motility monitoring. Am J Gastroenterol 1992; 87:562–567.
47. Jacob P, Kahrilas PJ, Vanagunas A. Peristaltic dysfunction associated with nonobstructive dysphagia in reflux disease. Dig Dis Sci 1990; 35:939–942.
48. Geisinger KR. Endoscopic biopsies and cytological brushings of the esophagus are diagnostically complementary. Am J Clin Pathol 1995; 103:295–299.
49. Alexander LN, Wilcox CM. A prospective trial of thalidomide for the treatment of HIV-associated idiopathic esophageal ulcers. AIDS Res Hum Retroviruses 1997; 13:301–304.
50. Clayton F, Clayton CH. Gastrointestinal pathology in HIV-infected patients. Gastroenterol Clin North Am 1997; 26:191–240.
51. Maillot C, Riachi G, Francois A, Ducrotte P, Lerebours E, Hemet J, Colin R. Digestive manifestations in an immunocompetent adult with varicella. Am J Gastroenterol 1997; 92:1361–1363.
52. Choi JH, Yoo JH, Chung IJ, Kim DW, Han CW, Shin WS, Min WS, Park CW, Kim CC, Kim DJ. Esophageal aspergillosis after bone marrow transplant. Bone Marrow Transplant 1997; 19:293–294.
53. Simon MR, Houser WL, Smith KA, Long PM. Esophageal candidiasis as a complication of inhaled corticosteroids. Ann Allergy Asthma Immunol 1997; 79:333–338.
54. Kikendall JW, Johnson LF. Pill-induced esophageal injury. In: Castell DO, ed. The Esophagus. Boston: Little, Brown, 1995.
55. Boyce HW. Drug induced esophageal damage: diseases of medical progress. Gastrointest Endosc 1998; 47:547–550.
56. Kikendall JW. Pill-induced esophageal injury. Gastroenterol Clin North Am 1991; 20:835–846.
57. Yamaoka K, Takenawa H, Tajiri K, Yamane M, Kadowaki K, Marumo F, Sato C. A case of esophageal perforation due to a pill-induced ulcer successfully treated with conservative measures. Am J Gastroenterol 1996; 91:1044–1045.
58. Simko V, Joseph D, Michael S. Increased risk in esophageal obstruction with slow-release medications. J Assoc Acad Minor Phys 1997; 8:38–42.
59. de Groen PC, Lubbe DF, Hirsch LJ, Daifotis A, Stephenson W, Freedholm D,

Pryor-Tillotson S, Seleznick MJ, Pinkas H, Wang KK. Esophagitis associated with the use of alendronate. N Engl J Med 1996; 335:1016–1021.

60. Ribeiro A, DeVault KR, Wolfe JE III, Start ME. Alendronate associated esophagitis: endoscopic and pathologic features. Gastrointest Endosc 1998; 47:525–528.
61. Sugawa C, Takekuma Y, Lucas CE, Amamoto H. Bleeding esophageal ulcers caused by NSAID's. Surg Endosc 1997; 11:143–146.
62. Katz PO, Codario R, Castell DO. Approach to the patient with unexplained chest pain. Comprehens Ther 1997; 23:249–253.
63. Braunwald E. Examination of the patient. In: Braunwald E, ed. Heart Disease, 5th ed. Philadelphia: WB Saunders, 1997:1–14.
64. Epstein SE, Talbot TL. Dynamic coronary tone in precipitation, exacerbation and relief of angina pectoris. Am J Cardiol 1981; 48:797–803.
65. Prinzmetal M, Kennamer R, Merliss R, et al. A variant form of angina pectoris. Am J Med 1959; 27:375.
66. Mehta AJ, de Caestecker JS, Camm AJ, Northfield TC. Gastro-oesophageal reflux in patients with coronary disease: how common is it and does it matter? Eur J Gastroenterol Hepatol 1996; 8:973–978.
67. Singh S, Richter JE, Hewson EG, Sinclair JW, Hackshaw BT. The contribution of gastroesophageal reflux to chest pain in patients with coronary artery disease. Ann Intern Med 1992; 117:824–830.
68. Voskuil JH, Cramer MJ, Breumelhof R, Timmer R, Smout AJ. Prevalence of esophageal disorders in patients with chest pain newly referred to a cardiologist. Chest 1996; 109:1210–1214.
69. Goyal RK. Changing focus on unexplained esophageal chest pain. Ann Intern Med 1996; 124:1008–1011.
70. Pasricha PJ. Noncardiac chest pain: from nutcracker to nociceptors. Gastroenterology 1997; 112:309–310.
71. Rao SS, Gregersen H, Hayek B, Summers RW, Christensen J. Unexplained chest pain: the hypersensitive, hyperactive, and poorly compliant esophagus. Ann Intern Med 1996; 124:950–958.
72. Mehta AJ, DeCaestecker JS, Camm AJ, Northfield TC. Sensitization to painful distention and abnormal sensory perception in the esophagus. Gastroenterology 1995; 108:311–319.
73. Achem SR, Kolts BE, Richter JE, Castell DO. Treatment of acid related chest pain: a double-blind, placebo controlled trial of omperazole vs. placebo. Gastroenterology 1993; 104:A29.
74. Ho KY, Kang JK, Yeo B, Ng WL. Non-cardiac, non-oesophageal chest pain: the relevance of psychological factors. Gut 1998; 43:105–110.
75. Spechler SJ. Barrett's esophagus. Curr Opinion Gastroenterol 1988; 4:535–541.
76. Spechler SJ, Schimmel EM. Gastrointestinal tract bleeding of unknown origin. Arch Intern Med 1982; 142:236–240.
77. Spechler SJ. Epidemiology and natural history of gastro-oesophageal reflux disease. Digestion 1992; 51:24–29.
78. Silverstein FE, Gilbert DA, Tedesco FJ, Buenger NK, Persing J. The national ASGE survey on upper gastrointestinal bleeding. II. Clinical and prognostic factors. Gastrointest Endosc 1981; 27:80–93.

79. Murphy PP, Ballinger PJ, Massey BT, Shaker R, Hogan WJ. Discrete ulcers in Barrett's esophagus: relationship to acute gastrointestinal bleeding. Endoscopy 1998; 30:367–370.
80. Kelly JP, Kaufman DW, Jurgelon JM, Sheehan J, Koff RS, Shapiro S. Risk of aspirin-associated major upper-gastrointestinal bleeding with enteric-coated and buffered product. Lancet 1996; 348:1413–1416.
81. Duchini A, Sessoms SL. Gastrointestinal hemorrhage in patients with systemic sclerosis and CREST syndrome. Am J Gastroenterol 1998; 93:1453–1456.
82. Weston AP. Hiatal hernia with Cameron ulcers and erosions. Gastrointest Endosc Clin North Am 1996; 6:671–679.
83. Maziak DE, Todd TR, Pearson FG. Massive hiatus hernia: evaluation and surgical management. J Thorac Cardiovasc Surg 1998; 115:53–60.
84. Lundell L, Ruth M, Sandberg N, Bove-Nielsen M. Does massive obesity promote abnormal gastroesophageal reflux? Dig Dis Sci 1995; 40:1632–1635.
85. Castell DO. Obesity and gastro-oesophageal reflux: is there a relationship? Eur J Gastroenterol Hepatol 1996; 8:625–626.
86. Savary M, Ollyo J-B. L'oesophagite par reflux et ses complications: ulcere, stenose, endobrachy-oesophage. Encycl Med Chir (Paris, France) ORL 1986; 20822A10: 16.
87. Kahrilas PJ. Gastroesophageal reflux disease. JAMA 1996; 276:983–988.
88. A Gallup Survey on Heartburn Across America. Princeton, NJ: Gallop Organization, 1988.
89. Ollyo J-B, Monnier P, Fontolliet C, Savary M. The natural history, prevalence and incidence of reflux oesophagitis. Gullet 1993; 3(suppl):3–10.
90. Ollyo J-B, Ferrarini F, Morselli Labate AM, Barbara L. Prevalence of esophagitis in patients undergoing routine upper endoscopy: a multicenter survey in Italy. In: DeMeester TR, Skinner DB, eds. Esophageal Disorders: Pathophysiology and Therapy. New York: Raven Press, 1985:213–219.
91. Collen MJ, Abdulian JB, Chen YK. Gastroesophageal reflux disease that requires aggressive therapy. Am J Gastroenterol 1995; 90:1053–1057.
92. Howard PJ, Heading RC. Epidemiology of gastro-esophageal reflux disease. World J Surg 1992; 16:288–293.
93. Rex JC, Anderson HA, Bartholomew LG, Cain JC. Esophageal hiatial hernia—a 10 year study of medically treated cases. JAMA 1961; 178:117–120.
94. Wienbeck M, Barnert J. Epidemiology of reflux disease and reflux esophagitis. Scand J Gastroenterol 1989; 156(suppl):7–13.
95. Spechler SJ, Sperber H, Doos WG, Schimmel EM. The prevalence of Barrett's esophagus in patients with chronic peptic esophageal strictures. Dig Dis Sci 1983; 28:769.
96. Spechler SJ, Goyal RK. Barrett's esophagus. N Engl J Med 1986; 315:362–371.
97. Winters C Jr, Spurling TJ, Chobanian SJ, Curtis DJ, Esposito RL, Hacker JF III, Johnson DA, Spurling TJ, Cruess DF, Cotelingam JD, Gurney MS, Cattau EL. Barrett's esophagus: a prevalent, occult complication of gastroesophageal reflux disease. Gastroenterology 1987; 92:118–124.
98. Corder AO, Jones RH, Sadler GH, Daniels P, Johnson CD. Heartburn, oesophagitis

and Barrett's esophagus in self-medicated patients in general practice. Br J Clin Pract 1996; 50:245–248.
99. Johnston BT, Gunning J, Lewis SA. Health care seeking by heartburn sufferers is associated with psychosocial factors. Am J Gastroenterol 1996; 91:2500–2504.
100. Tew S, Jamieson GG, Pilowsky I, Myers J. The illness behavior of patients with gastroesophageal reflux disease with and without endoscopic esophagitis. Dis Esoph 1997; 10:9–15.
101. Pace F. Santalucia F, Bianchi Porro G. Natural history of gastro-oesophageal reflux disease without esophagitis. Gut 1991; 32:845–848.
102. Isolauri J, Loustarinen M, Isolauri E, Reinikainen P, Viljakka M, Keyrilainen O. Natural course of gastroesophageal reflux disease: 17–22 year follow-up of 60 patients. Am J Gastroenterol 1997; 92:37–41.
103. Cameron AJ, Zinsmeister AR, Ballard DJ, Carney JA. Prevalence of columnar-lined (Barrett's) esophagus. Gastroenterology 1990; 99:918–922.
104. Klinkenberg-Knol EC, Festen HP, Jansen JB, et al. Long-term treatment with omperazole for refractory reflux esophagitis: efficacy and safety. Ann Intern Med 1994; 121:161–169.
105. Ollyo J-B, Lang F, Fontolliet CH, Monnier PH. Savary-Miller's new endoscopic grading of reflux-oesophagitis: a simple, reproducible, logical, complete and useful classification. Gastroenterology 1990; 98:100A.
106. Silverstein FE, Tytgat GNJ. Esophagus I and II. In: Silverstein FE, Tytgat GNJ, eds. Gastrointestinal Endoscopy, 3rd ed. Philadelphia: Mosby-Wolfe, 1997:29–89.
107. Eisenberg RL. Esophageal ulceration. In: Eisenberg RL, ed. Gastrointestinal Radiology: A Pattern Approach, 3rd ed. Philadelphia: Lippincott-Raven, 1996:45–69.
108. Vincent ME, Robbins AH, Spechler SJ, Schwartz R, Doos WG, Schimmel EM. The reticular pattern as a radiographic sign of Barrett esophagus: an assessment. Radiology 1984; 153:333–335.
109. Wolf BS, Brahms SA, Khilnani MT. The incidence of hiatus hernia in routine barium meal examination. J Mt Sinai Hosp 1959; 26:598–600.
110. Palmer ED. The hiatus hernia-esophagitis-esophageal stricture complex. Twenty-year prospective study. Am J Med 1968; 44:566–579.
111. El-Serag HB, Sonnenberg A. Associations between different forms of gastro-oesophageal reflux disease. Gut 1997; 41:594–599.
112. El-Serag HB, Sonnenberg A. Association of esophageal strictures with diseases treated with nonsteroidal anti-inflammatory drugs. Am J Gastroenterol 1997; 92: 52–56.
113. Ismail-Beigi, Horton PF, Pope CE 2nd. Histologic consequences of gastroesophageal reflux in man. Gastroenterology 1970; 58:163–174.
114. Ismail-Beigi, Pope CE 2nd. Distribution of histological changes of gastroesophageal reflux in the distal esophagus of man. Gastroenterology 1974; 66:1109–1113.

2

Risk Factors for Gastroesophageal Reflux Disease

Types and Mechanisms

John David Horwhat and Roy K. H. Wong
Walter Reed Army Medical Center, Washington, D.C.,
and Uniformed Services University of the Health Sciences,
Bethesda, Maryland

INTRODUCTION

Gastroesophageal reflux (GER) is a disease entity with a broad spectrum of manifestations and potential complications. From the occasional acute discomfort of pyrosis to the development of reflux esophagitis with peptic stricture to Barrett's esophagus with its increased risk of adenocarcinoma, gastroesophageal reflux is a common problem. The weekly prevalence of heartburn or acid regurgitation in the general population is 19.8%, with a yearly prevalence of up to 58.7% (1). In spite of our current understanding of the LES and crural diaphragm, transient lower esophageal sphincter relaxation (TLESR), and hiatal hernia in the pathophysiology of GERD, active research in this area persists.

In this chapter, we will review the current literature concerning risk factors for developing gastroesophageal reflux. We will discuss the mechanisms of how these risk factors affect GER and thoroughly review the clinical, experimental

The opinions or assertions contained herein are the private views of the authors and are not to be construed as official or as reflecting the views of the Department of the Army or the Department of Defense.

and epidemiological evidence that supports or refutes these risk factors as a cause of GER.

HIATAL HERNIA

As discussed in another chapter, hiatal hernia has been intensively researched and debated over the last 40 years with respect to its role in the etiopathogenesis and pathophysiology of gastroesophageal reflux (Table 1). Whether hiatal hernia raises the risk for GER, and to what extent, is still a topic of active research, despite advances in radiological and manometric modalities to demonstrate reflux. We have chosen to discuss hiatal hernia first as it holds a central position in understanding the mechanisms that lead to GERD. We will briefly review the normal function of the lower esophagus and the antireflux barrier created by the lower esophageal sphincters (LES) and crural diaphragm to contrast the normal state with the pathological state seen in hiatal hernia.

Herniation of part of the stomach through the diaphragmatic hiatus is not uncommon with an estimated prevalence of 5 per 1000 in the general population. There is no clear gender predominance and radiographic studies demonstrate that 50% of patients over the age of 50 have hiatal hernia (2). About 75–90% are of the sliding type in which a transient bulbous structure referred to radiographically as the phrenic ampulla or esophageal vestibule is seen when the esophagus shortens during swallowing and the gastric cardia moves proximally through the diaphragmatic hiatus into an intrathoracic location (3). Despite the movement of the cardia from a positive- to a negative-pressure intrathoracic location, gastroesophageal reflux rarely occurs. The anatomical features of the gastroesophageal junction discussed in another chapter normally act to maintain a competent antireflux barrier to the flow of gastroduodenal contents, even after swallow-induced LES relaxation.

In the normal state, the LES is composed of an area of thickened smooth muscle at the distal 4 cm of the esophagus. The right crus of the diaphragm forms the diaphragmatic hiatus and encircles the proximal 2 cm of the sphincter such that part of the sphincter lies normally within the intrathoracic esophageal hiatus while the remainder is normally intra-abdominal. The gastroesophageal junction maintains an effective antireflux barrier through the combination of the pressure exerted by the contraction of the smooth muscle of the LES as well as the contraction of the skeletal muscle of the crural diaphragm. The crural diaphragm contracts during inspiration with proportional increases in LES pressure and in doing so can fortify LES pressure during rapid increases in intragastric pressure such as with coughing, straining, or Valsalva maneuvers (4). Any of these maneuvers could promote gastroesophageal reflux down the pressure gradient exerted by

Table 1 Studies That Have Examined the Relationship Between Hiatal Hernia and Gastroesophageal Reflux

Study	Subjects (total number)	Modality				Conclusions
		EGD	EM	pH	BaS	
Cohen, 1971	75	−	+	−	+	No apparent effect of hiatal hernia on LES pressure.
Petersen, 1991	930	+	−	−	−	Severity of esophagitis was dependent ($p < 0.05$) on both presence and size of hiatal hernia.
Sontag, 1991	184	+	+	+	−	Hiatal hernia was more predictive of reflux than decreased LESP.
Sloan, 1991	36	−	+	+	+	GEJ competence was severely impaired in patients with nonreducing hiatal hernias.
Sloan, 1992	50	−	+	−	+	HH and low LESP compromise GEJ competence during increases in intra-abdominal pressure.
Kasapidis, 1995	60	−	+	+	−	Increased amount of reflux, prolonged acid clearance time, impaired esophageal peristalsis, and more severe esophagitis with nonreducing hiatal hernia.
Peck, 1995	57	−	+	+	−	Crural pressure is decreased in patients with hiatal hernia.
Ott, 1995	319	−	−	+	+	Patients with larger hiatal hernias (≥2 cm) were more likely to have abnormal esophageal pH results than patients without hiatal hernia.
Patti, 1996	95	+	+	+	+	Hiatal hernia size affects the degree of esophagitis.
Jones, 1998	75	+	+	+	−	Severity of esophagitis is dependent on hiatal hernia size, LESP, and male sex. Hiatal hernia was the strongest predictor of esophagitis severity.

BaS = barium swallow; DH = diaphragmatic hiatus; EGD = esophagogastroduodenoscopy; EM = esophageal manometry; GEJ = gastroesophageal junction; GER = gastroesophageal reflux; HH = hiatal hernia; LESP = lower-esophageal-sphincter pressure; pH = pH monitoring; UGI = upper gastrointestinal series.

high intra-abdominal pressure were it not for the contribution of the crural diaphragm on the LES.

The presence of a hiatal hernia is felt to raise the risk for GER through several different mechanisms. Decreased acid clearance (5), retrograde flow of retained gastroduodenal refluxate, and impairment of the sphincter-like action of the diaphragmatic crura on the esophagogastric junction (6) are all felt to contribute to the greater risk of reflux seen with hiatal hernia. Epidemiological evidence in support of this has been demonstrated in the higher prevalence of hiatal hernia among patients with moderate to severe manifestations of gastroesophageal reflux, as 50–60% of patients with hiatal hernia have endoscopic esophagitis, but >90% with endoscopic esophagitis have hiatal hernia (7).

Sloan and Kahrilas studied the impairment of esophageal emptying in hiatal hernia using videofluoroscopy and manometry during barium esophagogram in 22 patients with axial hiatal hernia and 14 volunteer subjects (8). The two groups were analyzed with respect to hiatal hernia length. Controls were those subjects with maximal phrenic ampullary length <2 cm while the other two groups analyzed were patients or volunteers with ≥2-cm reducing hernias and patients with nonreducing hernias. Statistically significant ($p < 0.05$) differences in esophageal emptying and acid clearance times were noted. Complete esophageal emptying without retrograde flow was noted in 86% of the controls, 66% of the reducing-hernia group, and 32% of the nonreducing-hernia group. The nonreducing group also had longer acid clearance times than the controls ($p < 0.05$). A pattern of early retrograde flow of gastric contents immediately after swallow-induced LES relaxation was seen in 48% of the patients with nonreducing hernia in contrast to the control subjects and the patients with reducing hernias, who had no evidence of early retrograde flow. Furthermore, the nonreducing-hernia patients demonstrated manometric evidence of a weakened LES mechanism. The inspiratory augmentation normally seen as a result of the contraction of the crural diaphragm, which serves to prevent retrograde gastroesophageal flow, was evident in the control and reducing-hernia groups but was absent or markedly diminished in the nonreducing group. This radiographic and manometric evidence allowed the authors to conclude the competence of the gastroesophageal junction was severely impaired among patients with nonreducing hernias. The study also demonstrated that the normal mechanism of esophageal emptying was dependent on the distal esophageal segment being surrounded by intra-abdominal pressure with the diaphragmatic crura acting as a one-way valve during respiration.

In another study, 34 patients with endoscopic evidence suggesting hiatal hernia and 16 asymptomatic volunteers were evaluated to demonstrate the effects of abrupt increases in intra-abdominal pressure on gastroesophageal competence (9). This study measured the size of hiatal hernia from videotaped barium esophagogram examinations and measured LES pressures immediately before increases in intra-abdominal pressure. Nonreducing hiatal hernias on videotaped barium swallows were defined upon noting gastric folds or a hernia pouch above the diaphragm between or during swallows. Barium swallow noted that 20 of the 34 patients and none of the asymptomatic volunteers had hiatal hernias. The provocative maneuvers utilized included the Valsalva and Müller maneuvers, leg lifts to 30 degrees, 10 successive coughs, and the gradual inflation of an abdominal cuff placed below the ribs to 100 mmHg. Barium reflux into the esophagus during a maneuver was considered a positive test with an overall reflux score calculated. Esophagitis was statistically more prevalent in the patients with hernias than the patients without hernias (15/20 vs. 5/14, $p < 0.05$). A lower LES pressure was also noted in the group of patients with hernia compared to those without hernias (5.3 ± 4.3 vs. 12.9 ± 7.1 mmHg). Hernia size, LES pressure, and the relationship between these two factors were the major determinants of gastroesophageal junction competence. According to the model developed by this study, a patient with a hypotensive LES and a large hernia was several times more likely to experience GER during abrupt increases in intra-abdominal pressure than a patient with a hypotensive LES but no hiatal hernia. Furthermore, the study demonstrated that as hernia size increased, LES pressure diminished (Fig. 1).

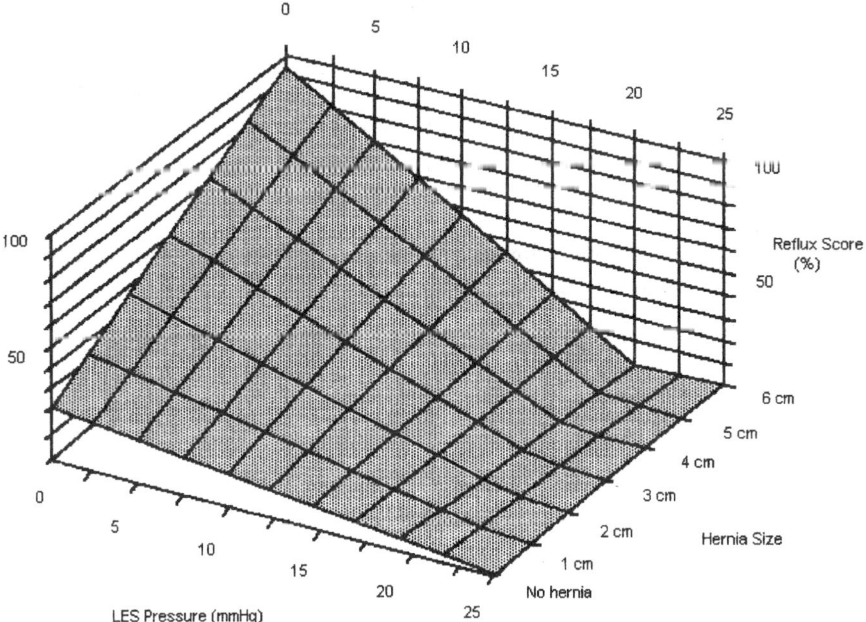

Figure 1 Relationship between LES pressure, hernia size, and gastroesophageal reflux. From Sloan, 1992.

Mittal questioned whether the reflux noted in response to the maneuvers originated from within the hiatal hernia or from the stomach below the diaphragm (10). This distinction is important because reflux originating from the hernia sac may occur in the presence of normal sphincteric closure of the crural diaphragm, whereas reflux originating below the diaphragm implies impaired sphincteric closure of the crural diaphragm and is one of the mechanisms that increase the risk of GER.

A study by Peck and colleagues measured the crural pressure in 57 patients with known reflux as documented by 24-h pH monitoring (11). Mean crural pressure in 41 patients with hiatal hernia was 5.0 mmHg compared with 15.0 mmHg in 16 patients without hiatal hernia ($p < 0.01$). These results demonstrate the importance of the diaphragmatic crura in maintaining the resting pressure of the LES at a level sufficient to protect against reflux.

The studies discussed above used the reflux of barium seen on videotaped barium esophagram as a means of determining whether gastroesophageal reflux had taken place. Although no diagnostic modality is 100% sensitive or specific for diagnosing gastroesophageal reflux, most authorities consider 24-h pH measurement the best means of documenting gastroesophageal reflux. A number of studies have been performed that used 24-h pH monitoring as a means of correlating hiatal hernia with the risk for gastroesophageal reflux (11–16).

In a well-designed study analyzing LES pressure, hiatal hernia, and esophagitis, Sontag and colleagues compared the endoscopic, histological, 24-h esophageal pH monitoring and manometric results to determine the importance of hiatal hernia in reflux esophagitis (12). Of 184 patients studied, LES pressure, acid contact time, and frequency of reflux episodes were all highly associated with hiatal hernias ($p < 0.003$). The authors concluded that the presence of a hiatal hernia, not LES pressure, was the most important predictor of reflux frequency, acid contact time, and esophagitis. Approximately 89% of patients with esophagitis and 64% of those without esophagitis had hiatal hernias. Using a hiatal hernia prevalence of 33% in healthy controls, it was determined that individuals with esophagitis had 16.5 times as many hiatal hernias when compared to healthy controls. Hiatal hernias were defined as gastric folds extending at least 2 cm above the diaphragmatic hiatus during quiet respiration. We know that the sphincter mechanism of the crural diaphragm may still be intact and able to guard against reflux esophagitis with a smaller or reducing hernia. Unfortunately, this study did not classify hernias according to whether they were reducible or nonreducible in terms of hernia size and therefore the degree of GER could not be assessed according to hernia characteristics.

Despite these convincing studies, some data continue to question the association of hiatal hernia with gastroesophageal reflux. In a recent retrospective radiological study, Ott et al. evaluated the correlation between heartburn, 24-h pH monitoring, and the radiographic examination of the esophagus (13). The prevalence of heartburn versus hiatal hernia was 37% and 63%, respectively. Seventy-one percent (94/132) of symptomatic patients had hiatal hernia, esophagitis, or stricture with only 41% (39/94) having abnormal pH studies. However, 95% of patients with abnormal 24-h pH had hiatal hernia plus esophagitis or stricture. Although this study showed that pH monitoring results did not correlate with the presence or absence of heartburn, a statistically significant higher percentage of abnormal 24-h pH results was demonstrated among those with hiatal hernia, esophagitis, or stricture compared to those with a radiographically normal esophagus. The study questioned the utility of 24-h monitoring as a gold standard for diagnosing GER, but the higher risk of GER in the setting of hiatal hernia versus a normal esophagus was still evident in this study.

The size of the hiatal hernia appears to be correlated with the risk for developing gastroesophageal reflux. Patti et al. evaluated 139 patients undergoing evaluation for GERD with upper endoscopy, esophageal manometry, and 24-h pH monitoring (14). Ninety-five patients from this total were found to have increased esophageal acid exposure and formed the study group. Hiatal hernias ($n = 51$) were subdivided according to hernia size with 31 being less than 3 cm in length, 14 between 3 and 5 cm, and 6 greater than 5 cm in axial length. These groups were compared with the remaining 44 patients without hernia who were found to have had increased esophageal acid exposure. Heartburn and regurgitation were found to be more common in the group with hernias larger than 5 cm. Patients with hernias greater than 3 cm had shorter LES with lower resting pressure and lower contraction amplitudes in the distal esophagus than patients with no hernia or hernias smaller than 3 cm. The patients with longer hernias also had more esophageal acid exposure and reduced acid clearance in comparison to those with small or no hernias.

Ott et al. have also published a large series of 319 patients who had undergone barium esophagogram and 24-h pH monitoring to determine the correlation between presence and size of hiatal hernia using 24-h pH monitoring as a measure of degree of gastroesophageal reflux (15). Hiatal hernias were documented radiographically and categorized as "minimal" or "larger" (≥2 cm axial length). A total of 199 patients (62%) had hiatal hernias; 104 (52%) were classified as minimal, 95 (48%) as larger. The mean total esophageal acid exposure was noted to be statistically significantly lower ($p < 0.05$) among patients without hernias (3.7% exposure time) than patients with larger hernias (6.6%). Overall, the patients without hiatal hernias had fewer abnormal 24-h pH studies than those with larger hernias (18% vs. 35%, $p < 0.05$). This study concluded that the presence and size of hiatal hernia raise the risk for gastroesophageal reflux; however, the results were most significant in those patients with larger hernias. Concerns were noted regarding the limitations of radiographically defining hiatal hernias while in the prone position since normal dynamic changes of the esophagogastric junction during this test can create a "physiological herniation" that would increase the number of hernias reported and lower the overall percent of acid exposure measured via 24-h pH monitoring.

Petersen et al. reported on the relationship between endoscopic hiatal hernia with and without concomitant esophagitis and GER symptoms (16). They studied 930 patients who had submitted to upper endoscopy secondary to any symptoms referable to the gastrointestinal tract. While 14% had esophagitis, 17% of patients had hiatal hernia. Of the patients with hiatal hernia, 49% had esophagitis, compared with 7% without hiatal hernia. Of the patients with esophagitis, 60% had hiatal hernias, compared with only 10% of those without esophagitis. After excluding patients with peptic ulcer or malignancy, it was found that patients with hiatal hernia as the only pathological finding had significantly ($p < 0.01$) more GER symptoms than the patients with no major endoscopic abnormality.

Finally, the most current evidence supports the role of hiatal hernia size as the principal determinant of esophagitis in patients with symptomatic gastroesophageal reflux (17). An evaluation of 66 symptomatic GER patients and nine controls demonstrated that hiatal hernia size was the strongest predictor of esophagitis severity. LES pressure and male sex were weaker, but equivalent, predictors. The study found that abnormalities in 24-h pH monitoring were strongly correlated with hiatal hernia size and not independent predictors of esophagitis in and of themselves.

OBESITY

While obesity is associated with numerous adverse affects on the gastrointestinal tract (18), it is unclear whether obesity increases the risk for GER. If there is an increased risk, is this related to differences in LES pressure, the gastroesophageal pressure gradient, esophageal and gastric emptying, or some other anatomical factors such as hiatal hernia? The lack of clarity between obesity and GER may also relate to the wide variation in patient populations studied, which have ranged from massively obese patients referred for gastric reduction surgery to mildly or moderately obese patients treated with low-calorie diets. Many of these studies were also conducted without control groups, which further impairs the data. The differences in patient populations and the paucity of research in this area have resulted in a poor understanding between obesity and gastroesophageal reflux (Table 2).

A review of gastroesophageal reflux and obesity by Beauchamp in the early 1980s centered on the role of surgery for obese patients with complicated reflux (19). Those patients with esophageal stenosis, hemorrhage, or severe esophagitis unresponsive to medical management (in the pre–proton pump era) defined complicated reflux. Of 102 patients evaluated for GER, 52 were selected for surgery for complicated reflux but only 13 of these 52 patients, all of whom were 21–

Table 2 Studies That Have Examined the Relationship Between Obesity and Gastroesophageal Reflux

Study	Subjects (total number)	Modality					Findings/conclusions
		GE	Cine	EGD	EM	pH	
Wright, 1983	77	+	−	−	−	−	No correlation of BSA and gastric emptying found.
Beauchamp, 1983	52	+	+	+	+	−	Selected study population was not indicative of obese patients in general.
Mercer, 1985	29	+	−	−	+	−	Mean GE pressure gradient significantly greater ($p < 0.01$) in obese refluxers vs. lean with no reflux. Prolonged esophageal transit in the obese increases mucosal acid exposure time.
Mercer, 1987	16	−	−	−	+	−	No difference in LESP between lean and obese. Greater GE pressure gradient in obese ($p < 0.001$), in spite of normal LESP, may facilitate reflux.
Stene-Larsen, 1988	224	−	−	+	−	−	Greater degree of obesity (>5% over IBW) seen in those with HH and with esophagitis.
Maddox, 1989	62	+	−	−	−	−	Delayed solid ($p < 0.001$) and liquid ($p < 0.02$) gastric meal emptying and delayed esophageal emptying ($p < 0.001$) compared to controls. Study did not specifically evaluate for (manifestations of) reflux.
Hutson, 1993	53	+	−	−	+	−	Similar gastric emptying of solids and liquids in both groups, which did not change despite mean weight reduction of 8.3%.
Rigaud, 1995	20	+	−	+	−	+	Total number of reflux events significantly correlated to BMI, fat intake, and delayed gastric emptying.
Lundell, 1995	50	−	−	+	−	+	No increase in prevalence of GER in the massively obese.
Kjellin, 1996	20	−	−	−	−	+	No reduction in subjective or objective manifestations of reflux despite weight loss of more than 10 kg.
Mathus-Vliegen, 1996	17	−	−	−	−	+	Median pH values were normal at baseline and did not change after weight loss.

BSA = body surface area; BMI = body mass index; Cine = cine-esophagram; EGD = esophagogastroduodenoscopy; EM = esophageal manometry; GES = gastric emptying scan; GER = gastroesophageal reflux; IBW = ideal body weight; pH = pH monitoring; UGI = barium upper gastrointestinal series.

38% over ideal weight, were included in the study group. All 13 of this select group had hiatal hernias with endoscopic esophagitis on preoperative evaluation. After Nissen fundoplication, no patient had endoscopic esophagitis or recurrence of reflux symptoms. Though preoperative LES manometry was seen to increase from a mean of 3 mmHg to a postoperative mean of 23.5 mmHg, the low LES pressure was likely related to the finding of hiatal hernia rather than obesity. The investigators did not study all obese patients undergoing surgery; therefore, one could not determine whether hiatal hernias were more common in obese versus nonobese patients.

Stene-Larsen and colleagues reported on the degree of obesity and its relationship to hiatal hernia and reflux esophagitis among 1224 patients referred for upper endoscopy over a 1-year period (20). The study reported the endoscopic findings of hiatal hernia, defined as circular extension of gastric mucosa more than 1.5 cm above the diaphragm, and endoscopic as well as histological esophagitis. Unfortunately, the incidence of GER in this population was not measured by the more sensitive method of 24-h pH monitoring. Overall, there was no statistically significant difference between the patients with esophagitis and those without esophagitis with regard to mean weight; however, the weight-for-height index calculated for each patient showed an average degree of obesity of approximately 5% for patients with esophagitis or hernia. Patients without esophagitis or hernia had normal body weight, while patients with coexisting reflux esophagitis and hiatal hernia were significantly more obese ($p < 0.01$) and represented the most obese group of patients. The study found a strong correlation of typical GER symptoms with esophagitis and found that hiatal hernia was more common in the setting of esophagitis; however, the study did not specifically analyze the data with regard to the presence of obesity. In doing so, the study suggested an association between obesity, hiatal hernia, and GER, but failed to present the data in a manner that clearly demonstrated a greater risk of reflux esophagitis with obesity. Several difficulties exist when comparing this seemingly positive study to future studies. One was the failure to document reflux by means of 24-h pH monitoring another was the failure to analyze the subgroups by the presence or absence of hiatal hernia with or without obesity. Finally, the low levels of obesity in the study population, wherein more than 10% over ideal weight was considered the most severely affected group, makes it difficult to compare the study with other studies in the massively obese.

Wilson and colleagues reported a similar, large, retrospective, case-control study that examined the relationship between obesity, hiatal hernia, and GER (21). After having performed upper endoscopy on 189 patients with esophagitis with 1024 controls and 151 patients with hiatal hernia with 1053 controls, the investigators stratified the patients by body mass index (thin = BMI < 20, normal = BMI 20–25, mildly obese = BMI 25–30, and obese = BMI > 30).

Multivariate analysis of the results found that BMI was significantly associated with the presence of both hiatal hernia ($p < 0.01$) and esophagitis ($p < 0.05$). Hiatal hernia was also significantly associated with esophagitis (odds ratio 4.2, 95% CI 2.9–6.1).

Studies from the mid-1980s sought to document mechanisms whereby obesity could increase the risk for prolonged acid exposure by increasing the gastroesophageal pressure gradient. Mercer and colleagues investigated whether elevated intra-abdominal pressure in obesity affected esophageal transit as measured by radionuclide scintigraphic technique (22). The study evaluated eight patients without reflux and five reflux patients who were 2–6% over ideal body weight versus 16 obese reflux patients who were 28% over ideal body weight. Esophageal manometry was used to assess esophageal peristalsis, GER, and gastroesophageal pressure gradient simultaneously. Subjects with known esophageal motility disorders were excluded from the study. No differences were noted between the lean reflux patients and the lean patients without reflux while obese reflux patients were significantly different in all measured parameters. Mean body mass, gastroesophageal pressure gradient, and mean transit time were significantly greater in the very obese versus the minimally obese group ($p < 0.01$–0.001). This study suggested that delayed transit of esophageal contents could result in prolonged exposure to gastroduodenal contents leading to a greater risk of mucosal injury.

A later study from 1989 evaluated radionuclide gastric and esophageal emptying in the obese to determine whether delayed emptying was related to body weight (23). This study evaluated 31 obese patients who were 40–174% over ideal body weight and 31 controls who were within 20% of ideal weight. Both gastric emptying of the solids ($p < 0.001$) and liquids ($p < 0.02$) in addition to esophageal emptying ($p < 0.001$) were delayed in the obese patients when compared to controls but there was no correlation between symptoms and the test results. Unfortunately, GER was not assessed. Other studies have failed to show differences in gastric emptying between obese and normal-weight subjects (18,24) or even abnormally rapid gastric emptying in obese subjects (25) thus adding to the controversy that GER results from delayed esophageal and gastric emptying in the obese.

Lundell et al. prospectively tested for GER by means of a standardized questionnaire, 24-h ambulatory pH monitoring, and endoscopy in 50 massively obese patients with a mean weight of 125.5 ± 17 kg (mean body mass index 42.5 kg/m^2) who were referred for weight-reduction gastroplasty (26). Symptomatically, mild heartburn and acid regurgitation were reported in 37% and 28%, respectively, while endoscopic esophagitis and pH studies showed no differences from the control population (mean weight 72.4 ± 11 kg). Multivariate linear regression analysis was performed between body weight, waist-to-hip ratio, BMI, and percent total, upright, and supine reflux time. No measure of obesity was associated with an increased acid reflux into the esophagus and unpublished 1-year follow-up data noted no reduction in acid reflux despite gastroplasty-related weight reduction.

Finally, Kjellin et al. reported that GER in obese patients did not decrease with weight reduction (27). In this study, obese patients had a mean body mass index of 31.4 kg/m^2 (range 28–42 kg/m^2) while the normal range was defined as 19–25 kg/m^2. Twenty patients with proven 24-h pH reflux and symptoms requiring daily medication were divided into two groups with one receiving a very-low-caloric diet and the other a normal diet. The treated group lost 10.8 ± 1.4 kg whereas the control group gained 0.6 ± 0.7 kg ($p < 0.001$). No reduction in GER was noted by pH monitoring and the subjects remained symptomatic. Likewise, when the control group lost weight (9.7 ± 1.6 kg), reflux persisted with patients remaining on medication for reflux.

In an interesting commentary that reviewed yet another investigation in which there was no detectable relationship between massive obesity and GER (28), Castell (29) reminds us of the role that dietary fat plays in lowering LES pressure and increasing TLESRs. A study by Rigaud and colleagues (30) of 20 morbidly obese patients had also correlated more frequent reflux events with fat intake. Before we assume that our obese patients suffer from GER as a result of their body habitus, we should first be cognizant of the important role that diet plays in all patients.

The concept that GER is more commonly seen in obese individuals and that weight loss in obese patients results in improvement of GER is widely accepted as part of the pathophysiology of GERD (31) despite the different conclusions from some of the studies discussed. Perhaps the image of an obese patient with heartburn is so prevalent among health care providers we have accepted this connection as fact without the proof of valid scientific study. On the other hand, the degree of GERD in obese patients may be so severe that our measurable parameters are too insensitive to note changes following weight reduction. Clearly, continued careful research in obesity needs to be performed.

ALCOHOL USE

In contrast to the poor correlation between obesity and GER, there is more evidence that links alcohol use to GER. Hogan et al. demonstrated that normal subjects had impaired propulsive motor activity of the esophagus and a reduction in LES pressure following the administration of 350 mL of bourbon (104 g alcohol) suggesting that one could be susceptible to GER with substantial alcohol ingestion (32). Keshavarzian et al. showed that 13 of 13 healthy controls demonstrated a transient decrease in LES pressure and in 10 of 13, a moderate decrease in esophageal contraction amplitude after the intravenous administration of 0.8 g/kg ethanol (33). The alcoholic group in this study had significantly less inhibition of LES pressure indicating a degree of tolerance. The esophageal contraction amplitude in the alcoholic group was actually increased compared to normals in agreement with prior studies of esophageal motor dysfunction in alcoholics (34). Alcohol has also been shown to reduce the normal clearing capacity of infused hydrochloric acid (35) and to diminish stimulated salivary output from the parotid glands (36,42), both of which could lead to more severe manifestations of GER.

In 1978, Kaufman and Kaye demonstrated that alcohol could cause GER in normal, healthy, young volunteers (37). Twelve patients without symptoms of GER were monitored with esophageal pH probes after consuming 180 mL of 100-proof vodka (90 g) versus consuming 180 mL of water. Eleven of the 12 patients had more GER following alcohol consumption and clearly demonstrated that at this ethanol dose, there was a measurable increase in GER. Vitale and colleagues (38) administered 120 mL of 80-proof scotch whiskey (48 g) to 17 healthy, young volunteers (average age 23.8 years) who underwent ambulatory 24-h pH monitoring pre– and post–alcohol ingestion. Seven of the 17 subjects had prolonged supine reflux episodes on the night of the alcohol ingestion while none of the subjects had reflux on the control night ($p < 0.01$). All of the prolonged reflux episodes occurred within 6 h of ingestion of the whiskey, while the subjects were asleep. The subjects were not aroused by the reflux episodes, and the subjects remained asymptomatic the following morning. The evidence for an increased risk of GER due to the ingestion of alcohol is well supported by these studies and is related to a decrement in LES pressure and decreased acid clearance from the esophagus.

Additionally, alcohol appears to differentially affect gastric acid secretion and serum gastrin depending upon the ethanol content of the alcohol ingested. With beer and wine (low ethanol content), ethanol stimulates acid secretion and gastrin release, while whiskey, gin, and cognac (high ethanol content) have little effect on these parameters (39). Unfortunately, resting LES pressure is probably not affected by physiological levels of serum gastrin. Mayer et al. reported that alcohol significantly inhibits the LES response to pharmacological doses of pentagastrin in a dose-dependent fashion whether the alcohol was given intravenously or by intraesophageal infusion (40). The authors felt that though not specifically investigated, a neural mechanism, rather than direct effects on the smooth muscle of the LES, mediated the observed effects. In contrast to these findings, Keshavarzian et al. used the cat model as a means of evaluating the effects of acute ethanol on esophageal motility (41). They found that both bilateral cervical vagotomy and the intravenous injection of the neurotoxin tetrodotoxin before the administration of ethanol did not prevent the effects of ethanol on the LES pressure. These results would argue for a direct effect of acute ethanol on muscle.

Based on the available literature in normal volunteers, the recommendation to avoid acutely imbibing more than 40–45 g of alcohol appears to prevent the induction of GER. In vitro studies using the cat model and clinical studies with humans (33,41,42) have demonstrated a decrease in LES pressure in response to the acute administration of ethanol. Interestingly, however, only a few studies have specifically evaluated the effects of alcohol on esophageal function and GER in chronic alcoholics. In fact, most studies in chronic alcoholics agree in demonstrating an elevated LES pressure, together with a higher incidence of esophageal motor dysfunction and changes in both salivary composition and flow rate (33,34,43,44), yet no specific studies of GER in this population have been performed. Finally, all of the studies that we evaluated studied normal, healthy control subjects. A need remains for studies evaluating the acute effects of alcohol in nonalcoholic patients with known GER.

CIGARETTE SMOKING

Long suspected of having an exacerbating role in GER, the effects of tobacco smoking on the esophagus and LES became more clearly understood as a result of work performed by Dennish and Castell in the early 1970s (45) (Table 3). They evaluated six normal male volunteers who were chronic cigarette smokers but had no symptoms of GERD. Esophageal manometry demonstrated a significant ($p < 0.001$) decrement in LES pressure from baseline while smoking two consecutive cigarettes with LES pressure returning to normal within 2–3 min of finishing the cigarettes. Puffing on an unlit cigarette revealed no change in LES pressure from baseline. These results suggested an acute effect of cigarette smoking on lowering LES pressure.

Stanciu and Bennett used pH monitoring in addition to manometry to evaluate GER in 25 chronic smokers who complained of heartburn (46). All patients had symptoms characteristic of heartburn related to posture and the postprandial state; 14 had radiographic evidence of GER and all smoked 15–60 cigarettes daily at baseline. During the study, LES pressure fell significantly ($p < 0.01$) within 1–4 min of smoking and returned to the starting pressure within 3–8 min after finishing the cigarette. The number of reflux episodes as measured by pH monitoring rose significantly (one event every 156.6 min vs. one event every 13.9 min, $p < 0.001$) when compared prior to and during smoking. Puffing on an unlit cigarette as a control again found no significant change from basal LES pressure. Again, chronic smokers were found to have acute lowering of LES pressure as well as an increase in reflux events while smoking.

Chattopadhyay and colleagues also evaluated the effect of smoking on LES pressure in 10 asymptomatic volunteers and 10 subjects with symptoms of GER (47) 8/10 of whom had endoscopic esophagitis and 10/10 had sliding hiatal hernias found on barium swallow. There was a significant drop in LES pressure during smoking and a return to baseline upon finishing cigarette smoking al-

Table 3 Studies That Have Examined the Relationship Between Cigarette Smoking and Gastroesophageal Reflux

Study	Subjects (total number)	Modality				Conclusions
		ACT	EGD	EM	pH	
Dennish, 1971	6	−	−	+	−	Rapid decrease in LESP from baseline within 2–3 min of smoking.
Stanciu, 1972	25	−	−	+	+	Significant ($p < 0.01$) fall in LESP within 1–4 min of smoking.
Chattopadhyay, 1977	20	−	−	+	−	Reduction of LESP during cigarette smoking.
Schindlbeck, 1987	40	−	−	−	+	More reflux episodes (upright and supine) in smokers than absolute nonsmokers though percent time pH < 4 was similar in both groups.
Kahrilas, 1989	24	+	−	+	−	60% less titratable base secretion and 50% longer acid clearance times at baseline in smokers; worsening immediately upon smoking.
Waring, 1989	8	−	−	−	+	Immediate cessation of smoking did not affect total esophageal acid exposure.
Kahrilas, 1990	26	−	−	+	+	Probable exacerbation of GER via a direct increase in acid reflux and by lasting effects on lowering LESP.
Kadakia, 1995	14	−	+	+	+	Significant increase in upright reflux.
Pehl, 1997	280	−	−	−	+	Similar (high) percentage of abnormal pH studies (50–53%) suggesting GER with no differences seen between the groups.

ACT = acid clearance test; EM = esophageal manometry; GER = gastroesophageal reflux; LESP = lower-esophageal-sphincter pressure; pH = intraesophageal pH monitoring.

though the study did not identify whether any of the subjects were chronic smokers.

The majority of the early evidence regarding smoking and GER substantiated an increased risk based on effects at the LES and an accompanying increase of reflux events. As we know that the manifestations of GER, such as esophagitis, are dependent on the extent of acid contact time, there appeared to be little room to dispute this relationship. One of the first studies to dispute the relationship between smoking and reflux was reported by Shindlbeck et al. in 1987 (48). In this study, the effect of smoking on GER was studied in 30 healthy volunteers (15 chronic smokers, 15 nonsmokers) and 10 smokers with known GER. The authors reported a significant increase in reflux episodes in the smokers compared to the nonsmokers though the percentage of time with $pH < 4$ and the duration of reflux episodes was similar in both groups. Abstaining from smoking for 24 h did not affect the results of repeat 24-h pH studies in smokers. The authors stated that it was ''questionable whether abstaining from smoking has a beneficial effect in patients with reflux disease.''

In a well-designed study, Kahrilas and Gupta reported a study involving eight nonsmoking volunteers and 16 chronic cigarette smokers (49). The aim was to define and compare the immediate effects of cigarette smoking on esophageal acid clearance time and salivary function—two additional parameters that determine the severity of GER. In chronic smokers, the acute effect of smoking resulted in a significant ($p < 0.05$) prolongation of acid clearance time. A similar finding was noted when smokers who refrained from smoking were compared to the nonsmokers ($p < 0.05$) suggesting an acute and lasting effect of smoking on acid clearance time. Because the oral stimulation inherent in smoking was felt to potentially counteract nicotine's pharmacological effect of hyposalivation, the after-smoking period was analyzed and revealed a slight reduction in salivary titratable base secretion. Smokers who did not smoke during the experiment showed lower ($p < 0.05$) salivary base excretion than the nonsmokers indicating that reduced salivary function in chronic smokers contributed to a decrease in acid clearance time compared to a nonsmoking control group.

Despite earlier studies demonstrating that healing of esophagitis is impaired in smokers (50), Waring et al. suggested that the cessation of smoking did not significantly affect esophageal acid exposure among patients with symptoms and endoscopic evidence of GERD (51). Subjects smoked 20 cigarettes one day and no cigarettes on the following day while undergoing 24-h pH monitoring. Significant improvement in upright reflux was noted with the cessation of smoking as the number of smoking-induced transient LES relaxations decreased; however, as in Shindlbeck's study (48), the total reflux time did not significantly change. The authors concluded that recommending cessation of smoking was reasonable but questioned whether improvement in overall esophagitis would be noted.

In another study by Kahrilas and Gupta (52), esophageal manometry and pH monitoring were performed to determine the effect of smoking on LES function in eight normal nonsmokers, nine asymptomatic smokers, and nine smokers with hiatal hernia and endoscopic or histological evidence of esophagitis. Baseline manometry revealed that LES pressures were lowest in the smokers with GERD, higher in asymptomatic smokers, and highest in the nonsmoking controls. No correlation was seen between duration of smoking and baseline LES pressure. Manometric studies during smoking could not be meaningfully interpreted because of frequent swallowing, coughing, and respiratory artifact. An increase in the mean hourly rate of transient LES relaxations (TLESR) was noted in both groups of smokers, though most of these events were not associated with acid reflux by the pH electrode. When acid reflux events did occur, they were associated with coughing and deep inspiration, especially in patients with low LES pressure. Reflux events noted in the nonsmokers were entirely due to TLESR. The authors postulated that the increased rate of TLESRs in the smokers was a mechanism for venting the intragastric gas that had accumulated during smoking and not a dominant mechanism of GER as in the nonsmoking group.

To clarify the controversy regarding cigarette smoking and gastroesophageal reflux, Kadakia and colleagues studied 14 patients with daily heartburn, endoscopic esophagitis, and a smoking habit of 20 or more cigarettes per day (53). Each subject had ambulatory 24-h pH monitoring first after a 48-h washout period of no smoking and then resumed smoking for 48 h and had a repeat study while smoking at least 20 cigarettes over a 14-h period. In contrast to Waring and Shindlbeck's studies (48,51), Kadakia et al. found that the total reflux time was significantly increased ($p < 0.007$) during the 24 h of smoking, especially in the upright position where a 114% increase in daytime heartburn following reflux events was seen. Prior studies probably failed to show a significant change in acid exposure because of a short washout period that resulted in incomplete washout of serum nicotine. This study by Kadakia et al. reaffirmed the finding that cigarette smoking raised the risk for symptomatic reflux and clarified some important controversies in this area.

Most recently, Pehl and colleagues (54) studied 280 patients with various symptoms suggesting reflux to see if smoking influenced the results of 24-h pH monitoring. Of these 280 patients, 78 were smokers and 202 were nonsmokers. Forty-five of the 78 smokers continued to smoke during the pH study while 33 abstained. No difference in reflux episodes or the fraction of pH time <4 was noted among the various groups, including those whose pH studies were consistent with GER. No mention of degree of smoking (packs per day), no standardization of the number of cigarettes smoked during the study, nor nicotine washout period was obtained, making it difficult to determine the full extent of the influence that smoking had in these patients. Interestingly, while a high percentage of patients from each group (50–53%) had pH monitoring indicating GER, none of them appeared to have severe GER and the only within-group comparison made was based on three 10-min periods. Whether smoking contributed to this high percentage is not given in the presentation of the data. Despite these potential shortcomings, the investigators concluded that neither smoking nor abstaining from smoking affected GER as measured by pH monitoring.

The evidence that cigarette smoking raises the risk for GER does not enjoy a unanimous opinion; however, the majority of the studies that we have discussed favor an increased risk of GER with smoking. Numerous pathophysiological mechanisms have been discussed in the literature (55) and include reduced LES pressure with increases in reflux from coughing or inhalation of smoke, increase in TLESRs, reduction in salivary base secretion, decreased acid clearance times, and possible irritant effects on the esophageal epithelia (56) from cigarette smoke. The literature is replete with evidence to demonstrate an increased prevalence of complicated reflux such as erosive esophagitis and the sequelae of severe reflux such as Barrett's esophagus and adenocarcinoma of the esophagus in smokers. We feel that it is prudent to continue to urge current smokers toward cessation especially in symptomatic GER.

NASOGASTRIC INTUBATION

The association between a nasogastric tube (NGT) and GER has been studied since the late 1950s (Table 4) although evidence of associated esophagitis has been noted since the 1930s. These early studies were retrospective, uncontrolled case reports, often from autopsy findings or in severely ill, hospitalized patients. In addition, the presence of multiple confounding factors such as preexisting GER, recumbency, vomiting, surgical trauma, or comorbid illness could also be reasons for esophagitis in these patients. In 1936, Butt and Vinson showed that 31% of 213 patients with autopsy-proven esophagitis had been previously intubated with an NGT and that the history of severe vomiting also correlated with esophagitis (57). In another postmortem study of 82 patients, Bartels disagreed, noting no greater prevalence of esophagitis in previously intubated patients (58).

Nagler and colleagues, in 1960, studied whether a rubber Levin tube placed in the stomach was associated with gastroesophageal reflux during a standard barium upper gastrointestinal study (59). No evidence of gastroesophageal reflux of barium was noted during the time of the study or immediately following the removal of the nasogastric tube.

The same authors then studied the effects of prolonged (3 h) NGT intubation while the patient remained in the supine position (60). At baseline, esophageal pH only transiently fell below 4.0; however, the pH decreased for 2 h immediately following the instillation of 300 mL of 0.1 N hydrochloric acid into the stomach with the patients complaining of progressively severe heartburn. Subcu-

Table 4 Studies That Have Examined the Relationship Between Nasogastric Intubation and Gastroesophageal Reflux

Study	Subjects	Modality used	Tube type	Length of time tube in place	Outcome
Nagler, 1960	20 normals	Barium upper-GI cineroentgenography	Levin	During the radiographic study only	No reflux seen
Nagler, 1963	3, all symptomatic	pH monitor	pH electrode	3 h	Supine reflux when tube across GEJ and acid instilled in stomach
Vinnik, 1964	12 normals	pH monitor	16-Fr Levin tube	Up to 72 h	Reflux in 7/12
Fisher, 1976	30, all with known GER	GE scintiscan	2-lumen NGT	Not specified	No difference in GE reflux with or without NG tube
Satiani, 1978	146 surgical patients	Visual inspection of indigo carmine dye pre and post endotracheal tube placement	14-Fr NGT	45 min–8 h	GER in 5/81 (6.2%) with the NGT, GER in 8/65 (12.3%) without an NGT
Emde, 1989	7 normals	Ambulatory 24-h pH monitor	3-mm pH electrode	24 h	No influence on GER with 3-mm cable across the GEJ
Singh, 1992	10 normals, 10 with GER	Ambulatory 24-h pH monitor	3-mm pH electrode	24 h	Increase in supine reflux in 3/10 normals and 9/10 GER patients with tube across GEJ
Ibañez, 1992	70 critically ill, mechanically ventilated patients receiving enteral nutrition	Technetium 99m sulfur colloid scintiscan	5.5-mm NGT	NGT in place at least 48 h, scan done after tube clamped for 2 h	GER in 37/54 (74%) with NGT in place, GER in 7/20 (35%) without NGT
Dotson, 1994	11 normals	Radioisotope scintiscan	8-Fr and 14-Fr NGT	1 h	No effect of tube on GER
Kuo, 1995	8 normals	pH monitor	2.1-mm pH probe and 3.8-mm NGT	6 h	No effect on GER with either tube, or both
Orozco-Levi, 1995	15 critically ill mechanically ventilated patients	Technetium 99m sulfur colloid scintiscan	5-mm NGT	NGT in place at least 48 h	Increase in GER seen after 5 h of monitoring

Fr = French size; GE = gastroesophageal; GEJ = gastroesophageal junction; GER = gastroesophageal reflux; GI = gastrointestinal; NGT = nasogastric tube.

taneous histamine also caused heartburn and at no time was there a change in LES pressure or associated esophageal spasm. When the subjects were restudied in the sitting position, no change in intraesophageal pH was seen even after the intragastric instillation of 300 mL 0.1 N hydrochloric acid. When the NGT was positioned 5 cm proximal to the LES, no reflux was noted despite the instillation of acid into the stomach and with the patient being in the supine position. Finally, when the subjects were studied in the supine position and at 10, 30, 45, and 90 degrees, esophageal reflux was seen only in the supine position. These authors concluded that the following conditions must be present for NGT-associated GER: a sufficient amount of acid must be available for reflux, the patient must be supine, and the NGT must cross the LES. Despite their findings, the authors were unable to describe the mechanism by which gastric intubation induced reflux since LES integrity was normal and reflux by capillary action could not be invoked as reflux did not occur in any of the upright positions. They postulated that transient relaxations allowed acid to become trapped around the tube with impaired acid clearance due to the presence of the tube.

Vinnik and Kern (61) performed a similar study in which 12 normal subjects had a 16-Fr Levin NGT placed for 48 h. In seven of 12 subjects, the pH fell below 4 with resolution of reflux following the NGT removal. Persistent reflux of 6 and 14 h was noted in two subjects despite NGT removal. It was suggested that the NGT might cause a transient alteration in the competency of the sphincter though no specific mechanisms were elucidated by this study.

In contrast to these studies, a prospective randomized study conducted on 146 surgical patients evaluated the incidence of gastric regurgitation and aspiration during general anesthesia and found that regurgitation was actually less common (6% vs. 12%) in the presence of a nasogastric tube (62). After evacuation of the gastric contents with a 14-Fr sump NGT, regurgitation was evaluated following the intragastric instillation of 2 cc of indigo carmine dye. Patients were randomized to tube removal or tube retention and the presence of the dye was sought in the oropharyngeal or endotracheal location just prior to and after the removal of the endotracheal tube. This study was limited by its design because esophageal regurgitation could not be assessed, gastric contents were aspirated from the stomach, and 2 cc of dye could have easily emptied from the stomach during the surgery.

Emde et al. (63) determined that a 3-mm pH probe placed across the LES and into the stomach did not increase intraesophageal acid exposure in normal subjects. However, Singh and Richter (64) noted that three of 10 healthy volunteers had increases in their supine acid exposure times when a pH electrode crossed the LES. In patients with known GER, a significant ($p = 0.01$) increase in supine esophageal acid exposure time was measured when the electrode was across the LES compared to intraesophageal-placed electrodes (12.1% vs. 4.4%). Interestingly, 5/9 initially had normal supine parameters, becoming abnormal only after the electrode was passed beyond the LES. These data suggested that poor acid clearance was the cause of the patients' increased supine acid exposure times and that even the presence of a 3-mm-diameter pH electrode across the LES could promote GER, primarily in the supine position.

NGT diameter has been specifically studied to determine its effect on GER. Two separate studies (65,66) noted that NGT size was not an important determinant of GER. These studies were small, with 11 and eight normal subjects, and of short duration (1 h and 6 h). The first study (65) evaluated GER by technetium 99m sulfur colloid scintigraphy at baseline and after passage of an 8-Fr and 14-Fr NGT in the supine position. An abdominal binder was inflated from 0 to 100 mmHg in 20-mmHg increments to provoke reflux in these subjects but no GER was noted. The second study (66) randomly measured esophageal pH at baseline without an NGT tube, with a 2.1-mm pH probe across the gastroesophageal junction, and with a 3.8-mm NGT attached to a 2.1-mm pH probe traversing the GE junction. No abnormal reflux was demonstrated during the 6 h that these normal volunteers were in the supine position.

The effect of patient position while intubated with an NGT has also been specifically studied to determine its impact on the tendency to reflux (67,68). These studies were performed on critically ill patients, the majority of whom were being mechanically ventilated in an intensive-care setting. Both studies overwhelmingly concluded that GER was more common in patients with orotracheal intubation and nasogastric intubation; however, the influence of confounding factors made it very difficult to determine the relative contribution of each variable.

In summary, it seems that NGT can cause GER if the following conditions are met: (1) the patient is in the supine position, (2) there is a fairly large amount of acid in the stomach (300 mL or more), and (3) the NGT remains in the patient for a protracted period (72 h or more). Patients with preexisting GER are more prone to NGT-associated GER, and while the exact causative factor for GER is not known in intubated subjects, GER seems to be a common problem in the patient with an NGT.

MEDICATIONS

The gastroesophageal effects of medications that contribute to a higher risk of GER may include alterations in LES pressure, esophageal motility, or gastric emptying. Medications may also cause caustic or inflammatory changes to the esophageal mucosa resembling reflux or pill-induced esophagitis. It is imperative that physicians know what medications predispose one to GER so that symptoms may be ameliorated by discontinuing the offending agent. In this section, we will review the agents that are felt to contribute to GER.

Anticholinergics

The major cholinergic neurotransmitter, acetylcholine, exerts a direct effect that increases the pressure of the smooth-muscle LES. Likewise, metoclopramide, domperidone, and cisapride act by releasing acetylcholine and indirectly increasing LES pressure. An antagonist of acetylcholine such as atropine should decrease LES pressure and increase the risk of GER. Brock-Utne et al. in 1977 (69) studied the effects of hyoscine and atropine on LES tone in normal human subjects, noting a decrease in LES pressure of approximately 11 cm H_2O ($p < 0.01$), and increased GER on pH monitoring. In another study (70), a similar decrement in LES pressure by an anticholinergic agent was reversed by domperidone.

While these anticholinergic agents were known to reduce the pressure of the LES, it had not been clearly shown that their therapeutic or diagnostic use led to increased GER. Hyoscine butylbromide is an anticholinergic agent known to reduce the pressure of the LES and is used as a hypotonic agent during upper-gastrointestinal examinations. McLoughlin et al. evaluated 112 consecutive patients for the presence or absence and the severity of GER before and after the injection of this agent (71) and found no significant difference in the overall occurrence ($p = 0.41$) or degree ($p = 0.81$) of reflux before and after injection of hyoscine butylbromide. Mittal et al. (72) reported similar results in 1995 when evaluating 13 normal subjects to determine the effects of atropine on LES pressure. They found that atropine reduced the basal LES pressure (16.4 $\pm$ 3 to 8.7 $\pm$ 2 mmHg) but that the frequency of reflux actually decreased ($p < 0.05$) after the injection of atropine compared to the control period. When GER did occur during periods of atropine-induced low LES pressure, TLESR and inhibition of the crural diaphragm were found to be the major mechanisms. Overall, atropine-induced low LES pressure did not predispose to GER in normal subjects, but instead reduced the frequency of reflux by inhibiting the TLESRs. The results demonstrated that a reduction in LES pressure in normal subjects did not necessarily cause pathological reflux and that other physiological effects of the pharmacological agent may actually reduce the amount of reflux seen in normal patients—wherein TLESRs are felt to be the mechanism responsible for the majority of reflux episodes. This study did not address patients with low to low-normal LES pressure or those with known GER. Lidums et al. reported a subsequent study with 15 reflux patients in 1998 (73), and again demonstrated that atropine inhibits reflux through the inhibition of TLESR and swallow induced LES relaxation.

Theophylline

The most common xanthines to adversely affect GER are caffeine and theophylline. Stein et al. in 1980 (74) compared the effects of theophylline on LES pressure in a group of normal volunteers and a group of asthmatics with symptoms of GER. Esophageal manometry was performed on four normal subjects and six asthmatics with symptoms of GER at baseline and after intravenous aminophylline was infused to obtain therapeutic levels. All four controls and five of the six asthmatics had a significant mean decrease ($p < 0.02$) in the LES pressure from baseline although GER was not evaluated.

A randomized, double-blind study (75) measured the effect of oral theophylline on acid reflux in 24 normal adults. Fifteen were randomized to receive theophylline and nine were given placebo. All of the theophylline patients demonstrated a 14% reduction in LES pressure, while only two of nine (22%) adults given placebo demonstrated such numbers. Thirteen of the 15 patients given theophylline had normal acid reflux tests at baseline. Eight of these 13 (61.5%) developed positive acid reflux tests by pH monitoring in comparison to none of the eight patients with normal baseline tests given placebo. One of nine (11%) placebo subjects reported heartburn compared to 11 of 15 (73%) theophylline subjects. The study concluded that oral theophylline inhibited LES pressure and induced GER in otherwise normal adults.

Johannesson et al. (76) provided additional evidence that theophylline also stimulated gastric secretion (77), which could contribute to GER in the setting of a relaxed LES. They compared the effects of another antiasthmatic xanthine, enprofylline, with theophylline using LES manometry and gastric acid secretory studies in eight normal, healthy volunteers. The study found that both medications lowered LES pressure to the same extent, but only theophylline stimulated gastric secretion via a mechanism independent of gastrin stimulation.

In a randomized, double blind, crossover study, Hubert and colleagues (78) compared the effects of theophylline (mean dose 9.8 ± 1.6 mg/kg/day) and placebo on the incidence of GER in 16 adult patients with asthma. Nocturnal intraesophageal pH monitoring (15 h) was performed after 1 week in each arm of the study. There was a trend for the number of reflux episodes to be higher with theophylline than placebo, which was very close to statistical significance ($p = 0.051$).

The evidence is clear that theophylline will lower the tone of the LES and increase gastric secretion. Obviously these effects will not lead to uniform reflux in all patients who use these medications, but it is worthwhile reminding patients with severe GER and asthma that theophylline is a medication that may worsen the manifestations of reflux.

Calcium Channel Blockers

The family of medications known as calcium channel antagonists comprises three structurally separate groups of medications: the benzothiazepines, represented by diltiazem; the diphenylalkylamines, represented by verapamil; and the dihydropyridines, represented by nifedipine. Each of these groups has different affinities for different types of smooth muscle and has come to occupy its own therapeutic niche for various medical disorders.

Although these medications could relieve the discomfort associated with esophageal motility disorders, the question remained as to whether decreased LES pressure could lead to GER and pain from esophagitis. If so, this class of medications might represent a double-edged sword, curing esophageal chest pain from dysmotility on one side, but raising the risk of GER and esophagitis on the other.

The ability of these medications to lower the LES pressure was reviewed by Richter et al. in 1985 (79). In this review it was mentioned that diltiazem decreased LES pressure in achalasia patients but had no effect in healthy volunteers or patients with the ''nutcracker esophagus.'' Nifedipine, however, had been shown to demonstrate a dose-related decrease in LES pressure in normal volunteers and patients with the nutcracker esophagus, in addition to its effects in achalasia (79,80).

An Italian study published in 1992 reported on ''oesophageal angina'' in patients with angina pectoris (81). In this study, the authors evaluated 18 subjects in whom nitrates and calcium channel antagonists did not improve or prevent angina-like chest pain. Eighteen patients with underlying angina pectoris underwent endoscopy, manometry, acid perfusion testing, and 24-h ambulatory pH monitoring of the esophagus. Ten of the 18 subjects had severe esophageal motility disorders, the most common of which was diffuse esophageal spasm. Basal LES tone was significantly lower than normal in all subjects and pathological GER was demonstrated in 14/18. It was postulated that the chronic use of nitrates and calcium channel antagonists might lead to angina-like chest pain by virtue of their ability to promote GER or esophageal motility disorders.

These studies indicate that in patients with preexisting GER, or in patients with other risk factors that would raise their risk independent of these medications, the calcium channel antagonists should be avoided if at all possible. If a calcium channel antagonist must be used for other indications, e.g., angina pectoris, diltiazem is the agent with the least effect on the LES in normal patients.

Other Pharmacological Agents

Other medications have been investigated with regard to their effects on the LES and the associated risk that gastroesophageal reflux might be induced or exacerbated. Singh et al. reported on the effect of the benzodiazepine alprazolam on esophageal motility and acid reflux in 1992 (82). They evaluated 10 healthy volunteers in a randomized, placebo-controlled study while administering alprazolam three times a day or placebo. While alprazolam had no significant effect on LES pressure or motility in the esophagus, one-third of the subjects had abnormal nocturnal acid reflux as measured by 24-h pH during the alprazolam phase of the study. The researchers felt that the alprazolam depressed the central nervous system resulting in deeper sleep levels with difficulty arousing to clear refluxed acid. The researchers pointed out that alprazolam interferes with arousal from sleep and therefore acid clearance is diminished. Though not specifically studied, commonly prescribed benzodiazepines such as diazepam, midazolam, and temazepam affect sleep and depress the central nervous system and one should be cautious in prescribing these agents to patients with GERD.

Nonsteroidal anti-inflammatory drugs (NSAIDs) have been implicated in a myriad of gastrointestinal complaints including inflammation, erosion and ulceration, pill-induced injury, and GER. Prior studies (83) have shown that PGE_2 inhibits LES pressure and decreases esophageal contractions while $PGF_2\alpha$ has the opposite effect. Hence, the administration of NSAIDs could interfere with the synthesis of both classes of prostaglandins and lead to an increase or decrease in LES pressure. One prior study, in which a single rectal dose of indomethacin increased LES pressure, demonstrated a beneficial influence on potential GER (84).

To determine whether NSAIDs could induce GER, Scheiman et al. studied the effects of naproxen on reflux parameters and esophageal function (85). Nine healthy volunteers received either naproxen 500 mg orally twice a day or placebo for 1 week followed by esophageal manometry and 24-h pH monitoring. After a 14-day washout period, the patients were crossed over and repeat studies were performed after a week on the other drug. Although reflux did increase in some subjects while taking naproxen, the NSAID had no significant effect on motility parameters nor did it induce GER in normal subjects. Prior endoscopic studies demonstrated that NSAID users had less esophagitis than gastric or duodenal injury. This suggested that a local irritative toxicity, rather than esophageal reflux, was the probable mechanism of action behind esophageal symptoms in NSAID users. Based on these results, the researchers postulated that pyrosis experienced during NSAID use might not even arise from the esophagus or might reflect an alteration in esophageal mucosal sensitivity secondary to NSAIDs. They suggested that the effects of NSAIDs on individuals with an increased risk for reflux be further studied.

Premedications used in patients undergoing general anesthesia have been studied with regard to GER and pulmonary aspiration. During induction of anesthesia, the loss of airway protection is unavoidable. Hall et al. (86) studied the effects of morphine sulfate, pethidine hydrochloride, and diazepam in 35 human volunteers and eight rhesus monkeys using esophageal manometry and esophageal pH probe. All three medications lowered LES pressure and were therefore felt to increase the probability of reflux in both monkey and human. Penagini and Bianchi (87) noted the opposite effect with morphine after evaluating eight healthy subjects and eight patients with reflux disease. Esophageal pH, LES, and esophageal pressures were simultaneously recorded for 30-min periods at baseline, after morphine, and after naloxone. Morphine reduced the number of reflux episodes ($p < 0.02$) and the time at pH < 4 ($p < 0.05$) in the reflux patients but not in the healthy controls. Morphine did not affect LES pressure in this study, but was seen to markedly reduce the number of transient LES relaxations ($p < 0.05$) in the reflux patients, in whom TLESRs were found to be the major mechanism responsible for reflux. Naloxone completely reversed the effects of morphine.

Rattan and Goyal published a study of the deleterious effects of intravenous dopamine on the tone of the LES of the opossum in 1976 (88), but when this agent was studied in normal humans (89) neither dopamine nor normal saline changed the LES pressure or raised the risk for clinically evident reflux.

Though not considered medications, enteral nutritional solutions are used as a source of nutrition in hospitalized, critically ill patients. The effects of intravenously and intragastrically administered amino acids (vs. saline control) on the LES pressure and frequency of TLESRs were studied by Gielkens et al. (90) using esophageal manometry and pH monitoring in six healthy volunteers. No significant changes in LES pressure or esophageal pH were seen in response to an intravenous or intragastric saline infusion; however, intravenous amino acid infusion caused a rapid and sustained decrease in LES pressure. Intragastric infusion of amino acids had a similar, but more gradual and temporary effect on LES pressure. The frequency of TLESRs, number of GER episodes, and duration of reflux did not differ between the baseline study, the two infusions of amino acids, or saline. The authors presented a discussion of the possible mechanisms whereby amino acids could influence GER to include LES relaxation resulting from the effects of nitric oxide donated from L-arginine. Whether amino acid infusion would lead to increased reflux in patients with a less competent antireflux barrier remains unanswered.

Finally, the effects of transdermal nicotine also merit discussion as to their impact on gastroesophageal reflux. Rahal and Wright presented data on 20 volunteers (91). Twelve were smokers, eight subjects were nonsmokers, and none had any history of GER. All were studied with a 24-h pH/motility apparatus while wearing a placebo patch followed by 24-h wearing a 21-mg nicotine patch. Smokers were not permitted to use any tobacco products during the study period though no prior washout period was performed. The study demonstrated a significant increase in acid exposure while wearing the nicotine patch compared to placebo with the differences noted during the supine period rather than upright. There was no significant difference in esophageal motility in response to nicotine.

Kadakia et al. evaluated 10 healthy, nonsmoking volunteers (92). Baseline esophageal manometry was performed followed by repeat manometry after wearing a 15-mg nicotine patch for 12 h. Plasma nicotine and cotinine levels were drawn prior to the two studies and demonstrated undetectable levels at baseline followed by significantly elevated levels after 12 h. LES pressure fell by 31% when measured by rapid pull-through technique and 27% by station pull-through after 12 h of the patch. No effects on motility of the esophageal body were demonstrated. The study concluded that transdermal delivery of nicotine resulted in significant reductions in LES pressure in healthy adult subjects. While pH monitoring was not performed, the demonstrated decrease in LES pressure provides a mechanism to explain de novo gastroesophageal reflux in healthy subjects as well as an explanation for more severe reflux in patients with preexisting GER. In their discussion, the authors highlighted the fact that further studies of the effects of transdermal nicotine in smokers with and without GER remain to be performed.

In this subsection, we have discussed various medications that have been linked with an increased risk of GER. As demonstrated by a review of the literature, the mechanisms by which medications lead to symptoms of heartburn or frank GER are often not entirely known. It appears unlikely that a single mechanism or common chemical mediator such as nitric oxide is involved in mediating GER, though this is still an area of active research. We should remind ourselves, our patients, and our colleagues of the possible effects that seemingly innocuous medications and substances can have on worsening underlying GER as well as the potential for development of de novo GER in otherwise asymptomatic patients.

PREGNANCY

The physiological changes that accompany the normal gravid state include effects involving the gastrointestinal system. GER is probably the most commonly seen gastrointestinal condition associated with pregnancy. Reports of the frequency of reflux have ranged from 48% (93) to 79% (94) in various studies with the true incidence of GER during pregnancy difficult to determine owing to a lack of large investigational studies to document its occurrence. Obstetricians are reluctant to place an expectant mother or her fetus at unnecessary risk such as that attendant to conscious sedation and especially radiographic studies. As a consequence, it is difficult to perform statistically relevant studies in this patient population.

Owing to the difficulty in performing procedures on pregnant patients in research protocols, much of the data regarding the prevalence of GER in pregnancy has come from questionnaires and other noninvasive techniques. One of the largest studies was a self-administered questionnaire given to 607 pregnant women at an antenatal clinic by Marrero et al. (95). This study reported an increase in the prevalence of heartburn with gestational age (22% in the first trimester, 39% in the second, and 72% in the third), though the symptom of pharyngeal regurgitation did not increase at the same rate. The researchers postulated that a hormone-related impairment on distal esophageal clearance was most likely involved in the higher incidence with time. Mechanical compression from the fetus was less likely as evidenced by the lack of improvement after fetal head descent.

Earlier theories concerning the pathophysiology of pregnancy-induced heartburn were a reflection of the state of technical expertise and the presumed psychic influence on pregnancy. Subsequent studies paralleled the expanding knowledge about the pathophysiology of GER and focused on the role of the LES in maintaining a competent antireflux barrier, the actions of gestational hormones on the esophagus, and the role of increased intra-abdominal pressure from the growing fetus.

One of the earliest studies to examine the role of the LES was done by Nagler and Spiro in 1961 (96). This study evaluated 39 pregnant women—20 with heartburn and 19 asymptomatic controls. Symptomatic patients were found to have a hypotensive LESP that progressively decreased with gestation and returned to normal after delivery. A later study by Van Theil and colleagues evaluated four pregnant women at 12, 24, and 36 weeks of gestation and again at 1–4 weeks postpartum (97). Again, LES pressure was seen to progressively fall during pregnancy and return to normal postpartum (Fig. 2).

These trends in reduction of LES pressure and increase in heartburn paralleled known increases in the female sex hormones with pregnancy (Fig. 3) and stimulated further research to specifically evaluate the role of estrogen and progesterone in pregnancy-related GER. Animal research using the opossum model

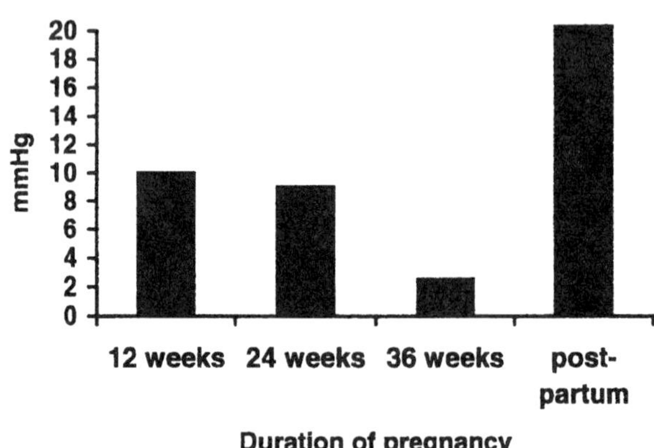

Figure 2 Measurement of LES pressure (mean values) in four women during pregnancy and in the postpartum period. Adapted from Van Thiel, 1977.

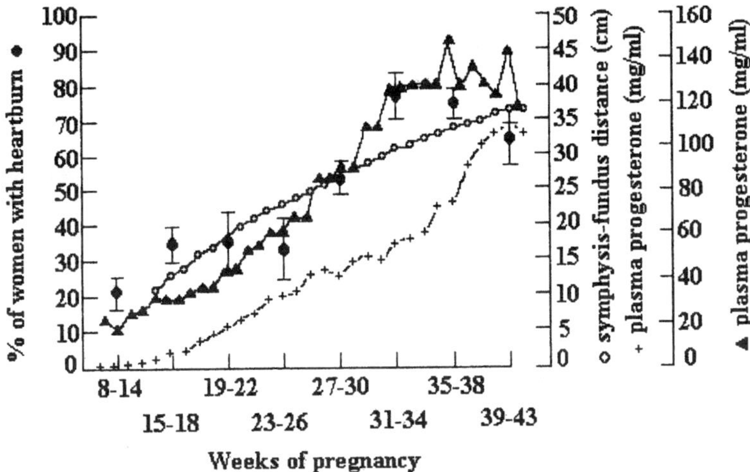

Figure 3 Relationship among prevalence of heartburn, symphysis-fundus height, plasma progesterone and urinary oestriol excretion with gestational age. Adapted from Marrero, 1992.

had demonstrated that the combination of estrogen and progesterone led to more pronounced decrements in LES muscle function than either estrogen or progesterone alone (98,99). Van Thiel and colleagues carried out similar human studies (100). They evaluated the effects of sequential estrogen and progesterone on LES pressure and found no change in LES pressure from baseline when estrogen was taken alone, but demonstrated a significant decrease in LES pressure on the days that both estrogen and progesterone were given. Further evidence was contributed by Filippone et al. in an interesting abstract published in 1983 (101). They studied five male transsexuals during a control period before hormone administration and while taking estrogen and progesterone in combination. The combination of hormones led to a significant decrease in resting LES pressure from baseline (11.2 ± 2.1 to 5.0 ± 0.7 mm Hg, $p < 0.02$), while neither hormone alone influenced changes significantly different from baseline (estrogen 11.0 ± 1.8 mmHg, progesterone 8.5 ± 1.7 mmHg, $p > 0.05$).

The commonly held belief regarding increased abdominal pressure (secondary to the enlarging gravid uterus) in the pathophysiology of pregnancy-related GER may be a misperception. It was originally felt that the enlarging uterus could increase gastric pressure, increase reflux down a gradient favoring retrograde flow across the gastroesophageal junction, and mechanically delay gastric emptying. A study in 1967 by Spence et al. examined intragastric pressures during anesthesia in 23 men, 36 children, 43 nonpregnant women, and 31 pregnant women (102). They found that intragastric pressure in the pregnant patients was twice that of the other groups and decreased immediately after delivery, suggesting the responsible role of the gravid uterus. On the other hand, a study by Lind and others in 1968 evaluated 10 nonpregnant asymptomatic controls, nine pregnant patients without heartburn, and 11 pregnant patients with heartburn (103). All of the pregnant women had been asymptomatic prior to pregnancy and none of the nonpregnant women were receiving hormonal therapy. The study demonstrated a normal increase in LES pressure in the controls with abdominal compression. Both groups of pregnant patients demonstrated an elevated baseline intragastric pressure equivalent to that obtained with abdominal compression in the normal controls. The interesting finding, however, was the differences in the maximal LES pressure measurements between the three groups. The pregnant patients without heartburn had a maximal sphincter pressure of 44.8 cm H_2O, which was significantly higher than the pressure of 34.8 cm H_2O found in the normal controls ($p < 0.02$). The symptomatic pregnant patients had a decreased maximal sphincter pressure of 23.8 cm H_2O, which was statistically significantly lower than that of both comparison groups. These findings demonstrated that asymptomatic pregnant patients were able to increase the maximal LES pressure over normal to compensate for an increased intragastric pressure while those women who could not generate this compensatory greater LES pressure had symptoms of heartburn. Postpartum studies conducted on some of the symptomatic women revealed a return toward normal control values. The authors did not offer an explanation why some pregnant women developed incompetent sphincter mechanisms and some did not, despite the fact that all were experiencing the same stressor in the form of an enlarged gravid uterus.

In an interesting study to isolate the true contribution of the gravid uterus as a potential mechanism in increasing reflux, Van Thiel and Wald studied LES pressure in 10 cirrhotic men with tense ascites before and after diuresis (104). None of the men had heartburn or evidence of acid reflux before or after diuresis. The tense ascites was felt to represent a pseudopregnant state in which abdominal pressure was increased to a level analogous to that of a pregnant woman at term and offered the opportunity to study the potential for GER due to this mechanism. The authors found that LES pressure was increased prior to diuresis when intra-abdominal pressure was increased. After diuresis, when intra-abdominal pressure had normalized, LES pressure returned to normal. At no time did increased abdominal pressure lead to symptoms of reflux. These data are similar to those generated by the asymptomatic pregnant women studied by Lind et al. (103) in which LES pressure increased with pregnancy (tense ascites) but returned to normal postpartum (after diuresis). The simplicity of this study strengthened the case against the role of increased abdominal pressure in the pathogenesis of pregnancy-related GER and refocused importance on the role of progesterone in pregnancy-associated reflux.

The role of delayed gastric emptying as a mechanism of GER in pregnancy has yet to be extensively studied. One small study by Wald et al. demonstrated delayed mouth-to-cecum transit using breath hydrogen testing in 15 women in the third trimester and at 4 weeks postpartum (105). This delay could not be clearly attributed to alterations in gastric or small bowel transit. A study by Braverman and colleagues, however, evaluated the postpartum restoration of prolonged intestinal transit using lactulose hydrogen breath tests in 10 women in the third trimester and at postpartum days 2 and 4 and compared these results with those of eight control women (106). These authors were able to demonstrate that intestinal transit improves early and is related to the fall in serum progesterone at delivery. These results suggest that the delayed transit measured by Wald et al. (105) was of intestinal rather than gastric origin. Another small study evaluated gastric emptying between 16 and 19 weeks of gestation and at 6 weeks after therapeutic abortion (107). Despite the relaxant effects of progesterone on smooth muscle, no difference in gastric liquid emptying was observed when the subjects were compared to themselves or to normal menstruating controls. None of these studies (105–107) evaluated the relationship between alterations in gastrointestinal motility and GER in these patients.

It now appears evident that GER in pregnancy is related to the effects of progesterone on the LES. These effects increase throughout the duration of pregnancy as progesterone levels rise and return to normal at parturition when levels return to normal. Previously held beliefs in the contribution of psychic factors and mechanical effects of the gravid uterus have largely been dismissed as our understanding of GER in general has evolved. We conclude this section with a reminder of the effects of estrogen and progesterone replacement in monopausal women. While the cardiovascular and bone-mineral-enhancing effects of these medications are of undisputed importance, the wary clinician should use these medications with caution in the patient with severe GERD.

PROGRESSIVE SYSTEMIC SCLEROSIS (SCLERODERMA)

Scleroderma is a systemic connective tissue disease of unknown etiology characterized by excessive deposition of collagen in the skin and internal organs. Involvement of the gastrointestinal tract was originally described in 1903 by Ehrmann (108), and has since been found to be the second most common manifestation of this disorder following Raynaud's phenomenon. Esophageal abnormalities such as decreased or absent peristalsis in the distal two-thirds (smooth-muscle portion) of the esophagus and reduced LES pressure have been reported in up to 90% of patients with scleroderma. To the extent that these abnormalities are known to contribute to GER, symptoms and manifestations of GER are correspondingly increased in this patient population. Some studies that reported on the symptoms of heartburn and dysphagia in the scleroderma esophagus focused on deranged motility and decreased peristalsis of the distal esophagus secondary to smooth muscle atrophy, while others highlighted the contribution of acid reflux in the pathogenesis of these symptoms. Other pathophysiological mechanisms in this population include decreased clearance of refluxed acid and reduced acid-neutralizing capability secondary to associated sicca syndrome (109). Interest in qualifying the relative importance of motility versus reflux has grown with the introduction of histamine receptor antagonists, promotility agents, and proton pump inhibitors as effective medical treatments for GERD. Several studies over the last 20 years have specifically addressed GER in systemic sclerosis.

A 1976 study by Orringer and colleagues evaluated 53 patients with scleroderma using history, barium swallow, and a battery of esophageal function tests to define the extent of esophageal involvement with scleroderma (110). While abnormal motility, manifest by diminished primary peristalsis on barium swallow, was seen in 43 subjects (81%), GER was radiographically evident in only nine subjects (17%). The battery of esophageal function tests were more sensitive, revealing abnormal motility in 51 (96%), abnormal acid clearance in 50 (94%), and moderate to severe acid reflux by pH testing in 38 (72%). The findings of abnormal acid clearance and abnormal motility in 50 and 51 patients, respectively, correlated well with the reported presence of esophageal symptoms in 48 of the 53 patients. The results argued strongly for the importance of the combined roles of acid reflux, poor clearance from diminished peristalsis, and increased mucosal acid contact time in the pathogenesis of esophagitis in scleroderma. The study demonstrated that GER, and not just abnormal peristalsis, was an important major contributor to the esophagitis seen in scleroderma and stressed the importance of an antireflux regimen in this population.

Hendel and colleagues further demonstrated the important relationship between symptomatic acid reflux and the endoscopic finding of esophagitis in scleroderma 10 years later (111). In their study, 18 scleroderma patients with symptomatic GER were treated with ranitidine 150 mg twice daily for 6 weeks and then randomized to 3 months of continued therapy at the same dose or placebo. These authors evaluated subjects by interview of symptoms, esophageal manometry, esophageal pH measurement, and endoscopy at baseline, after 6 weeks, and after 3 months. After 6 weeks of ranitidine, the investigators found an improvement in symptoms of heartburn in 16 (two unchanged, $p < 0.01$), improvement in mucosal appearance at endoscopy in 15 (three unchanged, $p < 0.01$), and improvement in dysphagia in three (15 unchanged, NS). Six of the eight subjects randomized to receive placebo noted an aggravation of their heartburn symptoms with a corresponding worsening of the esophageal mucosal appearance in seven. Of the 10 subjects who continued to use ranitidine, eight had no change or an improvement in symptoms of heartburn. Mucosal appearance at endoscopy was unchanged or improved in seven while dysphagia was unchanged in all 10 treated subjects. Esophageal motility and pH studies were unchanged in response to the treatment with ranitidine or placebo. The study concluded that acid suppression was effective in relieving heartburn symptoms and in healing esophageal mucosa in the scleroderma population but did not affect esophageal motility or relieve dysphagia.

A 1987 study by the same authors sought to determine whether esophageal manometry or esophageal pH monitoring was of superior diagnostic ability over the other in selecting scleroderma patients for antireflux therapy (112). Fifty-five unselected patients with scleroderma were evaluated for GER using esophageal manometry, 12-h pH monitoring, and symptom questionnaires. The investigators found that only 30 patients had pathological GER by pH monitoring despite reported symptoms of GER from 39. Forty-six (84%) of the patients had impaired motility of the distal two-thirds of the esophagus. There were 13/39 with reflux symptoms who did not have pathological GER and 4/16 without symptoms who did have pathological GER (33% false positives, 25% false negatives). When all three study methods (manometry, pH, and symptoms) were combined, a positive correlation of 60% was found in patients with reduced distal esophageal peristalsis and GER. The investigators concluded that manometry alone was too insensitive to determine who had pathological GER and that sensitive esophageal pH monitoring should be performed in all scleroderma patients to ensure proper detection of pathological GER.

In contrast to this, a study by Zamost and colleagues published the same year suggested that esophageal manometry was the best test to identify those who required further evaluation for esophagitis (113). These investigators evaluated 53 scleroderma patients with endoscopic biopsy and found erosive esophagitis in 32 (60%). All patients with erosive esophagitis had an aperistaltic distal esophagus, including five asymptomatic patients. None of the patients with normal esophageal motility had erosive esophagitis. Those with erosive esophagitis had significantly more frequent episodes of heartburn and dysphagia, more frequent episodes of reflux, and single episodes of reflux of longer duration than those subjects without erosive esophagitis. Although supine pH was significantly lower in those with erosive esophagitis than in those without, upright reflux did not differ. The data suggested that acid clearance in the aperistaltic patients was hampered to a greater degree when supine and that these circumstances were critical in combining to promote the development of erosive esophagitis. In this regard, esophageal manometry was crucial in its ability to demonstrate which patients were aperistaltic and therefore at greatest risk for developing more severe esophagitis.

Along similar lines, a study by Murphy et al. (114) reported that decreased distal esophageal smooth-muscle peristalsis appeared to be the most important factor in determining the degree of acid exposure and esophageal injury seen in scleroderma. The group studied seven scleroderma patients with known severe esophagitis using simultaneous intraesophageal pH monitoring and scintigraphy following a radiolabeled meal. They compared the findings from the scleroderma patients to those from nine patients with identical endoscopic findings but with no evidence of a connective-tissue disorder. The investigators sought to determine whether decreased clearance of reflux events and/or increased frequency of reflux events was primarily responsible for the postprandial reflux seen in scleroderma patients. The study found that scleroderma patients had significantly fewer reflux events ($p < 0.01$), but the events that did occur were of significantly longer duration ($p < 0.01$). By using scintigraphy and pH monitoring together, the investigators demonstrated that additional reflux events were able to occur before complete clearance of the preceding reflux event. The prolonged clearance in the scleroderma patients was predominantly due to decreased peristaltic contractions. An additional contribution secondary to diminished salivary neutralization of acid from sicca syndrome could not be dismissed. This study focused on the important role that prolonged acid clearance played in the pathogenesis of esophagitis in scleroderma and demonstrated a lessor role for increased reflux events due to an incompetent LES.

Subsequent studies (115) have supported the findings of Zamost et al. (113) and Murphy et al. (114) in reporting that the severity and extent of GER and esophagitis in scleroderma are most closely influenced by the integrity of distal esophageal peristalsis. If one accepts that a weakened peristaltic wave would hinder expulsion of the majority of the acid refluxate and delay delivery of neutralizing saliva to the residual acid remaining in the distal esophagus (116), the factors responsible for the high incidence of esophagitis in scleroderma can be more easily understood. That abnormally delayed esophageal emptying plays a key role in the degree of GER experienced by progressive systemic sclerosis (PSS) patients is also highlighted by the fact that the outcome of antireflux surgery in this group of patients is usually poor. The pathogenesis of gastroesophageal reflux in the scleroderma patient is therefore appreciated in a different light than that of the nonscleroderma patient wherein the competency of the LES and frequency of TLESRs play a more central role.

ZOLLINGER-ELLISON SYNDROME

While the Zollinger-Ellison syndrome (ZES) is characterized by severe ulcer disease, gastric acid hypersecretion, and hypergastrinemia, the relationship between GERD and ZES must be examined separately from the effects of gastrin on the LES.

The relationship between gastrin, the LES, and GERD was intensively studied in the late 1960s and early 1970s. For a time, gastrin was believed to play a major role in determining LES pressure. Several early studies demonstrated marked increases in LES pressure in response to pharmacological stimulation or intravenous administration of gastrin, while others demonstrated sphincteric hypotension in the setting of diminished levels of endogenous gastrin (117–122). The finding of an increased LES pressure in a small study of six ZES patients compared to eight control subjects added to the early evidence supporting gastrin's importance as a regulator of LES pressure (123). Contradictory evidence was later presented, however, when McCallum and Walsh demonstrated similar basal LES pressures among patients with ZES versus normals (124) and when Snyder and Hughes demonstrated similar basal LES pressure in ZES- versus non-ZES-related duodenal ulcer patients (125). The possible correlation between LES pressure and gastrin was further questioned when studies failed to demonstrate a significant relationship between these two factors in GER patients (126–128).

As part of an effort to clarify the controversy regarding the physiological versus pharmacological effects of gastrin on LES competence, further studies evaluating ZES emerged. Earlier literature on the ZES had suggested that esophageal involvement was rare because of the presumed protection afforded by the hypergastrinemia-enhanced LES pressure. In fact, Ellison's 1964 review of 260 registered cases of ZES described esophageal ulceration in only two of 166 patients. Symptoms of heartburn and dysphagia, however, were not specifically mentioned in the study (129). A later review from the Mayo clinic in 1978 again failed to mention esophageal symptoms, though it did report endoscopic esophagitis in four of 27 patients (130).

The first study that specifically evaluated for the presence of GERD in the ZES was published by Richter and colleagues in 1981 (131). Fifteen patients with known ZES were evaluated using questionnaire, acid reflux test, Bernstein test, esophageal manometry, endoscopy, and esophageal suction biopsy via Rubin tube. Interestingly, five patients had originally presented with esophageal disease as the initial manifestation of the ZES. Despite ongoing long-term use of cimetidine, 6/15 patients reported heartburn, while 9/15 had objective evidence for reflux disease. LES pressure was significantly higher in the total group of ZES patients versus controls (25.2 ± 2.8 vs. 18.3 ± 0.6 mmHg, $p < 0.001$). Though ZES patients with heartburn were found to have significantly lower LES pressure than asymptomatic ZES patients (16.8 ± 1.7 vs. 30.8 ± 3.4 mmHg, $p < 0.001$), their LES pressure remained significantly higher than in those with idiopathic GER (16.8 ± 1.7 vs. 5.4 ± 0.4 mmHg, $p < 0.01$) (Fig. 4). No correlation was seen between LES pressure and fasting serum gastrin concentration in the ZES patients.

A retrospective review of the medical and radiographic records of 18 patients with ZES by Agha (132) demonstrated esophageal disease in six (33%). Esophagogram, endoscopy, or histopathological evaluation of esophageal biopsy

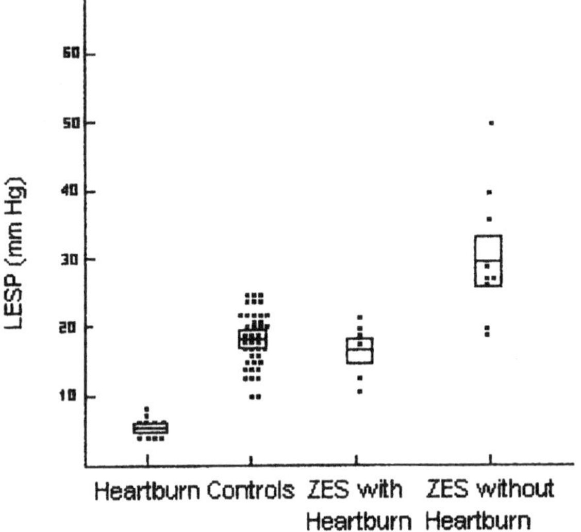

Figure 4 Comparison of LES pressure in patients with GER, controls and subjects with Zollinger-Ellison syndrome (with and without heartburn). Data points are individual LES pressures. From Richter, 1981.

material established the diagnosis of esophageal involvement. Four of the 18 patients (22%) had had symptoms of heartburn or dysphagia from 6 months to 3 years prior to the diagnosis of ZES.

A larger study of 122 ZES patients from the National Institutes of Health by Miller and colleagues (133) reported esophageal symptoms of heartburn or dysphagia in 55 (45%), endoscopic abnormalities of esophagitis, stricture, or Barrett's esophagus in 51 (42%), or a combination of both in 74 (61%). As in Richter's study (131), all patients were on histamine H_2-receptor antagonists at entry into the study. Following an initial endoscopy, histamine H_2-receptor antagonist or proton pump antagonist medications were given at doses sufficient to completely eradicate signs or symptoms of esophageal disease and patients were reassessed in 2 weeks. Of the 52 patients with reflux esophagitis on initial endoscopy, 40 (77%) had complete mucosal healing with reduction of gastric acid output to <10 mEq/h at 2 weeks. Twenty patients had partial improvement with reduction in gastric acid output to <10 mEq/h and required increased doses of histamine H_2-receptor antagonist (19 patients) or proton pump antagonist (one patient) to reduce acid output to <5 mEq/h. Twelve of the 19 had persistent abnormalities after 2 weeks at this higher dose and required further suppression of gastric acid output to <1 mEq/h with omeprazole before resolving the signs or gaining control of the symptoms of esophageal disease. Not only did this study demonstrate a high incidence of esophageal involvement in ZES, it also demonstrated that some patients with ZES will only have their esophagitis controlled after being rendered virtually achlorhydric with a proton pump antagonist.

Having demonstrated that gastrin levels and LES competence were unrelated and that the incidence of esophageal involvement in ZES was at least as great as 61% (probably higher if one considers that all patients were on histamine H_2-receptor antagonists at entry), the task of explaining the pathophysiology of esophageal involvement in ZES remains. Strader and colleagues evaluated 92 patients with ZES (66 with active disease, 26 disease-free after curative resection) to determine whether the high prevalence of esophageal disease was due to gastric acid hypersecretion alone or to additional abnormalities in esophageal motility or LES function (134). At entry, all patients had had acid secretion normalized by antisecretory medications or surgery for at least 5 weeks to ensure that no changes were due to gastric acid hypersecretion or secondary to acid-reflux-induced esophageal damage. No correlation was noted between LES pressure, esophageal manometry, fasting serum gastrin, or basal or maximal acid output levels. Esophageal manometry and LES pressure were similar in active ZES patients and those who were disease-free. The investigators concluded that the high prevalence of reflux disease in ZES was primarily due to gastric acid hypersecretion. A multivariate analysis of the pathophysiological factors in idiopathic reflux esophagitis showed that peak acid output was one of three significant independent parameters along with esophageal acid clearance and LES pressure (135). An additional report by Straathof and colleagues (135a) studied the effect of gastrin-17 on the LES in nine healthy controls to determine the effect of this hormone on TLESR. While the frequency and duration of TLESR were not affected by the gastrin infusion (15 pmol/kg/h), the percentage of TLESRs associated with reflux was significantly higher ($p < 0.05$) in response to gastrin. Further study comparing TLESR in ZES patients, GER patients, and normals is necessary to determine whether this finding is truly relevant.

DELAYED GASTRIC EMPTYING

Reflux Patients

Does delayed gastric emptying predispose an individual to GERD, or does GER itself lead to delayed gastric emptying? Is delayed gastric emptying merely one manifestation of a broader motility disorder that also affects GER? Could delayed gastric emptying protect against reflux esophagitis? Are there any medications or medical conditions associated with delayed gastric emptying that correspond to a higher incidence of GER? In the following section, we will discuss delayed gastric emptying as it pertains to GERD and will attempt to answer the questions raised by reviewing some of the conditions clinically associated with delayed gastric emptying.

The medical literature contains evidence that supports and refutes an association between delayed gastric emptying and GER. Little et al. (136) evaluated 50 patients with GER diagnosed on the basis of abnormal 24-h esophageal pH. Twenty-six had esophagitis, while 24 had no esophagitis and there were 15 normal controls. Gastric emptying was significantly delayed in patients with esophagitis compared to those without esophagitis and normal subjects. Upright refluxers were found to have rapid emptying compared to controls in contrast to the delayed emptying seen in patients with supine or combined reflux. Manometry showed no difference in LES characteristics between the groups with and without esophagitis. In esophagitis patients, there was decreased esophageal acid clearance and more reflux episodes lasting longer than 5 min. The investigators proposed three possible mechanisms whereby delayed gastric emptying increased GER: (1) delayed gastric emptying results in an increase in gastric contents and overflow into the esophagus, (2) the higher intragastric pressure may overcome LES pressure, and (3) gastric dilatation could conceivably cause LES shortening, sphincter incompetence, and GER.

Other studies have shown that postprandial gastric distension can change fundic gastric wall tension and lead to increased TLESRs (137,138) and more frequent reflux events (139,140). Excessive GER by any mechanism could also lead to severe esophagitis and scarring with subsequent esophageal dysmotility and delayed acid clearance (136). Biancani et al. (141) noted that esophagitis in cats led to decreased esophageal contractile amplitude. This decrease was related to increased prostaglandins associated with inflammation, which then interfered with storage and transfer of calcium into smooth-muscle cells. Extension of the inflammatory process to involve vagal fibers leading to the stomach could lead to gastric emptying abnormalities furthering this vicious cycle.

Studies by Shay et al. (142), Schwizer et al. (143), and Keshavarzian et al. (144) all concluded that delayed gastric emptying did not play a major role in the pathophysiology of gastroesophageal reflux in most patients. These three groups studied a total of 119 patients and 67 controls. GER was defined by abnormal 24-h intraesophageal pH monitoring in all patients ($n = 43$) in the Shay and Keshavarzian studies. Patients were entered into the Schwizer study based on symptoms; however, once enrolled, all patients ($n = 76$) underwent 24-h pH monitoring. While 25/76 (33%) had no evidence of abnormal exposure to acid on 24-h pH, they were still analyzed within the patient group with results significantly different from control in all parameters ($p < 0.0001$). All three studies found no difference in gastric emptying rates between controls or patients with or without reflux. Moreover, the Schwizer study found that delayed emptying was associated with less esophagitis than found in those with normal gastric emptying, suggesting that the presence of food within the stomach may have a protective role in buffering gastric acidity.

It is worth mentioning that Little's 1980 study (136) was one of few early studies that defined the reflux group by abnormal 24-h pH. Previous studies that reported delayed gastric emptying in "reflux" patients defined GER by symptoms, radiography, or Bernstein testing (145–147) and may have included a more heterogeneous group of patients than those with pure GER. The possible inclusion of patients with nonulcer dyspepsia or other disease states with symptoms that mimic GER might have affected the results of prior studies as delayed gastric emptying might be more prevalent in these groups of patients than in those suffering from isolated GER. Methodological differences in scintigraphic techniques for measuring gastric emptying have also been implicated in interpretative discrepancies between studies. A 1996 study from Benini and colleagues (148) used real-time ultrasonography to evaluate whether a mixed meal emptied more slowly in 25 patients with 24-h proven reflux. Although gastric emptying was significantly delayed in reflux patients compared to control, there was no correlation between delayed emptying and either pH monitoring or the presence of esophagitis. Esophageal acid exposure in the postprandial period was similar in patients with normal and delayed gastric emptying. These results argue against a direct causal link between delayed emptying and reflux and suggest the presence of a broader motility disorder in certain patients with GER.

A recent pediatric study by Cucchiara and colleagues (149) evaluated the relationship between gastric electrical activity by electrogastrography (EGG) and gastric emptying by antral ultrasonography in 42 reflux patients. Gastric dysrhythmias were detected more frequently in patients than controls ($p < 0.01$) and were associated with delayed gastric emptying. Soykan and colleagues (150) evaluated 30 adult reflux patients with EGG and radionuclide gastric emptying and found that 52% had gastric motor or myoelectric abnormalities that contributed to the pathogenesis of their GER. While these two studies provided evidence that gastric motor abnormalities were prevalent in GER patients, neither study used esophageal pH nor was able to demonstrate a direct etiological link between these abnormalities and GER.

A 1991 study by Cunningham and colleagues (151) evaluated the relationship between autonomic nerve dysfunction, esophageal motility, and gastric emptying in 48 patients with GER. They found that 21/48 (44%) had abnormal autonomic nerve function with delayed solid food emptying in 46% and delayed esophageal transit in 28%. Contrary to the suggestion that vagal nerve impairment was secondary to severe esophagitis, the study revealed that autonomic nerve impairment was also unrelated to the degree of esophagitis and therefore a primary phenomenon leading to delayed esophageal transit, abnormal esophageal peristalsis, and GER. No significant relation was found between autonomic nerve dysfunction and delayed gastric emptying or between endoscopic grade of esophagitis and gastric emptying. The investigators concluded that a high prevalence of autonomic nerve dysfunction in GER might be of pathogenic importance by its relation to delayed esophageal transit and abnormal peristalsis.

Diabetes Mellitus

It is well known that delayed gastric emptying may be found in the setting of the autonomic neuropathy of diabetic gastropathy. A prevalence of 27% was seen in a study of 30 chronic insulin-requiring patients (152). While those with autonomic neuropathy secondary to advanced disease are felt to be at greatest risk, even physiological hyperglycemia has been shown to slow gastric emptying in both normal subjects and diabetics (153). A study by Samsom and colleagues (154) demonstrated that hyperglycemia reduced antral contractile activity in eight type I diabetics with autonomic neuropathy.

Though hyperglycemia has been shown to induce delayed gastric emptying, there are no studies in the literature that have specifically investigated the relationship between diabetes, gastric emptying, and gastroesophageal reflux. A 1987 study of 20 diabetics (14/20 insulin dependent) by Murray and colleagues (155) evaluated the relationship between esophageal function, GER, and peripheral neuropathy; however, the relationship between diabetic peripheral neuropathy, autonomic neuropathy, and gastric emptying was not explored. One must therefore make assumptions or borrow from the results of other studies that have investigated gastric emptying and GER to draw any conclusions about the risk of esophageal reflux in the setting of autonomic neuropathy, delayed gastric emptying, and diabetes.

Parkman and Schwartz (156) retrospectively evaluated the prevalence of gastrointestinal disorders associated with diabetic gastroparesis in 20 patients who had been hospitalized for intractable nausea and vomiting. Nine (45%) of these patients had normal upper endoscopy and only four (20%) had erosive esophagitis on endoscopy, but no patients had 24-h pH monitoring to evaluate for GER.

While previous investigators had suggested that diabetics with autonomic neuropathy secreted less gastric acid and therefore had less gastroesophageal reflux (157), we now have evidence that shows this to be untrue (153). Until investigations are performed to evaluate whether diabetic gastroparesis/autonomic neuropathy leads to gastroesophageal reflux, this question remains unanswered.

Intestinal Pseudo-Obstruction

In 1959, Murley (158) first described intestinal pseudo-obstruction (IP) as a degenerative neuromuscular disorder affecting intestinal motility presenting with features of intestinal obstruction in the absence of a true mechanical obstruction. IP can be seen in scleroderma with intestinal involvement and had been thought to be the consequence of an underlying systemic disorder. Subsequent research revealed that the difference between scleroderma and IP was the degree of muscle fibrosis seen in IP versus collagen replacement in scleroderma, suggesting a primary role of muscle fibrosis rather than collagenous replacement in IP (159). While the intestinal manifestations of this disorder have been well characterized, little has been published with regard to gastroesophageal involvement. Schuffler and Pope (160) noted that five IP patients undergoing esophageal manometry had complete esophageal aperistalsis in two patients and distal aperistalsis in the remaining three. This pattern resembled classic achalasia in three patients and ''vigorous'' achalasia in two and was distinctly different from the manometric findings of scleroderma of the esophagus.

A 1988 study by Mayer and colleagues (161) evaluated gastric emptying of solids and liquids in 11 patients with IP and noted that 8/11 had abnormal gastric emptying. Although specific studies of GER were not part of the evaluation, esophageal manometry noted 4/9 patients with abnormal or absent esophageal peristalsis. One patient had a hiatal hernia and decreased peristalsis and the other a stricture and esophageal ulceration on the upper-gastrointestinal tract.

These studies demonstrate IP as a heterogeneous disorder, involving the esophagus as well as segments all along the intestinal tract. When GER is present, possible contributing factors include delayed gastric emptying or poor acid clearance secondary to an aperistaltic esophagus.

Medications

While we can demonstrate that medications possess pharmacological properties that affect smooth muscle, vagal tone, or gastric motility, there is a paucity of evidence that has specifically evaluated the role of these medications in delaying gastric emptying and an etiological or exacerbating contribution to GER. As a consequence, much of what we know about the risk of medications exacerbating GER via a delayed gastric emptying mechanism is derived from observing that these medications can influence radionuclide studies and translating this knowledge to the evidence regarding delayed gastric emptying in general. Medications that are commonly implicated in delayed gastric emptying are shown in Table 5 (162,166).

Progressive Systemic Sclerosis (PSS/Scleroderma)

The esophagus is the gastrointestinal organ most frequently involved by PSS while the stomach is usually the last gastrointestinal organ to be involved by dysmotility in scleroderma (110). In 1984, a study by Maddern and colleagues

Table 5 Causes of Delayed Gastric Emptying

	Medications
Alcohol (high concentration)	Octreotide
Aluminum antacids	Opiates
Anticholinergics	Phenothiazines
Beta agonists	Potassium salts
Calcium channel blockers	Progesterone
Fenfluramine[a]	Sucralfate
L-Dopa	Tricyclic antidepressants
Nicotine	
	Mechanical Causes
Peptic ulcer disease	Postoperative stenosis
Gastric ulcer	Stricture
Pyloric channel ulcer	Gastroenterostomy intussusception
Duodenal ulcer	Gastroenterostomy edema
Inflammatory	Transverse mesocolon obstruction of Billroth II
Crohn's disease	Complications of obesity surgery
Cholecystitis	Other
Pancreatitis	Annular pancreas
Neoplasm	Bezoar
Gastric cancer	Caustic stricture
Gastric polyps	Duodenal webs
Duodenal polyps	Hypertrophic pyloric stenosis
Ampullary carcinoma	Superior mesenteric artery syndrome
Pancreatic carcinoma	
Metastatic carcinoma	

[a] Ref. 162a.

(163) noted that seven of 12 patients had abnormal esophageal and gastric emptying and symptomatic correlation of dysphagia and GER with these results. This study and results of other investigations (164,165) have concluded that delayed gastric emptying may be an important factor in the pathogenesis of GERD in PSS.

Others (164) have also shown that patients with more severe GER had more delayed gastric emptying and more severe alterations in interdigestive gastric motility compared to those with mild GER. Though only these few studies have specifically investigated the relationship between esophageal and gastric emptying in patients with PSS, they all agree that delayed gastric emptying is seen almost exclusively in those with abnormal esophageal emptying (165).

Gastric Outlet Obstruction

Gastric outlet obstruction, previously a complication of long-standing peptic ulcer disease, is now seen less frequently as diagnosis and treatment of peptic ulcer disease and *Helicobacter pylori* has improved over the last decade. Malignancy now accounts for the major cause of gastric outlet obstruction. Regardless of the underlying cause (Table 5) (162,166), gastric atony can develop after prolonged obstruction and lead to gastric retention. The resultant stasis of gastric contents can increase both the available volume and potential contact time for these contents to reflux into the esophagus. In addition, hypergastrinemia, which can also delay gastric emptying, can develop due to the gastric distension and retained food. As such, a high prevalence of GER as well as a more severe degree of esophagitis might be expected in this population of patients; however, despite an exhaustive review of the literature, no published studies have investigated this potential relationship.

Helicobacter pylori

A number of studies (167–174) have examined the possible relationship between *H. pylori* and GERD (Table 6) and have stimulated a number of reviews discussing this pathogen's putative role in GERD (175–177). While the majority of studies demonstrate no association or a protective role for *H. pylori* in GERD, features of this pathogen, per Vicari et al. (176), suggest mechanisms whereby this organism could cause or aggravate preexisting reflux disease. First, a study by El-Omar and colleagues (178) demonstrated that in *H. pylori*–infected duodenal ulcer patients, there was an elevated basal acid output, which decreased back toward the levels found in *H. pylori*–negative volunteers 1 year following *H. pylori* eradication. The observed increase in acid secretion relates to increased gastrin secretion as a consequence of the *H. pylori* infection decreasing somatostatin release (with subsequent loss of the inhibition of gastrin release). Second, *H. pylori*–induced inflammation of the cardia might trigger vagally mediated receptors, stimulating TLESR and increased GER. Third, cytotoxins elaborated by *H. pylori* might cause esophageal mucosal injury. Evidence later published by Vicari and colleagues showed that CagA positivity was protective of GERD (173). Finally, *H. pylori* gastritis might cause GER via delayed gastric emptying. Though a subset of patients with GER secondary to delayed gastric emptying may exist (147), numerous studies of gastric emptying of solids and liquids suggest that *H. pylori* has no effect on this mechanism (179–181).

While the review by Vicari and colleagues described mechanisms by which *H. pylori* might contribute to the pathogenesis of GER, current experimental and epidemiological evidence supports a protective role for *H. pylori*. Epidemiological studies demonstrate that where *H. pylori* CagA+ infection rates are high [China (>80%) (182)], the corresponding incidence of esophagitis is low (<5%) (183). Furthermore, complications of GER such as Barrett's esophagus and esophageal adenocarcinoma are significantly more common in whites than blacks or Asians, despite the higher prevalence of *H. pylori* in Asians (184, 185).

Table 6 Studies That Have Examined the Relationship Between *H. pylori* and Gastroesophageal Reflux

Study	Purpose/design	Methods/outcome	Comments
O'Connor, 1994	Prospective evaluation of relationship between *H. pylori* (HP) and GER.	93 symptomatic patients with endoscopic evidence of GER 50 (54%) HP+ve on antral biopsy.	No association seen between HP infection and grade of esophagitis. No control group.
Kuipers, 1996	Prospective cohort study to determine effects of omeprazole and fundoplication in GER patients with and without HP.	59/105 (56%) patients in the omeprazole cohort and 31/72 (43%) in the fundoplication cohort were HP+ve.	Though a substantial percentage of GER patients were HP+ve, the intent was not directed at a correlation between GER and HP and no control group was studied.
Werdmuller, 1997	Prospective, controlled study to determine prevalence of HP in patients with GER and/or hiatal hernia and Barrett esophagus.	74/240 (30%) patients and 204/399 (51%) controls were HP+ve ($p < 0.001$).	HP has no role in the pathogenesis of reflux esophagitis.
Labenz, 1997	Prospective evaluation to determine rate of development of reflux esophagitis in duodenal ulcer patients with HP.	244 patients cured of HP and 216 with persistent HP underwent EGD at 1-yr intervals or when GER symptoms developed.	New reflux esophagitis seen in 12.9% of persistently HP+ve patients vs. 25.8% of those HP−ve. Severity of corpus gastritis precure correlated with postcure esophagitis.
Csendes, 1997	Prospective, controlled comparison of prevalence of HP and degree of endoscopic esophagitis.	236 patients (55 without endoscopic esophagitis, 81 erosive esophagitis, 100 Barrett), 190 controls and 24-h pH and biopsy from duodenal bulb, antrum, fundus, and distal esophagus.	Prevalence of antral HP was similar in controls and all 3 patient groups (range 20–25%). No evidence for a pathogenic role for HP in chronic reflux.

Newton, 1997	Prospective, controlled evaluation of prevalence and distribution of HP in various patient groups with GER.	9/25 (36%) controls, 13/36 (36%) erosive esophagitis, 15/16 (94%) duodenal ulcer (DU) alone, 6/15 (40%) esophagitis and DU, and 4/16 (25%) Barrett were HP+ve.	HP is not more common in those with esophagitis compared with control.
Goldblum, 1998	Prospective, controlled evaluation of relationship between carditis, HP, and cardial intestinal metaplasia in patients with and without GER.	N = 85, 58 with GER, 27 controls. All had EGD with biopsy of distal esophagus, cardia, fundus, and antrum.	No difference in prevalence of HP (48% control, 41% GER) or carditis (41% control, 40% GER). More esophagitis in GER (33%) than control (7%). Carditis (96–100% HP+ve) does not appear to be a marker of GER.
Vicari, 1998	Prospective, controlled study to determine prevalence of CagA-positive (CagA+) HP strains in patients with GER.	153 patients (GER, Barrett, Barrett with dysplasia or adenocarcinoma) and 57 controls. 34% HP+ve patients vs. 45.6% controls (p = 0.15). Decreasing prevalence of CagA+ strains as severity of GER increased. Nonerosive GER 41.2%, erosive GER 30.8%, Barrett 13.3%, Barrett with dysplasia, or adenocarcinoma 0%.	Lower (not significant) prevalence of HP in GER than controls. CagA+ patients may be protected against complications of GER such as Barrett with dysplasia or adenocarcinoma.
Varanasi, 1998	Prospective study to determine if HP is associated with lower rates of esophagitis in patients with and without GER and a subgroup with peptic ulcer disease.	30.7% reflux esophagitis patients HP+ve versus 42% without esophagitis (p = 0.039). Duodenal ulcer patients with esophagitis 36.4% HP+ve versus 69.2% DU without esophagitis (p = 0.018).	*H. pylori* is significantly less prevalent in patients with reflux esophagitis with even more dramatic findings in duodenal ulcer patients.

DU = duodenal ulcer; EGD = esophagogastroduodenoscopy. GER = gastroesophageal reflux; HP+ve = *H. pylori*–positive.

A review by Labenz and Malfertheiner (175) described mechanisms by which *H. pylori* might protect against GER. First, *H. pylori* infection lowers intragastric acidity by generating large amounts of ammonia, which acts as a potent neutralizing agent. Second, *H. pylori*, especially CagA+ strains, might lead to more severe corpus gastritis, leading to multifocal atrophic gastritis, destruction of gastric glands, and eventually, hypochlorhydria. This relationship (186) suggested that decreased acid secretion (or increased ammonia production) secondary to severe *H. pylori*–related gastritis was protective against reflux esophagitis as reflux esophagitis was seen in 12.9% when infected with *H. pylori*, rising to 25.8% within 3 years of cure.

Clearly, the presence of *H. pylori* is cause for concern when found on serological or histopathological evaluation of the patient with upper gastrointestinal symptoms. The importance of the patient's CagA status, whether this has prognostic implications for the development of future gastrointestinal pathology and whether it should be routinely sought after, is quite uncertain. Conceivably, if certain strains of this organism prevent reflux esophagitis, current treatment strategies concerning the eradication of this pathogen may change.

SUMMARY

The purpose of this chapter has been to present and discuss the evidence that currently exists regarding the known risk factors for GER. We have discussed various types of risk factors as well as the mechanisms by which they are felt to act. From anatomical considerations such as hiatal hernia to volitional habits such as cigarette smoking and alcohol consumption to medical conditions beyond our control such as the ZES and progressive systemic sclerosis, the factors that are able to contribute to a greater risk of GER are quite diverse. Some risk factors, such as medications, nasogastric intubation, or pregnancy, may only be a temporary or transient concern to the affected individual, knowing that manifestations of GER will resolve at delivery, after removal of the NGT, or once the offending medication is discontinued. Other risk factors, such as cigarette smoking or alcohol consumption, appear to raise the risk of GER, yet are not universally successful in provoking GER in those who partake of these substances. Perhaps there is a dose-response relationship that has not yet been determined or an individual susceptibility that is merely unmasked by these substances. The answers to these questions remain unanswered by the available evidence. As we have found in our review of the literature, the evidence that currently exists is flawed in many areas by study design and lack of sophisticated or sensitive techniques to measure GER (such as 24-h pH monitoring). While we may have provided answers to many of the readers' questions, we hope we have also provoked new questions that remain to be answered by future studies.

REFERENCES

1. Locke GR, Talley NJ, Fett SL, Zinmeister AR, Melton LJ. Prevalence and clinical spectrum of gastroesophageal reflux: a population-based study in Olmsted County, Minnesota. Gastroenterology 1997; 112:1448–1456.
2. Wienbeck M, Barnert J. Epidemiology of reflux disease and reflux esophagitis. Scand J Gastroenterol 1989; 24(suppl 156):7–13.
3. McArthur KE. Hernias and volvulus of the gastrointestinal tract. In: Feldman M, Scharschmidt BF, Sleisenger MH, eds. Sleisenger and Fordtran's Gastrointestinal and Liver Disease Pathophysiology/Diagnosis/Management. Philadelphia: WB Saunders, 1998:318.
4. Mittal RK. Hiatal hernia: myth or reality? Am J Med 1997; 103:33S–39S.
5. Mittal RK, Lange RC, McCallum RW. Identification and mechanism of delayed acid clearance in subjects with hiatus hernia. Gastroenterology 1987; 92:130–135.
6. Mittal RK, Rochester DF, McCallum RW. Electrical and mechanical activity in the human lower esophageal sphincter during diaphragmatic contraction. J Clin Invest 1988; 81:1182–1189.
7. Holloway RH, Dent J. Pathophysiology of gastroesophageal reflux: lower esophageal sphincter dysfunction in gastroesophageal reflux disease. Gastroenterol Clin North Am 1990; 19:517–535.
8. Sloan S, Kahrilas PJ. Impairment of esophageal emptying with hiatal hernia. Gastroenterology 1991; 100:596–605.
9. Sloan S, Rademaker AW, Kahrilas PJ. Determinants of gastroesophageal junction incompetence: hiatal hernia, lower esophageal sphincter, or both? Ann Intern Med 1992; 117:977–982.
10. Mittal RK. Hiatal hernia and gastroesophageal reflux: another attempt to resolve the controversy. Gastroenterology 1993; 105:941–943.
11. Peck N, Callander N, Watson A. Manometric assessment of the effect of the diaphragmatic crural sling in gastro-oesophageal reflux: implications for surgical management. Br J Surg 1995; 82:798–801.
12. Sontag SJ, Schnell TG, Miller TQ, Nemchausky B, Serlovsky R, O'Connell S, Chejfec G, Seidel UJ, Brand L. The importance of hiatal hernia in reflux esophagitis compared with the lower esophageal sphincter pressure or smoking. J Clin Gastroenterol 1991; 13:628–643.
13. Ott DJ, McManus CM, Ledbetter MS, Chen MYM, Gelfand DW. Heartburn correlated to 24-hour pH monitoring and radiographic examination of the esophagus. Am J Gastroenterol 1997; 92:1827–1830.
14. Patti MG, Goldberg HI, Arcerito M, Bortolasi L, Tong J, Way LW. Hiatal hernia affects lower esophageal sphincter function, esophageal acid exposure, and the degree of mucosal injury. Am J Surg 1996; 171:182–186.

15. Ott DJ, Glauser SJ, Ledbetter MS, Chen MYM, Koufman JA, Gelfand DW. Association of hiatal hernia and gastroesophageal reflux: correlation between presence and size of hiatal hernia and 24-hour pH monitoring of the esophagus. Am J Roentgenol 1995; 165:557–559.
16. Petersen H, Johannessen T, Sandvik AK, Kleveland PM, Brenna E, Waldum H, Dybdahl JD. Relationship between endoscopic hiatus hernia and gastroesophageal reflux symptoms. Scand J Gastroenterol 1991; 26:921–926.
17. Jones MP, Sloan S, Kahrilas PJ, Chen M, Rabine JC. Hiatal hernia (HH) size is the principal determinant of esophagitis in patients with symptomatic gastroesophageal reflux disease (abstr). Gastroenterology 1998; 114:A163.
18. Lieverse RJ, Jansen JBMJ, Masclee AAM, Lamers CBHW. Gastrointestinal disturbances with obesity. Scand J Gastroenterol 1993; 28(suppl 200):53–58.
19. Beauchamp G. Gastroesophageal reflux and obesity. Surg Clin North Am 1983; 63:869–876.
20. Stene-Larsen G, Weberg R, Frøyshov Larsen I, Bjørtuft Ø, Hoel B, Berstad A. Relationship of overweight to hiatus hernia and reflux esophagitis. Scand J Gastroenterol 1988; 23:427–432.
21. Wilson LJ, Ma W, Hirschowitz BI. Association of obesity with hiatal hernia and esophagitis. Am J Gastroenterol 1999; 94:2840–2844.
22. Mercer CD, Rue C, Hanelin L, Hill LD. Effect of obesity on esophageal transit. Am J Surg 1985; 149:177–181.
23. Maddox A, Horowitz M, Wishart J, Collins P. Gastric and oesophageal emptying in obesity. Scand J Gastroenterol 1989; 24:593–598.
24. Hutson WR, Wald A. Obesity and weight reduction do not influence gastric emptying and antral motility. Am J Gastroenterol 1993; 88:1405–1409.
25. Wright RA, Krinsky S, Fleeman C, Trujillo J, Teague E. Gastric emptying and obesity. Gastroenterology 1983; 84:747–751.
26. Lundell L, Ruth M, Sandberg N, Bove-Nielsen M. Does massive obesity promote abnormal gastroesophageal reflux? Dig Dis Sci 1995; 40:1632–1635.
27. Kjellin A, Ramel S, Rössner S, Thor K. Gastroesophageal reflux in obese patients is not reduced by weight reduction. Scand J Gastroenterol 1996; 31:1047–1051.
28. Mathus-Vliegen LM, Tytgat GN. Twenty-four-hour pH measurements in morbid obesity: effects of massive overweight, weight loss and gastric distension. Eur J Gastroenterol Hepatol 1996; 8(7):635–640.
29. Castell DO. Obesity and gastro-oesophageal reflux: is there a relationship? Eur J Gastroenterol Hepatol 1996; 8(7):625–626.
30. Rigaud D, Merouche M, Le Moel G, Vatier J, Paycha F, Cadiot G, Naoui N, Mignon M. Factors of gastroesophageal acid reflux in severe obesity. Gastroenterol Clin Biol 1995; 19(10):818–825.
31. Mercer CD, Wren SF, DaCosta LR, Beck IT. Lower esophageal sphincter pressure and gastroesophageal pressure gradients in excessively obese patients. J Med 1987; 18:135–146.
32. Hogan WJ, Viegas de Andrade SR, Winship DH. Ethanol induced acute esophageal motor dysfunction. J Appl Physiol 1972; 32:755–760.

33. Keshavarzian A, Polepalle C, Iber FL, Durkin M. Esophageal motor disorder in alcoholics: result of alcoholism or withdrawal? Alcohol Clin Exp Res 1990; 14: 561–567.
34. Keshavarzian A, Iber FL, Ferguson Y. Esophageal manometry and radionuclide emptying in chronic alcoholics. Gastroenterology 1987; 92:651–657.
35. Kjellen G, Tibbling L. Influence of body position, dry and wet swallows, smoking and alcohol on esophageal clearing. Scand J Gastroenterol 1978; 13:283–288.
36. Kissin B, Kaley MM. Alcohol and cancer. In: Kissin B, Begleiter H, eds. The Biology of Alcoholism. New York: Plenum Publishing Corp., 1974:481–511.
37. Kaufman SE, Kaye MD. Induction of gastro-oesophageal reflux by alcohol. Gut 1978; 19:336–338.
38. Vitale GC, Cheadle WG, Patel B, Sadek SA, Michel ME, Cuschieri A. The effect of alcohol on nocturnal gastroesophageal reflux. JAMA 1987; 258:2077–2079.
39. Chari S, Teyssen S, Singer MV. Alcohol and gastric acid secretion in humans. Gut 1993; 34:843–847.
40. Mayer EM, Grabowski CJ, Fisher R. Effects of graded doses of alcohol upon esophageal motor function. Gastroenterology 1978; 75:1133–1136.
41. Keshavarzian A, Urban G, Sedghi S, Willson C, Sabella L, Sweeny C, Anderson K. Effect of acute ethanol on esophageal motility in cat. Alcohol Clin Exp Res 1991; 15:116–121.
42. Keshavarzian A, Muska B, Sundaresan R, Urban G, Fields J. Ethanol at pharmacologically relevant concentrations inhibits contractility of isolated smooth muscle cells of cat esophagus. Alcohol Clin Exp Res 1996; 20:180–184.
43. Silver LS, Worner TM, Korsten MA. Esophageal function in chronic alcoholics. Am J Gastroenterol 1986; 81:423–427.
44. Dutta SK, Orestes M, Vengulekur S, Kwo P. Ethanol and human saliva: effect of chronic alcoholism on flow rate, composition, and epidermal growth factor. Am J Gastroenterol 1992; 87:350–354.
45. Dennish GW, Castell DO. Inhibitory effect of smoking on the lower esophageal sphincter. N Engl J Med 1971; 284:1136–1137.
46. Stanciu C, Bennett JR. Smoking and gastro-oesophagus reflux. Br Med J 1972; 3: 793–795.
47. Chattopadhyay DK, Greaney MG, Irvin TT. Effect of cigarette smoking on the lower oesophageal sphincter: assessment of normal and symptomatic patients using rapid pull-through technique of oesophageal manometry. Gut 1977; 18:833–835.
48. Shindlbeck NE, Heinrich C, Dendorfer A, Pace F, Müller-Lissner SA. Influence of smoking and esophageal intubation on esophageal pH-metry. Gastroenterology 1987; 92:1994–1997.
49. Kahrilas PJ, Gupta RR. The effect of cigarette smoking on salivation and esophageal acid clearance. J Lab Clin Med 1989; 114:431–438.
50. Koelz HR, Birchler R, Bretholz A, Bron B, Capitaine Y, Delmore G, Fehr HF, Fumigalli I, Gehrig J, Gonvers JJ, Halter F, Hammer B, Kayasseh L, Kobler E, Miller G, Munst G, Pelloni S, Realini S, Schmid P, Voirol M, Blum AL. Healing and relapse of reflux esophagitis during treatment with ranitidine. Gastroenterology 1986; 91:1198–1205.

51. Waring JP, Eastwood TF, Austin JM, Sanowski RA. The immediate effects of cessation of cigarette smoking on gastroesophageal reflux. Am J Gastroenterol 1989; 84:1076–1078.
52. Kahrilas PJ, Gupta RR. Mechanisms of acid reflux associated with cigarette smoking. Gut 1990; 31:4–10.
53. Kadakia SC, Kikendall JW, Maydonovitch C, Johnson LF. Effect of cigarette smoking on gastroesophageal reflux measured by 24-h ambulatory esophageal pH monitoring. Am J Gastroenterol 1995; 90:1785–1790.
54. Pehl C, Pfeiffer A, Wendl B, Nagy I, Kaess H. Effect of smoking on the results of esophageal pH measurement in clinical routine. J Clin Gastroenterol 1997; 25: 503–506.
55. Kahrilas PJ. Cigarette smoking and gastroesophageal reflux disease. Dig Dis 1992; 10:61–71.
56. Orlando RC, Bryson JC, Powell DW. Effect of cigarette smoke on esophageal epithelium of the rabbit. Gastroenterology 1986; 91:1536–1542.
57. Butt HR, Vinson PP. Esophagitis. II. Pathologic and clinical study. Arch Otolaryngol 1936; 23:550–572.
58. Bartels EC. Acute ulcerative esophagitis. Arch Pathol 1935; 20:369–378.
59. Nagler R, Wolfson AW, Lowman RM, Spiro HM. Effect of gastric intubation on the normal mechanisms preventing gastroesophageal reflux. N Engl J Med 1960; 262:1325–1326.
60. Nagler R, Spiro HM. Persistent gastroesophageal reflux induced during prolonged gastric intubation. N Engl J Med 1963; 269:495–500.
61. Vinnik IE, Kern F. The effect of gastric intubation on esophageal pH. Gastroenterology 1964; 47:388–394.
62. Satiani B, Bonner JT, Stone HH. Factors influencing intraoperative gastric regurgitation: a prospective random study of nasogastric tube drainage. Arch Surg 1978; 113:721–723.
63. Emde C, Cilluffo T, Bauerfeind P, Blum AL. Combined esophageal and gastric pH-metry in healthy volunteers: influence of cable through LES and effect of misoprostol. Dig Dis Sci 1989; 34:79–82.
64. Singh S, Richter JE. Effects of a pH electrode across the lower esophageal sphincter. Dig Dis Sci 1992; 37:667–672.
65. Dotson RG, Robinson RG, Pingleton SK. Gastroesophageal reflux with nasogastric tubes: effect of nasogastric tube size. Am J Respir Crit Care Med 1994; 149:1659–1662.
66. Kuo B, Castell DO. The effect of nasogastric intubation on gastroesophageal reflux: a comparison of different tube sizes. Am J Gastroenterol 1995; 90:1804–1807.
67. Ibanez J, Penafiel A, Raurich JM, Marse P, Jorda R, Mata F. Gastroesophageal reflux in intubated patients receiving enteral nutrition: effect of supine and semirecumbent positions. J Parenter Enteral Nutr 1992; 16:419–422.
68. Orozco-Levi M, Torres A, Ferrer M, Piera C, El-Ebiary M, Puig De La Bellacasa J, Rodriguez-Roisin R. Semirecumbent position protects from pulmonary aspiration but not completely from gastroesophageal reflux in mechanically ventilated patients. Am J Respir Crit Care Med 1995; 152:1387–1390.
69. Brock-Utne JG, Rubin J, McAravey R, Dow TG, Welman S, Dimopoulos GE,

Moshal MG. The effect of hyoscine and atropine on the lower oesophageal sphincter. Anaesth Intens Care 1977; 5:223–225.
70. Brock-Utne JG. Domperidone antagonizes the relaxant effect of atropine on the lower esophageal sphincter. Anesth Analg 1980; 59:921–924.
71. McLoughlin RF, Mathieson JR, Chipperfield PM, Grymaloski MR, Wong AD. Effect of hyoscine butylbromide on gastroesophageal reflux in barium studies of the upper gastrointestinal tract. Can Assoc Rad J 1994; 45:452–454.
72. Mittal RK, Holloway R, Dent J. Effect of atropine on the frequency of reflux and transient lower esophageal sphincter relaxation in normal subjects. Gastroenterology 1995; 109:1547–1554.
73. Lidums I, Checklin H, Mittal RK, Holloway RH. Effect of atropine on gastro-oesophageal reflux and transient lower oesophageal sphincter relaxations in patients with gastro-oesophageal reflux disease. Gut 1998; 43:12–16.
74. Stein MR, Towner TG, Weber RW, Mansfield LE, Jacobson KW, McDonnell JT, Nelson HS. The effect of theophylline on the lower esophageal sphincter pressure. Ann Allergy 1980; 45:238–241.
75. Berquist WE, Rachelefsky GS, Kadden M, Siegel SC, Katz RM, Mickey MR, Ament ME. Effect of theophylline on gastroesophageal reflux in normal adults. J Allergy Clin Immunol 1981; 67:407–411.
76. Johannesson N, Andersson K, Joelsson B, Persson CGA. Relaxation of lower esophageal sphincter and stimulation of gastric secretion and diuresis by antiasthmatic xanthines: role of adenosine antagonism. Am Rev Respir Dis 1985; 131:26–31.
77. Krasnov S, Grossman MJ. Stimulation of gastric secretion in man by theophylline ethylenediamine. Proc Soc Exp Biol Med 1949; 71:335–336.
78. Hubert D, Gaudric M, Guerre J, Lockhart A, Marsac J. Effect of theophylline on gastroesophageal reflux in patients with asthma. J Allergy Clin Immunol 1988; 81:1168–1174.
79. Richter JE, Dalton CB, Buice RG, Castell DO. Nifedipine: a potent inhibitor of contractions in the body of the human esophagus. Studies in healthy volunteers and patients with the nutcracker esophagus. Gastroenterology 1985; 89:549–554.
80. Hongo M, Traube M, McAllister RG, McCallum RW. Effects of nifedipine on esophageal motor function in humans: correlation with plasma nifedipine concentration. Gastroenterology 1984; 86:8–12.
81. Bortolotti M, Labriola E, Baccheli S, Degli Esposti D, Sarti P, Brunelli F, Del Campo L, Barbara L. ''Oesophageal angina'' in patients with angina pectoris: a possible side effect of chronic therapy with nitroderivatives and Ca-antagonists. Ital J Gastroenterol 1992; 24:405–408.
82. Singh S, Bailey RT, Stein HJ, DeMeester TR, Richter JE. Effect of alprazolam (Xanax) on esophageal motility and acid reflux. Am J Gastroenterol 1992; 87:483–488.
83. Occhipinti M. Prostaglandins and gastrointestinal function. Adv Pediatr 1978; 25:205–221.
84. Dilawari JB, Newman A, Poleo J, Misiewicz JJ. Response of the human cardiac sphincter to circulating prostaglandins F_{2a} and E_2 and to anti-inflammatory drugs. Gut 1975; 16:137–143.

85. Scheiman JM, Patel PM, Henson EK, Nostrant TT. Effect of naproxen on gastroesophageal reflux and esophageal functions: a randomized, double-blind, placebo-controlled study. Am J Gastroenterol 1995; 90:754–757.
86. Hall AW, Moossa AR, Clark J, Cooley GR, Skinner DB. The effects of premedication drugs on the lower oesophageal high pressure zone and reflux status of rhesus monkeys and man. Gut 1975; 16:347–352.
87. Penagini R, Bianchi PA. Effect of morphine on gastroesophageal reflux and transient lower esophageal sphincter relaxation. Gastroenterology 1997; 113:409–414.
88. Rattan S, Goyal RK. Effect of dopamine on the esophageal smooth muscle in vivo. Gastroenterology 1976; 70:377–381.
89. Berges W, Wienbeck M, Strohmeyer G. Does dopamine predispose to gastroesophageal reflux? Z Gastroenterol 1979; 17:681–684.
90. Gielkens HAJ, Lamers CBHW, Masclee AAM. Effect of amino acids on lower esophageal sphincter characteristics and gastroesophageal reflux in humans. Dig Dis Sci 1998; 43:840–846.
91. Rahal PS, Wright RA. Transdermal nicotine and gastroesophageal reflux. Am J Gastroenterol 1995; 90:919–921.
92. Kadakia SC, Renom De La Baume H, Shafer RT. Effects of transdermal nicotine on lower esophageal sphincter and esophageal motility. Dig Dis Sci 1996; 41:2130–2134.
93. Nagler R, Spiro HM. Heartburn in pregnancy. Am J Dig Dis 1962; 7:648–655.
94. Bassey OO. Pregnancy heartburn in Nigerians and Caucasians with theories about aetiology based on manometric recordings from the oesophagus and stomach. Br J Obstet Gynaecol 1977; 84:439–443.
95. Marrero JM, Goggin PM, de Caestecker JS, Pearce JM, Maxwell JD. Determinants of pregnancy heartburn. Br J Obstet Gynaecol 1992; 99:731–734.
96. Nagler R, Spiro HM. Heartburn in late pregnancy: manometric studies of esophageal motor function. J Clin Invest 1961; 40:954–970.
97. Van Thiel DH, Gavaler JS, Joshi SN, Sara RK, Stremple J. Heartburn of pregnancy. Gastroenterology 1977; 72:666–668.
98. Fisher RS, Roberts GS, Grabowski CJ, Cohen S. Inhibition of lower esophageal sphincter circular muscle by female sex hormones. Am J Physiol 1978; 234:E234–E237.
99. Schulze K, Christensen J. Lower sphincter of the opossum esophagus in pseudopregnancy. Gastroenterology 1977; 73:1082–1085.
100. Van Thiel DH, Gavaler JS, Stremple J. Lower esophageal sphincter pressure in women using sequential oral contraceptives. Gastroenterology 1976; 71:232–234.
101. Filippone M, Malmud L, Kryston L, Antonucci J, Bottger J, Fisher RS. Esophageal and lower esophageal sphincter pressures (LESP) in male transsexuals treated with female sex hormones. Clin Res 1983; 31:282A.
102. Spence AA, Moir DD, Finlay WEI. Observations on intragastric pressure. Anaesthesia 1967; 22:249–256.
103. Lind JF, Smith AM, McIver DK, Coopland AT, Crispin JS. Heartburn in pregnancy—a manometric study. Can Med Assoc J 1968; 98:571–574.
104. Van Thiel DH, Wald A. Evidence refuting a role for increased abdominal pressure

in the pathogenesis of the heartburn associated with pregnancy. Am J Obstet Gynecol 1981; 140:420–422.

105. Wald A, Van Thiel DH, Hoechstetter L, Gavaler JS, Egler KM, Verm R, Scott L, Lester R. Effect of pregnancy on gastrointestinal transit. Dig Dis Sci 1982; 27: 1015–1018.
106. Braverman DZ, Herbet D, Goldstein R, Persitz E, Eylath U, Jacobsohn WZ. Postpartum restoration of pregnancy-induced cholecystoparesis and prolonged intestinal transit time. J Clin Gastroenterol 1988; 10:642–646.
107. Schade RR, Pelekanos MJ, Tauxe WN, Van Thiel DH. Gastric emptying during pregnancy. Gastroenterology 1984; 86:1234.
108. Ehrmann S. Ueber die Bieziehung der Sklerodermie Zu den Autotoxichen erythemen. Ubien Med Wochenschr 1903; 53:1097–1159.
109. Rose S, Young MA, Reynolds JC. Gastrointestinal manifestations of scleroderma. Gastroenterol Clin North Am 1998; 27:563–594.
110. Orringer MB, Dabich L, Zarafonetis CJD, Sloan H. Gastroesophageal reflux in esophageal scleroderma: diagnosis and implications. Ann Thorac Surg 1976; 22: 120–129.
111. Hendel L, Aggestrup S, Stentoft P. Long-term ranitidine in progressive systemic sclerosis (scleroderma) with gastroesophageal reflux. Scand J Gastroenterol 1986; 21:799–805.
112. Stentoft P, Hendel L, Aggestrup S. Esophageal manometry and pH-probe monitoring in the evaluation of gastroesophageal reflux in patients with progressive systemic sclerosis. Scand J Gastroenterol 1987; 22:499–504.
113. Zamost BJ, Hirschberg J, Ippoliti AF, Furst DE, Clements PJ, Weinstein WM. Esophagitis in scleroderma: prevalence and risk factors. Gastroenterology 1987; 92:421–428.
114. Murphy JR, McNally P, Peller P, Shay SS. Prolonged clearance is the primary abnormal reflux parameter in patients with progressive systemic sclerosis and esophagitis. Dig Dis Sci 1992; 37:833–841.
115. Yarze JC, Varga J, Stampfl D, Castell DO, Jimenez SA. Esophageal function in systemic sclerosis: a prospective evaluation of motility and acid reflux in 36 patients. Am J Gastroenterol 1993; 88:870–876.
116. Sjogren RW. Gastrointestinal motility disorders in scleroderma. Arthritis Rheum 1994; 37:1265–1282.
117. Giles GR, Mason MC, Humphries C, Clark CG. Action of gastrin on the lower oesophageal sphincter in man. Gut 1969; 10:730–734.
118. Castell DO, Harris LD. Hormonal control of gastroesophageal-sphincter strength. N Engl J Med 1970; 282:886–889.
119. Cohen S, Lipshutz W. Hormonal regulation of human lower esophageal sphincter competence: interaction of gastrin and secretin. J Clin Invest 1971; 50:449–454.
120. Lipshutz WH, Gaskins RD, Lukash WM, Sode J. Pathogenesis of lower-esophageal-sphincter incompetence. N Engl J Med 1973; 289:182–184.
121. Cohen S. Hypogastrinemia and sphincter incompetence. N Engl J Med 1973; 289: 215–217.
122. Lipshutz WH, Gaskins RD, Lukash WM, Sode J. Hypogastrinemia in patients with lower esophageal sphincter incompetence. Gastroenterology 1974; 67:423–427.

123. Isenberg J, Csindis A, Walsh JH. Resting and pentagastrin-stimulated gastroesophageal sphincter pressure in patients with Zollinger-Ellison syndrome. Gastroenterology 1971; 61:655–658.
124. McCallum RW, Walsh JH. Relationship between lower esophageal sphincter pressure and serum gastrin concentration in Zollinger-Ellison syndrome and other clinical settings. Gastroenterology 1979; 76:76–81.
125. Snyder N, Hughes W. Basal and calcium stimulated gastroesophageal pressure in patients with Zollinger-Ellison syndrome. Gastroenterology 1977; 72:1240–1243.
126. Farrell RL, Castell DO, McGuigan JE. Measurements and comparisons of lower esophageal sphincter pressures and serum gastrin levels in patients with gastroesophageal reflux. Gastroenterology 1974; 67:415–422.
127. Wright LF, Slaughter RL, Gibson RG, Hirschowitz BI. Correlation of lower esophageal sphincter pressure and serum gastrin level in man. Am J Dig Dis 1975; 20: 603–606.
128. McCallum RW, Holloway RH, Callachan C, Avella J, Walsh JH. Endogenous gastrin release and antral gastrin concentration in gastroesophageal reflux patients and normal subjects. Am J Gastroenterol 1983; 78:398–402.
129. Ellison EH, Wilson SD. Zollinger-Ellison syndrome: reappraisal and evaluation of 260 registered cases. Ann Surg 1964; 160:512–528.
130. Regan PT, Malagelada JR. A reappraisal of clinical, roentgenographic, and endoscopic features of the Zollinger-Ellison syndrome. Mayo Clin Proc 1978; 53:19–23.
131. Richter JE, Pandol SJ, Castell DO, McCarthy DM. Gastroesophageal reflux disease in the Zollinger-Ellison syndrome. Ann Intern Med 1981; 95:37–43.
132. Agha F. Esophageal involvement in the Zollinger-Ellison syndrome. Am J Roentgenol 1985; 144:721–725.
133. Miller LS, Vinayek R, Frucht H, Gardner JD, Jensen RT, Maton PN. Reflux esophagitis in patients with Zollinger-Ellison syndrome. Gastroenterology 1990; 98:341–346.
134. Strader DB, Benjamin SB, Orbuch M, Lubensky TA, Gibril F, Weber C, Fishbeyn VA, Jensen RT, Metz DC. Esophageal function and occurrence of Barrett's esophagus in Zollinger-Ellison syndrome. Digestion 1995; 56:347–356.
135. Cadiot G, Bruhat A, Riguad D, Coste T, Vuagnat A, Benyedder Y, Vallot T, Le Guludec D, Mignon M. Multivariate analysis of pathophysiologic factors in reflux oesophagitis. Gut 1997; 40:167–174.
135a. Straathof JWA, Lamers CBHW, Masclee AAM. Effect of gastrin-17 on lower esophageal sphincter characteristics in man. Dig Dis Sci 1997; 42:2547–2551.
136. Little AG, DeMeester TR, Kirchner PT, O'Sullivan DC, Skinner DB. Pathogenesis of esophagitis in patients with gastroesophageal reflux. Surgery 1980; 88:101–107.
137. Holloway RH, Hongo M, Berger K, McCallum RW. Gastric distention: A mechanism for postprandial gastroesophageal reflux. Gastroenterology 1985; 89:779–784.
138. Holloway RH, Kocyan P, Dent J. Provocation of transient lower esophageal sphincter relaxations by meals in patients with symptomatic gastroesophageal reflux. Dig Dis Sci 1991; 36:1034–1039.
139. Dodds WJ, Dent J, Hogan WJ, Helm JF, Hauser R, Patel GK, Egide MS. Mecha-

nisms of gastroesophageal reflux in patients with reflux esophagitis. N Engl J Med 1982; 307:1547–1552.
140. Dent J, Holloway RH, Toouli J, Dodds WJ. Mechanisms of lower esophageal sphincter incompetence in patients with symptomatic gastroesophageal reflux. Gut 1988; 29:1020–1028.
141. Biancani P, Barwick KW, Selling J, McCallum RW. Effects of acute experimental esophagitis on mechanical properties of the lower esophageal sphincter. Gastroenterology 1984; 87:8–16.
142. Shay SS, Eggli D, McDonald C, Johnson LF. Gastric emptying of solid food in patients with gastroesophageal reflux. Gastroenterology 1987; 92:459–465.
143. Schwizer W, Hinder RA, DeMeester TR. Does delayed gastric emptying contribute to gastroesophageal reflux disease? Am J Surg 1989; 157:74–81.
144. Keshavarzian A, Bushnell DL, Sontag S, Yegelwel EJ, Smid K. Gastric emptying in patient with severe reflux esophagitis. Am J Gastroenterol 1991; 86:738–742.
145. McCallum RW, Berkowitz DM, Lerner E. Gastric emptying in patients with gastroesophageal reflux. Gastroenterology 1981; 80:285–291.
146. Maddern GJ, Chatterton BE, Collins PJ, Horowitz M, Shearman DJC, Jamieson GG. Solid and liquid gastric-emptying in patients with gastro-oesophageal reflux. Br J Surg 1985; 72:344–347.
147. Fink SM, Barwick KW, DeLuca V, Sanders FJ, Kandathil M, McCallum RW. The association of histologic gastritis with gastroesophageal reflux and delayed gastric emptying. J Clin Gastroenterol 1984; 6:301–309.
148. Benini L, Sembenini C, Castellani G, Caliari S, Fioretta A, Vantini I. Gastric emptying and dyspeptic symptoms in patients with gastroesophageal reflux. Am J Gastroenterol 1996; 91:1351–1354.
149. Cucchiara S, Salvia G, Borrelli O, Ciccimarra E, Az-Zeqeh N, Rapagiolo S, Minella R, Campanozzi A, Riezzo G. Gastric electrical dysrhythmias and delayed gastric emptying in gastroesophageal reflux disease. Am J Gastroenterol 1997; 92:1103–1108.
150. Soykan I, Lin Z, Jones S, Chen J, McCallum RW. Gastric myoelectrical activity, gastric emptying and correlations with dyspepsia symptoms in patients with gastroesophageal reflux. J Invest Med 1997; 45:483–487.
151. Cunningham KM, Horowitz M, Riddell PS, Maddern GJ, Myers JC, Holloway RH, Wishart JM, Jamieson GG. Relations among autonomic nerve dysfunction, oesophageal motility, and gastric emptying in gastro-oesophageal reflux disease. Gut 1991; 32:1436–1440.
152. Keshavarzian A, Iber FL, Vaeth J. Gastric emptying in patients with insulin-requiring diabetes mellitus. Am J Gastroenterol 1987; 82:29–35.
153. Schvarz E, Palmer M, Aman J, Horowitz M, Stridsberg M, Berne C. Physiological hyperglycemia slows gastric emptying in normal subjects and patients with insulin-dependent diabetes mellitus. Gastroenterology 1997; 113:60–66.
154. Samsom M, Akkermans LMA, Jebbink RJA, van Isselt H, vanBerge-Henegouwen GP, Smout AJPM. Gastrointestinal motor mechanisms in hyperglycemia induced delayed gastric emptying in type I diabetes mellitus. Gut 1997; 40:644–646.
155. Murray FE, Lombard MG, Ashe J, Lynch D, Drury MI, O'Moore B, Lennon J, Crowe J. Esophageal function in diabetes mellitus with special reference to acid

studies and relationship to peripheral neuropathy. Am J Gastroenterol 1987; 82: 840–843.

156. Parkman HP, Schwartz SS. Esophagitis and gastroduodenal disorders associated with diabetic gastroparesis. Arch Intern Med 1987; 147:1477–1480.
157. Hosking DJ, Bennett T, Hampton JR. Diabetic autonomic neuropathy. Diabetes 1978; 27:1043–1055.
158. Murley RS. Painful enteromegaly of unknown etiology. Proc R Soc Med 1959; 52: 479.
159. Schuffler MD, Beegle RG. Progressive systemic sclerosis of the gastrointestinal tract and hereditary hollow visceral myopathy: two distinguishable disorders of intestinal muscle. Gastroenterology 1979; 77:664.
160. Schuffler MD, Pope CE. Esophageal motor dysfunction in idiopathic intestinal pseudoobstruction. Gastroenterology 1976; 70:677–682.
161. Mayer EA, Elashoff J, Hawkins R, Berquist W, Taylor IL. Gastric emptying of mixed solid-liquid meal in patients with intestinal pseudoobstruction. Dig Dis Sci 1988; 33:10–18.
162. Weber FH, McCallum RW. Gastric motor disorders. In: Snape WJ, ed. Consultations in Gastroenterology. Philadelphia: WB Saunders, 1996:247–259.
162a. Horowitz M, Collins PJ, Tuckwell V, Vernon-Roberts J, Shearman DJ. Fenfluramine delays gastric emptying of solid food. Br J Clin Pharmacol 1985; 19:849–851.
163. Maddern GJ, Horowitz M, Jamieson GG, Chatterton BE, Collins PJ, Roberts-Thomson P. Abnormalities of esophageal and gastric emptying in progressive systemic sclerosis. Gastroenterology 1984; 87:922–926.
164. Bortolotti M, Turba E, Tosti A, Sarti P, Brunelli F, Del Campo L, Barbara L. Gastric emptying and interdigestive antroduodenal motility in patients with esophageal scleroderma. Am J Gastroenterol 1991; 86:743–747.
165. Wegener M, Adamek RJ, Wedmann B, Jergas M, Altmeyer P. Gastrointestinal transit through esophagus, stomach, small and large intestine in patients with progressive systemic sclerosis. Dig Dis Sci 1994; 39:2209–2215.
166. Auslander M. Gastric outlet obstruction. In: Snape WJ, ed. Consultations in Gastroenterology. Philadelphia: WB Saunders, 1996:264–269.
167. O'Connor HJ, Cunnane K. *Helicobacter pylori* and gastro-oesophageal reflux disease: a prospective study. Ir J Med Sci 1994; 163:369–373.
168. Kuipers EJ, Lundell L, Klinkenberg-Knol E, Havu N, Festen HPM, Liedman B, Lamers CBHW, Jansen JBMJ, Dalenbock J, Snel P, Nelis GF, Meuwissen SGM. Atrophic gastritis and *Helicobacter pylori* infection in patients with reflux esophagitis treated with omeprazole or fundoplication. N Engl J Med 1996; 334:1018–1022.
169. Werdmuller BFM, Loffeld RJLF. *Helicobacter pylori* infection has no role in the pathogenesis of reflux esophagitis. Dig Dis Sci 1997; 42:103–105.
170. Csendes A, Smok G, Cerda G, Burdiles P, Mazza D, Csendes P. Prevalence of *Helicobacter pylori* infection in 190 control subjects and in 236 patients with gastroesophageal reflux, erosive esophagitis or Barrett's esophagus. Dis Esoph 1997; 10:38–42.
171. Newton M, Bryan R, Burnham WR, Kamm MA. Evaluation of *Helicobacter pylori* in reflux oesophagitis and Barrett's oesophagus. Gut 1997; 40:9–13.

172. Goldblum JR, Vicari JJ, Falk GW, Rice TW, Peek RM, Easley K, Richter JE. Inflammation and intestinal metaplasia of the gastric cardia: the role of gastroesophageal reflux and *H. pylori* infection. Gastroenterology 1998; 114:633–639.
173. Vicari JJ, Peek RM, Falk GM, Goldblum JR, Easley KA, Schnell J, Perez-Perez GI, Halter SA, Rice TW, Blaser MJ, Richter JE. The seroprevalence of CagA-positive *Helicobacter pylori* strains in the spectrum of gastroesophageal reflux disease. Gastroenterology 1998; 115:50–57.
174. Varanasi RV, Fantry GT, Wilson KT. Decreased prevalence of *Helicobacter pylori* infection in gastroesophageal reflux disease. *Helicobacter* 1998; 3:188–194.
175. Labenz J, Malfertheiner P. *Helicobacter pylori* in gastro-oesophageal reflux disease: causal agent, independent or protective factor? Gut 1997; 41:277–280.
176. Vicari J, Falk GW, Richter JE. *Helicobacter pylori* and acid peptic disorders of the esophagus: is it conceivable? Am J Gastroenterol 1997; 92:1097–1102.
177. Xia HH, Talley NJ. *Helicobacter pylori* infection, reflux esophagitis, and atrophic gastritis: an unexplored triangle. Am J Gastroenterol 1998; 93:394–400.
178. El-Omar EM, Penman ID, Ardill JES, Chittajallu RS, Howie C, McColl KEL. *Helicobacter pylori* infection and abnormalities of acid secretion in patients with duodenal ulcer disease. Gastroenterology 1995; 109:681–691.
179. Minocha A, Mokshagundam S, Gallo SH, Rahal PS. Alterations in upper gastrointestinal motility in *Helicobacter pylori*–positive nonulcer dyspepsia. Am J Gastroenterol 1994; 89:1797–1800.
180. Barnett J, Behler EM, Appelman HD, Elta GH. *Campylobacter pylori* is not associated with gastroparesis. Dig Dis Sci 1989; 34:1677–1680.
181. Scott AM, Kellow JE, Shuter B, Cowan H, Corbett AM, Riley JW, Lunzer MR, Eckstein RP, Hoschl R, Lam SK, Jones MP. Intragastric distribution and gastric emptying of solids and liquids in functional dyspepsia: lack of influence of symptom subgroups and *H. pylori*–associated gastritis. Dig Dis Sci 1993; 38:2247–2254
182. Mitchell HM, Hazell SL, Li YY, Hu PJ. Serologic response to specific *Helicobacter pylori* antigens: antibody to CagA antigen is not predictive of gastric cancer in a developing country. Am J Gastroenterol 1996; 91:1785–1788.
183. Chang CS, Poon SK, Lien HC, Chen GH. The incidence of reflux esophagitis among the Chinese. Am J Gastroenterol 1997; 92:668–671.
184. Hesketh PJ, Clapp RW, Doos WG, Spechler SJ. The increasing frequency of adenocarcinoma of the esophagus. Cancer 1989; 64:526–530.
185. Graham DY, Malaty HM, Evans DG, Evans DJ Jr, Klein PD, Adams E. Epidemiology of *Helicobacter pylori* in an asymptomatic population in the United States. Effect of age, race and socioeconomic status. Gastroenterology 1991; 100:1495–1501.
186. Labenz J, Blum AL, Bayerdörffer E, Meining A, Stolte M, Börsch G. Curing *Helicobacter pylori* infection in patients with duodenal ulcer may provoke reflux esophagitis. Gastroenterology 1997; 112:1442–1447.

3
Epidemiology of Gastroesophageal Reflux Disease

Dawn Provenzale
Duke University Medical Center, Durham, North Carolina

In this chapter the epidemiology of the two major forms of gastroesophageal reflux disease (GERD) is covered—that is, symptomatic (nonerosive) reflux disease and erosive esophagitis. In addition, the epidemiology of the esophageal complications of GERD is reviewed.

Although definitions vary, GERD encompasses a broad spectrum of pathology ranging from esophageal to extraesophageal disease. Moreover, the esophageal manifestations of GERD also vary considerably, from an asymptomatic condition to symptoms of heartburn, cough, and chest pain resulting from esophageal mucosal injury. With continued reflux, there is damage to the esophageal mucosa. The extent of damage depends on the duration and severity of the reflux, with reflux esophagitis reflecting histological and endoscopic damage, and esophageal stricture and Barrett's esophagus as sequelae of long-term reflux. The broad spectrum of findings reflects the variability in the clinical spectrum of the disorder, with most patients reporting occasional, intermittent symptoms that typically do not require medical intervention.

SYMPTOMATIC (NONEROSIVE) REFLUX

Data regarding the epidemiology of the esophageal manifestations of GERD are essentially based on reports of heartburn as the indicator of GERD. From this vantage point, the prevalence and incidence of GERD vary by region, with the highest prevalence in Western countries (1). A Gallup survey revealed that 44% of adult Americans experienced heartburn at least once a month in the United

Table 1 Prevalence of Reflux-Like Symptoms

Ref.	No. of subjects	Geographic/ ethnic origin	Frequency (%) Daily	Weekly	Monthly	Yearly	Other
2		American	44				
3	385	American	7	14	15		
4	1511	American		17.8/100		42.4/100 (heartburn)[a]	
				6.3/100		45/100 (acid regurgitation)[a]	
				19.8/100		58.7/100 (either)[a]	
7	313	American ≥ 62 yo		14			
10	3105	British Scottish					18 (6 mo)
11	1700	Finnish	10[b]	15[c]	25[c]	50[c]	
12	1486	Danish					12% heartburn[d] 9% acid regurgitation[d]
13	3600	Danish			12.5 women[e] 14.5 men[e]		54.3[f] 46.7[f]
14	337	Swedish					21 heartburn 20 acid regurgitation 12 chest pain

[a] Any episode in the last year.
[b] On the day of the questionnaire.
[c] In the last week, month, year.
[d] Last 6 months, 30% of each group had symptoms more than 10 days each month.
[e] Once per month or more.
[f] One-year period prevalence.

States (2), while a survey of presumed normal hospital employees found that 7% of individuals experienced daily heartburn, 14% experienced weekly heartburn, and 15% experienced heartburn once a month (3). A survey of residents of Olmsted County found that 42.4 per 100 residents experienced heartburn at least one time in the past year while 17.8 per 100 stated that they had heartburn at least once per week. Acid regurgitation for at least a year and at least once each week was reported by 45.0 and 6.3 per 100 residents, respectively. Notable is that 58.7 per 100 residents reported either symptom occurring in the last year, while weekly episodes were reported by 19.8 per 100 residents (4). In contrast to other studies that suggest a slight male predominance for GERD (1) and an increasing prevalence with increasing age (5–9), this survey found no significant differences by age or sex (4). The survey also demonstrated that heartburn, but not acid regurgitation, was inversely associated with increasing age (4).

There is substantial geographic variation in the prevalence of reflux, which may, in part, be explained by differences in definitions of GERD. A large postal survey in England and Scotland reported an 18% prevalence of reflux symptoms, but medical attention was sought by only one-quarter of respondents. Although symptom frequency decreased with age and was not associated with social class, the proportion seeking medical care increased with age and was greater among those in the lowest social class (10). A Finnish study found that among 1700 respondents, symptoms suggestive of reflux disease, including heartburn, regurgitation, dysphagia, upper abdominal, and chest pain, were experienced by more than half of respondents in the previous year, by more than 25% in the past month, by approximately 15% in the week before, and by 10% on the day they replied to the questionnaire. They noted that 16% of symptomatic individuals used medication and 5% sought medical advice for the problem in the last year (11). A Danish study found that 12% of the interviewees reported heartburn while 9% reported regurgitation in the previous 6 months; 61% and 64% used antacids, 19% and 23% used H_2-receptor antagonists, and 63% and 68% sought medical advice (12). Another Danish study noted that the 1-year prevalence of epigastric pain, heartburn, and acid regurgitation was 54.3% in men and 46.7% in women (13), while a Swedish population study reported heartburn in 21%, acid regurgitation in 20%, and noncardiac chest pain in 12% (14). This population was evaluated 10 years later and the prevalence of heartburn, acid regurgitation, and chest pain was essentially unchanged (15).

In summary, the prevalence of at least occasional reflux symptoms in the Western world ranges from approximately 12% to 54% (3–7,10,11,13,14). A Chinese study revealed a prevalence of acid regurgitation, heartburn, or belching of 16.9% among individuals presenting for routine physical examination (16), within the range reported by the Western studies.

Gastroesophageal reflux is a common problem among pregnant women, occurring in 48–81.5% of Caucasian women (17–20). While three studies have detected no racial variation in the incidence of pregnancy-associated heartburn in Britain or the United States (17,19,20), a study by Bassey (18) showed that both Nigerians living in Nigeria and those living in Britain for more than 2 years had a lower prevalence of heartburn (9.8%) than Caucasians living in Britain.

REFLUX (EROSIVE) ESOPHAGITIS

Reflux esophagitis, a sequela of chronic GERD, refers to mucosal injury characterized by epithelial erosions, ulceration, and hyperplasia associated with inflammation. Most patients are symptomatic, although esophagitis may occasionally occur without symptoms.

The reported prevalence of esophagitis among individuals who undergo endoscopy for GERD symptoms ranges from 30% to 79% (21–25) (Table 2), while the prevalence in the general population has been estimated at 2–4% (26). In one small series, histological esophagitis was found in up to 60% of individuals who did not have a history of reflux symptoms and who had no evidence of endoscopic esophagitis, suggesting that while histological evidence of esophagitis may be common, the utility of using criteria such as squamous hyperplasia and the presence of inflammatory cells in histological specimens for the diagnosis of esophagitis in the asymptomatic individual is questionable (27). The incidence of severe esophagitis (number of new cases in a specified time period) has been estimated at 4.5 per 100,000 population annually in a population in northeast Scotland (6), with a dramatic increase after the age of 50 (Fig. 1). The association between age and esophagitis has also been demonstrated by Zhu et al. (28), who found endoscopic grades III and IV esophagitis in 20.8% of patients 65–76 years old compared to 3.4% in patients younger than age 64.

Reflux esophagitis appears to be a disorder of predominantly Western populations, although the data are limited by a selection bias, in that it has been pre-

Table 2 Prevalence of Erosive Esophagitis Among Those Who Undergo Endoscopy for GERD

Ref.	No. of subjects	Geographic/ ethnic origin	Mean age (years)	Gender	Erosive esophagitis (%)
20	77	American	50	100% male	61
21	100	Swedish	52	36% male	35
22	1217	British	—	62% male	9.9
	8445	British	—	—	23
23	50	American	55.2	44% male	46

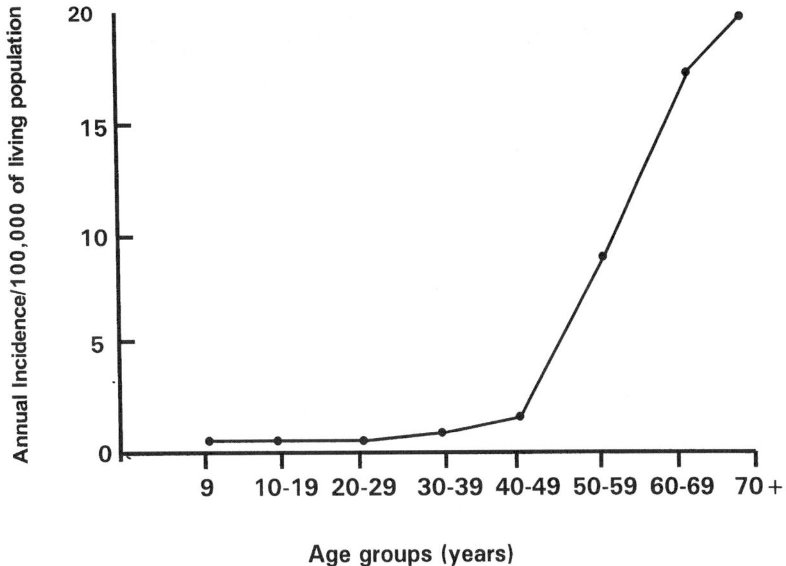

Figure 1 Severe peptic esophagitis. Annual incidence per 100,000 of living population in each age group.

dominantly patients in Western populations who have undergone endoscopy to document esophagitis. A report from Kashmir, however, found that 5.6% of symptomatic ulcer patients had endoscopic esophagitis compared to 1.1% of asymptomatic patients who also underwent endoscopy (29). The high prevalence of esophagitis in northern Iran and northern China, is not thought to be due to reflux, but up to 9% of those studied in Iran and 22% of those studied in China complained of typical reflux symptoms (30).

Gender Differences

Although there is an approximately equal sex ratio for symptomatic reflux from self-reported questionnaires, the ratio of men to women with esophagitis has generally been reported to range from 1.5:1 to 3:1 (31–34). There have been a few studies, however, that suggest a female predominance of both nonstenotic esophagitis (1:1.8) and peptic stricture (1:1.9) (6,35).

Genetic Factors

The role of genetic factors in GERD is unknown. However, Romero et al. found that reflux symptoms were significantly more prevalent among parents and sib-

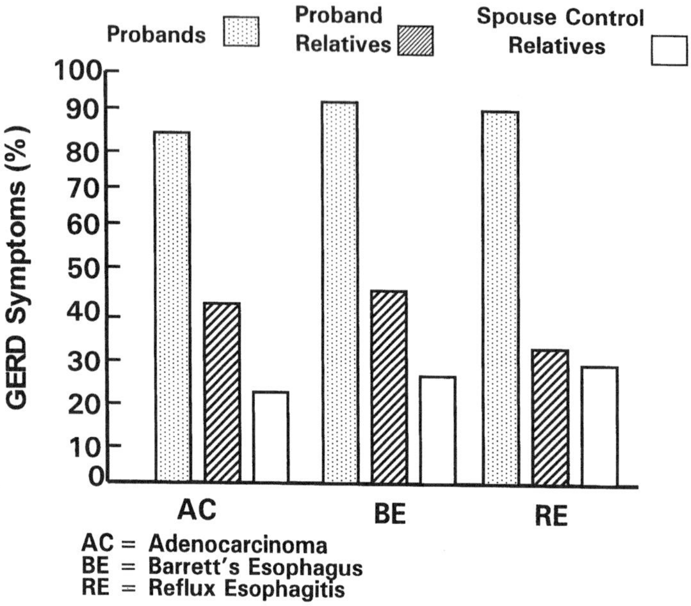

Figure 2 Prevalence of GERD symptoms among proband relatives and spouse control relatives of patients with adenocarcinoma, Barrett's esophagus, and reflux esophagitis.

lings of patients with adenocarcinoma than spouse control relatives (43% vs. 23%) (Fig. 2). They also found that patients with Barrett's esophagus had significantly more first-degree relatives with GERD symptoms than their spouse control relatives (46% vs. 27%). Of note is that first-degree relatives of patients with reflux esophagitis were not more likely to have significant reflux compared to spouse control relatives (33% vs. 29%). Reflux was more prevalent among siblings than among spouses of patients with Barrett's esophagus (41% vs. 12%) and adenocarcinoma (40% vs. 6%). There was, however, no difference in the prevalence of reflux symptoms among siblings and spouse control relatives of patients with reflux esophagitis (24% vs. 32%). The authors concluded that there may be a genetic predisposition to the development of reflux in families of patients with Barrett's esophagus and esophageal adenocarcinoma, but that environmental factors appear more important for uncomplicated reflux (36) (Fig. 2).

COMPLICATIONS OF GERD

The sequelae of chronic gastroesophageal reflux include esophagitis, esophageal strictures, and Barrett's esophagus. Few studies have evaluated methods for early identification of patients with these sequelae and those at increased risk for their development. We examined GERD complications among veterans to determine whether race was associated with sequelae of GERD such as esophagitis, stricture, esophageal ulcers, and Barrett's esophagus. The results suggested that males with GERD were 2.58 times more likely to have esophagitis (95% CI, 1.20–5.53). After adjusting for gender, Caucasians were more likely to have esophagitis OR 1.51 (95% CI, 1.11–2.04). We noted that dysphagia was the most common indication for endoscopy in those with esophagitis, esophageal ulcers, and strictures, and heartburn was the most common indication for endoscopy in patients with Barrett's esophagus (37) (Fig. 3). We also evaluated demographic and clinical parameters of patients with GERD to determine whether there was an association between patient characteristics, clinical symptoms, and Barrett's esophagus. We found that age greater than 40 (OR 4.86, 95% CI 1.50–15.80), the presence of heartburn or acid regurgitation (OR 4.12, 95% CI 1.26–17.00), and heartburn more than once each week (OR 3.01, 95% CI 1.35–6.73) were associated with endoscopically and histologically confirmed Barrett's esophagus, while duration of symptoms, race, alcohol, and smoking history were not associated with an increased prevalence of Barrett's esophagus (38). Although many series suggest that Barrett's esophagus is more likely to affect Caucasians than African-Americans (39,40), we found that race was not associated with an increased risk for Barrett's esophagus in this veteran population with GERD who were referred for endoscopy. While our study may have had insufficient power to detect all but a very large risk, our results may also reflect the severity of GERD symptoms in this population in that only those with the most severe and refractory disease were referred for endoscopy. This requires further prospective study.

Because there is currently no method to identify those with GERD who are at increased risk for the development of Barrett's esophagus, a decision model that examines the effectiveness and cost-effectiveness of screening for Barrett's

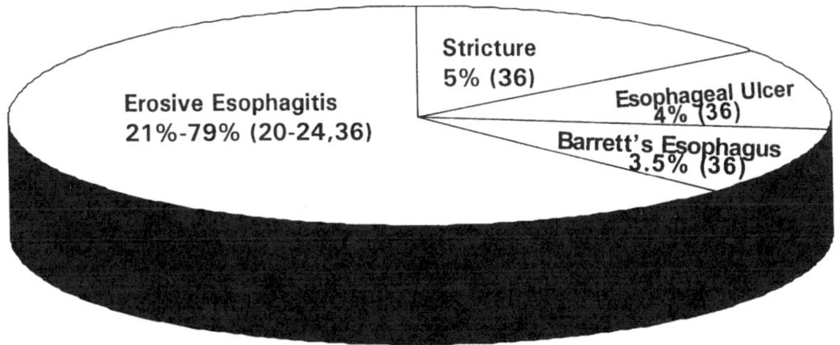

Figure 3 GERD complications in an asymptomatic Western population. Shown are proportions with erosive esophagitis, stricture, esophageal ulcer, and Barrett's esophagus.

esophagus among those with chronic heartburn has been developed. The decision model examines one-time screening for Barrett's esophagus in individuals with 5 or more years of GERD and compares this strategy with no screening (41). Using published literature on the rate of progression of Barrett's esophagus to dysplasia and cancer, the authors calculated the remaining quality-adjusted life expectancy for individuals in each strategy, and the cost. The model suggests that for a prevalence of Barrett's esophagus of 10% among those with GERD *and* an incidence of cancer of 1/75 patient-years (1.3% annually), one-time screening is less expensive and more effective than no screening. One-time screening is less costly than no screening because at this high prevalence of Barrett's esophagus (10%) and relatively high incidence of cancer (1.3%), it is less costly to screen patients with GERD, identify Barrett's patients, and place them into a surveillance program. Waiting for the development of symptomatic cancer among a proportion of those with Barrett's esophagus is more costly and less effective because symptomatic cancer is associated with a poor prognosis (5-year survival of 17% or less) and is expensive to treat (42). If Barrett's esophagus were present, surveillance every 2 years would provide the greatest gain in quality-adjusted life expectancy. The incremental cost-utility ratio for this strategy would be $82,000 per quality-adjusted life year gained, similar to the cost-effectiveness ratio for heart transplantation in patients less than 50 years of age with irremediable terminal cardiac disease (160,000/LY gained) (43). The results of the analysis are dependent upon the estimates for the prevalence of Barrett's esophagus among those with GERD and the incidence of cancer among those with Barrett's esophagus. Barrett's esophagus has been reported in up to 20% of individuals undergoing upper endoscopy, though recent estimates suggest that the prevalence of Barrett's esophagus is as low as 2% in those undergoing endoscopy (44) and approximately 3–5% in individuals with gastroesophageal reflux (45). The incidence of adenocarcinoma in patients with Barrett's esophagus, another critical parameter in this analysis, has been reported to be as low as 0.2% per year (46) and as high as 2.1% per year (47). The authors performed a sensitivity analysis on these parameters varying them over a broad range to examine their impact on the most effective strategy. The analysis showed that if the prevalence of Barrett's esophagus were only 4% or less among those with GERD, and the incidence of cancer in this group were 1/200 patient-years (0.5% annually) or less, similar to recent reports (45,48) then no screening would be less costly and more effective. Few patients who would undergo screening would actually have Barrett's esophagus, and in those who did, the development of cancer would be uncommon (0.5% annually). Therefore, the risks and costs of screening would outweigh any benefit in terms of cancer death prevented. This analysis identifies the uncertainties surrounding the management of patients with gastroesophageal reflux, particularly the incidence and prevalence of Barrett's esophagus in patients with GERD and the incidence of cancer in patients with Barrett's esophagus.

The management of patients with Barrett's esophagus, a known sequela of GERD, is controversial. The incidence of cancer, a critical parameter in management strategies for surveillance and subsequent esophagectomy, varies in published reports, reflecting the uncertainty about the cancer risk in this group (46,47). We developed a decision model that evaluates the impact of cancer risk on surveillance strategies in patients with Barrett's esophagus (42). The simulation model begins 1 year after a baseline endoscopic biopsy demonstrates Barrett's esophagus without evidence of dysplasia. The model evaluates surveillance every 1–5 years with esophagectomy performed for the development of high-grade dysplasia, and compares these strategies to no surveillance. To model the natural history of Barrett's esophagus, we included states for the possible development of dysplasia and cancer. The model assumes that cancer develops as a progression from Barrett's esophagus to low-grade dysplasia to high-grade dysplasia, and finally to cancer. Over time, patients with Barrett's esophagus and no evidence of dysplasia may remain in this health state or may progress toward cancer, and move to a low-grade dysplasia state, then to a high-grade dysplasia state, and finally to a cancer state; or they may die. The model includes published data on the incidence of dysplasia and cancer, the risks associated with endoscopy and esophagectomy, and the prognosis for those who develop esophageal cancer. The simulation also considers that patients may be willing to forgo some portion of their life to avoid the inconvenience of endoscopy, and the morbidity of an endoscopic complication or esophagectomy. We, therefore, adjusted for both the short- and long-term morbidity associated with the surveillance endoscopy and esophagectomy (49).

The model permits calculation of the average life expectancy, the cumulative incidence of cancer, and the number of endoscopic and surgical procedures for each strategy (42).

Costs for endoscopy, for endoscopy with a complication, for elective and urgent esophagectomy, and for follow-up of postesophagectomy patients and of those with esophageal cancer are included. The model records the costs as they occur during the lifetime of the patient, e.g., as procedures and surgery are performed, and calculates the average lifetime cost per patient for each strategy. The model also calculates the additional cost per quality-adjusted life-year gained (the incremental cost-utility ratio) for each strategy.

The results suggest that surveillance every 2–3 years with esophagectomy performed if high-grade dysplasia is diagnosed will increase quality-adjusted life expectancy by up to 1.2 years compared to no surveillance. When costs are considered, this strategy is dominated by less frequent surveillance because it costs more and yields a lower-quality-adjusted life expectancy than less frequent surveillance. Costs are higher and quality-adjusted life expectancy is lower because, on average, there are more endoscopies, endoscopic complications, and surgeries in this group (Fig. 4). Surveillance every 4 years provides the greatest gain in

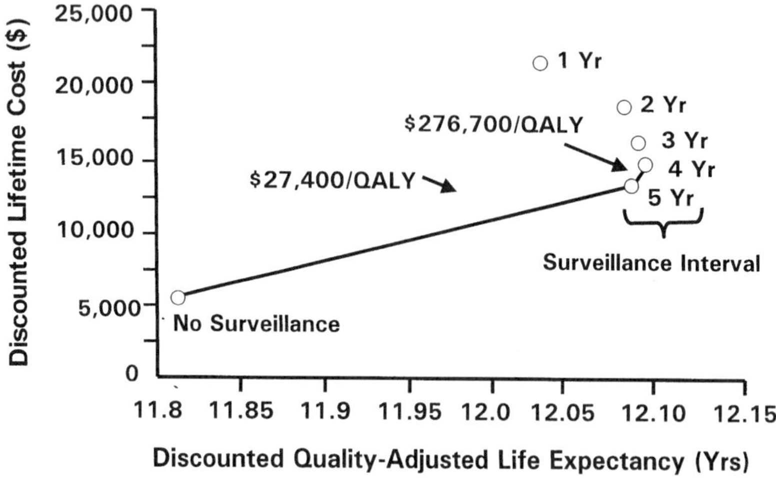

Figure 4 Cost-utility analysis. Average discounted lifetime cost per patient and discounted quality-adjusted life-years for each strategy. The incremental cost-utility ratio (addition cost/increase in quality-adjusted life expectancy) of moving to a more frequent surveillance strategy is shown above the line connecting the strategies. (See text for details.)

quality-adjusted life expectancy, and has an incremental cost-utility ratio of $276,700 per quality-adjusted life-year gained, similar to the incremental cost-effectiveness ratio for cervical cancer screening with pap smear every 3 years (250,000/LY gained) (50). Surveillance every 5 years also increases quality-adjusted life expectancy and, with an incremental cost-utility ratio of $27,400, is similar to breast cancer screening with mammography in women over the age of 50, which has an incremental cost-effectiveness ratio of $22,000 per life-year gained (51).

Because of the uncertainty surrounding the cancer risk in patients with Barrett's esophagus, we performed a sensitivity analysis in which we varied the parameter over the range of reported values [0.2% per year (46) to 2.1% per year (47)] (Fig. 5). The model suggests that for an incidence of cancer of less than 0.5% annually (1/200 patient-years) no surveillance is the preferred strategy. The risk of surveillance and esophagectomy outweighs any benefit in length and quality of life. If the cancer incidence is 1% or 1/99 patient-years, as reported in one summary (48), surveillance every 4 years would provide the greatest benefit. If, for any given population, the risk of cancer is less than 0.5% (1/200 patient years), however, no surveillance is the preferred strategy, because the risk of surveillance and esophagectomy outweighs any benefit in terms of length and

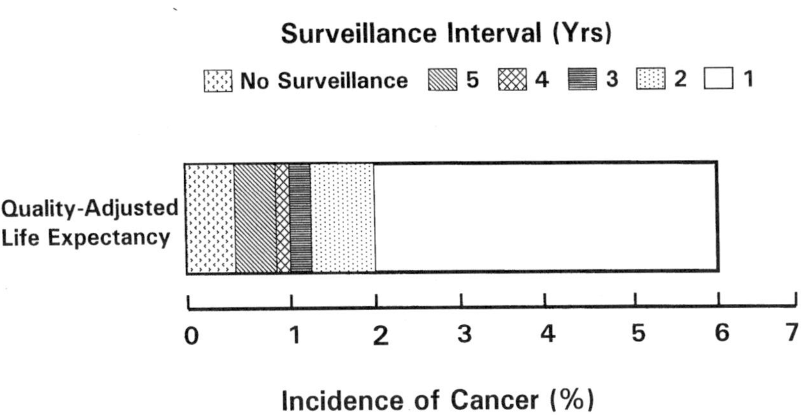

Figure 5 Effect of the cumulative incidence of cancer on surveillance with esophagectomy for high-grade dysplasia (considering both length and quality of life). As the incidence of cancer increases, more frequent surveillance provides a greater gain in quality-adjusted life expectancy.

quality of life. If the cancer risk approaches 2%, or the reported 1/52–1/56 patient-years (52–54), aggressive surveillance every 2 years is the preferred strategy. If, for any given population, the cancer incidence exceeds 2.0%, and is 1/48 patient-years as suggested by one report (47), surveillance every year is preferred (42).

Thus, as shown in Figure 5, the decision about surveillance depends on the cancer risk in those with Barrett's esophagus. To summarize, our model suggests that when costs are considered surveillance every 4 years will maximize quality-adjusted survival if the cancer incidence is 1%. For a cancer risk of 2%, surveillance every 2 years will maximize quality-adjusted survival. If the cancer incidence exceeds 2%, surveillance every year is optimal, but if the cancer risk falls below 0.5% annually, no surveillance is preferred.

SUMMARY

GERD is a diverse disorder ranging from occasional symptoms of heartburn without endoscopic evidence of mucosal damage, to esophagitis, strictures, and Barrett's esophagus. The epidemiology of the disorder is as diverse as its clinical spectrum, although most series report both an increased prevalence and incidence of symptoms in Western populations and an increased prevalence of symptoms among those with first-degree relatives with Barrett's esophagus and cancer (36).

While the prevalence appears to be approximately equal among men and women, GERD complications, including esophagitis and Barrett's esophagus, appear more common in men (26,55). Furthermore, increasing age, the presence of heartburn, and frequent heartburn (more than once each week) may be associated with Barrett's esophagus (38), although it has been difficult to identify a high-risk group for Barrett's esophagus among those with GERD. In the absence of well-defined risk factors for Barrett's esophagus, a decision analysis has been performed to examine the effectiveness and cost-effectiveness of screening for Barrett's esophagus among those with GERD. Screening and subsequent surveillance is both effective and cost-effective if the prevalence of Barrett's esophagus is 10% among those who undergo endoscopy for GERD symptoms and the incidence of cancer is at least 1/75 patient-years in patients with Barrett's esophagus (41). Because of the increased risk for the development of adenocarcinoma in patients with Barrett's esophagus, decision analysis has been employed to evaluate the most effective and cost-effective surveillance strategies for this group. Surveillance strategies are based on cancer risk. Surveillance is effective if the incidence of cancer is at least 0.5%. As the cancer risk increases, more frequent surveillance is warranted (42).

REFERENCES

1. Sonnenberg A. Epidemiologic und Spontanverlauf der Refluxkrankheit. In: Blum AL, Siewert JR, eds. Refluxtherapie. Gastroesophageale Refluxkrankheit: konservative und operative Therapie. Berlin: Springer-Verlag, 1981:85–106.
2. A Gallup Organization National Survey: Heartburn Across America. Princeton, NJ: Gallup Organization, 1988.
3. Nebel OT, Fornes MF, Castell DO. Symptomatic gastroesophageal reflux: incidence and precipitating factors. Am J Dig Dis 1976; 21(11):953–956.
4. Locke GR 3rd, Talley NJ, Fett SL, Zinsmeister AR, Melton LJ III. Prevalence and clinical spectrum of gastroesophageal reflux: a population-based study in Olmsted County, Minnesota. Gastroenterology 1997; 112(5):1448–1456.
5. Wienbeck M, Barnert J. Epidemiology of reflux disease and reflux esophagitis. Scand J Gastroenterol 1989; 24(suppl 156):7–13.
6. Brunnen PL, Karmody AM, Needham CD. Severe peptic oesophagitis. Gut 1969; 10:831–837.
7. Mold JW, Reed LE, Davis AR, Allen ML, Decktor DL, Robinson M. Prevalence of gastroesophageal reflux in elderly patients in a primary care setting. Am J Gastroenterol 1991; 86:965–970.
8. Heading RC. Epidemiology of oesophageal reflux disease. Scand J Gastroenterol 1989; 24(suppl 168):33–37.
9. Stoker DL, Williams JG, Leicester RG, Colin-Jones DG. Oesophagitis—a five year review. Gut 1988; 29:A1450.

10. Jones RH, Lydeard SE, Hobbs FDR, Kenkre JE, Williams EI, Jones SJ, Repper JA, Caldow JL, Dunwoodie WMB, Bottomley JM. Dyspepsia in England and Scotland. Gut 1990; 31:401–405.
11. Isolauri J, Laippala P. Prevalence of symptoms suggestive of gastroesophageal reflux disease in an adult population. Ann Intern Med 1995; 27(1):67–70.
12. Norrelund N, Pederson PA. Prevalence of gastro-oesophageal reflux-like dyspepsia. Int Congr Gastroenterol, 1988 (abstr). Rome, 4–10.
13. Kay L, Jörgensen T. Epidemiology of upper dyspepsia in a random population. Prevalence, incidence, natural history, and risk factors. Scand J Gastroenterol 1994; 29: 1–6.
14. Ruth M, Mansson I, Sandberg N. The prevalence of symptoms suggestive of esophageal disorders. Scand J Gastroenterol 1991; 26(1):73–81.
15. Ruth M, Mjörnheim A-C, Lundell L. Symptoms suggestive of esophageal disorders in a normal population—a 10 year follow up study. Gastroenterology 1997; 112(4): A41.
16. Chang CS, Poon SK, Lien HC, Chen GH. The incidence of reflux esophagitis among the Chinese. Am J Gastroenterol 1997; 92(4):668–671.
17. Nagler R. Heartburn of pregnancy. Am J Dig Dis 1962; 7:648–655.
18. Bassey OO. Pregnancy heartburn in Nigerians and Caucasians with theories about aetiology based on manometric recordings from the oesophagus and stomach. Br J Obstet Gynaecol 1977; 84:439–443.
19. Bainbridge ET, Temple JG, Nicholas SP, Newton JR, Boriah V. Symptomatic gastro-oesophageal reflux in pregnancy; a comparative study of white Europeans and Asians in Birmingham. Br J Clin Pract 1983; 37:53–57.
20. Atlay RD, Gillison EW, Horton AL. A fresh look at pregnancy heartburn. J Obstet Gynaecol Br Commonw 1973; 80:63–66.
21. Behar J, Biancani P, Sheahan DG. Evaluation of esophageal tests in the diagnosis of reflux esophagitis. Gastroenterology 1976; 71:9–15.
22. Johanson KE, Ask P, Boeryd B, Fransson SG, Tibbling L. Oesophagitis, signs of reflux and gastric acid secretion in patients with symptoms of gastro-oesophageal reflux disease. Scand J Gastroenterol 1986; 21:837–874.
23. Howard PJ, Heading RC. Epidemiology of gastro-esophageal reflux disease. World J Surg 1992; 16:288–293.
24. Blackstone MO. Endoscopic Interpretation—Normal and Pathologic Appearances of the Gastrointestinal Tract. New York: Raven Press, 1984:19.
25. Brown LF, Goldman H, Antonioli DA. Intraesophageal eosinophils in endoscopy biopsies of adults with reflux esophagitis. Am J Surg Pathol 1984; 8:899–905.
26. Richter JE. Severe reflux esophagitis. Gastro Endo Clin North Am 1994; 4(4):677–698.
27. Tabibian N, Morrison JM. Incidence of microscopic esophagitis in asymptomatic patients without endoscopic esophagitis. Am J Gastroenterol 1997; 92(9):A87.
28. Zhu H, Pace F, Sangaletti O, et al. Features of symptomatic gastroesophageal reflux in elderly patients. Scand J Gastroenterol 1993; 28:235–238.
29. Khuroo MS, Mahajan R, Zargar SA, Javid G, Munshi S. Prevalence of peptic ulcer in India: an endoscopic and epidemiological study in urban Kashmir. Gut 1989; 30: 930–934.

30. Hetzel DJ, Dent J, Reed WD, Narielvala FM, Mackinnon M, McCarthy JH, Mitchell B, Beveridge BR, Laurence BH, Gibson GG, Grant AK, Shearman DJC, Whitehead R, Buckle PJ. Healing and relapse of severe peptic esophagitis after treatment with omeprazole. Gastroenterology 1988; 95:903–912.
31. Palmer ED. The hiatus hernia-esophagitis-esophageal stricture complex: twenty-year prospective study. Am J Med 1968; 44:566–579.
32. Koelz HR, Birchler R, Bretholz A, Bron B, Capitaine Y, Delmore G, Fehr HF, Fumagalli J, Gehrig J, Gonvers JJ, Halter F, Hammer B, Kayasseh I, Kobler E, Miller G, Munst G, Pelloni S, Realini S, Schmid P, Voirol M, Blum AL. Healing and relapse of reflux esophagitis during treatment with ranitidine. Gastroenterology 1986; 91:1198–1205.
33. Dawson J, Barnard J, Delattre M. Cimetidine 800 mg at bed-time in reflux esophagitis: a multicenter trial. In: Siewert JR, Holscher AH, eds. Diseases of the Esophagus. Berlin: Springer-Verlag, 1987:1116–1119.
34. Wienbeck M, Barnert J. Epidemiology of reflux disease and reflux esophagitis. Gastroenterology 1989; 24(suppl 156):7–13.
35. Wesdorp ICE, Bartelsman JFWM, Den Hartog Jager FCA, Huibregtse K, Tytgat GN. Results of conservative treatment of benign esophageal strictures: a follow-up study of 100 patients. Gastroenterology 1982; 82:487.
36. Romero Y, Cameron AJ, Locke GR 3rd, Schaid DJ, Slezak JM, Branch CD, Melton LJ III. Familial aggregation of gastroesophageal reflux in patients with Barrett's esophagus and esophageal adenocarcinoma. Gastroenterology 1997; 113:1449–1456.
37. Eloubeidi M, Sloane R, Provenzale D. Racial variation in GERD complications among veterans. Gastroenterology 1998; 114(4):A11.
38. Eloubeidi M, Provenzale D. Can we predict Barrett's esophagus in GERD patients based on demographic characteristics and clinical symptoms? Am J Gastroenterol 1998; 1614:A22.
39. Spechler SJ. Epidemiology and natural history of gastroentero-oesophageal reflux disease. Digestion 1992; 51(suppl 1):24.
40. Skinner DB, Walther BC, Riddle RH, Schmidt H, Iascone C, DeMeester TR. Barrett's esophagus: Comparison of benign and malignant cases. Ann Surg 1983; 198: 554–566.
41. Heudebert G, Centor R, Marks R, Wilcox M. Endoscopy in chronic heartburn to screen for Barrett's esophagus (BE): can we really afford it? Am J Gastroenterol 1998; 93(9):A28.
42. Provenzale D, Kemp JA, Arora S, Wong JB. A guide for surveillance of patients with Barrett's esophagus. Am J Gastroenterol 1994; 89(5):670–680.
43. Pennock JL, Oyer PE, Reitz BA, Jamieson SW, Bieber CP, Wallwork J, Stinson EB, Shumway NE. Cardiac transplantation in perspective for the future survival, complications, rehabilitation, and cost. J Thorac Cardiovasc Surg 1982; 83(2):168–177.
44. Phillips RW, Wong RK. Barrett's esophagus. Natural history, incidence, etiology, and complications. Gastroenterol Clin North Am 1991; 20(4):791–816.
45. Cameron AJ. Epidemiology of columnar-lined esophagus and adenocarcinoma. In:

Spechler SJ, ed. Gastroenterology Clinics of North America: The Columnar-Lined Esophagus. Philadelphia: WB Saunders, 1997:487–494.
46. Cameron AJ, Ott BJ, Payne WS. The incidence of adenocarcinoma in columnar-lined (Barrett's) esophagus. N Engl J Med 1985; 313:857–859.
47. Skinner DB. The incidence of cancer in Barrett's esophagus varies according to series. In: Giuli R, McCallum RW, eds. Benign Lesions of the Esophagus and Cancer: Answer to 210 Questions. New York: Springer-Verlag, 1989:764–765.
48. Drewitz DJ, Sampliner RE, Garewal HS. The incidence of adenocarcinoma in Barrett's esophagus: a prospective study of 170 patients followed 4.8 years. Am J Gastroenterol 1997; 92(2):204–211.
49. United States Government. Federal Register: Rules and Regulations. Washington, DC: U.S. Government Printing Office, 1989, 169:36533–36546.
50. Eddy DM. Screening for cervical cancer. Ann Intern Med 1990; 113:214–226.
51. van der Maas PJ, de Koning HJ, van Ineveld BM, van Oortmarssen GJ, Habbema JD, Lubbe KT, Geerts AT, Collette HJ, Verbeek AL, Hendriks JH. The cost-effectiveness of breast cancer screening. Int J Cancer 1989; 43(6):1055–1060.
52. Robertson CS, Mayberry JF, Nicholson DA, James PD, Atkinson M. Value of endoscopic surveillance in the detection of neoplastic change in Barrett's oesophagus. Br J Surg 1988; 75(8):760–763.
53. Hameeteman W, Tytgat GN, Houthoff HJ, van den Tweel JG. Barrett's esophagus: development of dysplasia and adenocarcinoma. Gastroenterology 1989; 96:1249–1256.
54. Ovaska J, Miettinen M, Kivilaakso E. Adenocarcinoma arising in Barrett's esophagus. Dig Dis Sci 1989; 34:1336–1339.
55. Spechler SJ, Goyal RK. Barrett's esophagus. N Engl J Med 1986; 315:362–371.

4

Diagnostic Tests for Gastroesophageal Reflux Disease

W. Keith Fackler and Joel E. Richter
Cleveland Clinic Foundation, Cleveland, Ohio

A range of tests are available to the physician pursuing the diagnosis of gastroesophageal reflux disease (GERD). Many times, these studies are unnecessary as the history is sufficiently revealing to identify the presence of troubling reflux disease. However, this may not be the case and the clinician must decide which tests to choose to arrive at a diagnosis in a reliable, timely, and cost-effective manner. Furthermore, the various esophageal tests need to be selected carefully depending on the information desired. For example, identifying the presence of gastroesophageal reflux is different than proving that the patient's symptoms are due to the reflux episodes. Additionally, defining that acid reflux exists may not be enough. To tailor appropriate medical or surgical therapy requires knowing whether complications of GERD are present as well as the possible mechanisms by which abnormal GER occurs. A thorough and well-devised investigation strategy requires knowledge of testing procedures ranging from radiology and pathology to physiology and endoscopy. An informed background in these areas allows the clinician and investigator to address not only the presence of reflux and its correlation to patients' symptoms, but also the severity of esophageal injury and even the mechanism by which the damage is done. By using the available tests judiciously, one can increase the opportunity of making a correct diagnosis of GERD quickly while at the same time limiting the potential inconveniences or cost to the patient. This chapter will review the currently available diagnostic tests for GERD, categorizing them into the question each answers and addressing the advantages and disadvantages of each compared to other available tests.

CLINICAL HISTORY

The cardinal manifestation of GERD is the symptom of ''pyrosis,'' otherwise known as heartburn. Heartburn is typically described as a substernal burning sensation that migrates from the epigastrum upward into the chest and in the direction of the neck or throat. It is often associated with regurgitation, which is the sensation of a bitter or acid taste in the mouth due to the presence of gastric contents. These symptoms most often occur after meals and may be heightened by the ingestion of certain foods such as fats, alcohol, chocolate, or peppermint (1). Bending at the waist or lying supine may worsen the sensation, while antacids or other buffers such as water or bicarbonate tend to ease this discomfort. The frequency of symptoms may range anywhere from once or twice a year to multiple times a day.

Dysphagia is a symptom of GERD relating to the impaired movement of food through the esophagus. It tends to occur with solids but may slowly progress to affecting liquids. Dysphagia typically appears in patients who complain of heartburn for prolonged periods. When related to reflux disease, dysphagia often represents the formation of a peptic stricture. If symptoms are intermittent and nonprogressive, it may reflect the presence of a ring. Other less common etiologies for dysphagia in reflux patients include esophagitis, peristaltic dysfunction, and esophageal adenocarcinoma arising from a background of Barrett's esophagus. Odynophagia can signify the development of ulcerative esophagitis. However, it is a rare symptom arising from reflux alone and should prompt an investigation for other concurrent problems such as pill or infectious esophagitis, or bullous disease of the esophagus. Water brash, a salty or sour fluid in the mouth, results from excess salivary gland production in response to intraesophageal acid exposure. Other less common symptoms of GER include excessive belching, burping, chronic hiccups, nausea, and vomiting (2).

More recently, atypical symptoms of reflux disease are increasingly being recognized. Referred to as ''atypical'' or ''supraesophageal'' because of their extraesophageal location, these complaints are often initially evaluated by a cardiologist, pulmonologist, or otolaryngologist (3). Atypical symptoms include, but are not limited to, chest pain, asthma, hoarseness, chronic cough, sore throat, and globus sensation. Studies suggest these presentations of GERD may be very common. For example, in one study of 100 patients with chest pain, almost three-fourths (74%) had heartburn and two-thirds (67%) had acid regurgitation (4). Among asthmatics, studies suggest that 34–89% of patients may have some or all of their respiratory symptoms attributed to reflux disease. ENT patients are commonly diagnosed as having GERD. Of patients with unresponsive hoarseness, 55–79% are found to have abnormally high amounts of acid reflux. Reflux has been indicated as the precipitating factor in as many as 20% of individuals with chronic cough; other studies suggest reflux as the etiology for 25% and 50% of sore throat and globus complaints, respectively (1).

Unfortunately, not all patients with GERD are symptomatic. This is especially true in the elderly population (5). Possibly because of impaired acid production or attenuated perception of heartburn, elderly patients often are asymptomatic until they develop reflux complications such as dysphagia from a stricture, Barrett's esophagus, or adenocarcinoma. Furthermore, symptoms alone cannot distinguish between GERD patients with and without esophagitis. For example, studies show that only 50–65% of patients with esophagitis complain of frequent heartburn, while nearly 30% of patients with Barrett's esophagus are free of heartburn (1,6–8). Thus, the reflux of gastric material into the esophagus may lead to symptoms alone, esophagitis, both, or neither (Fig. 1) (9). This discordance

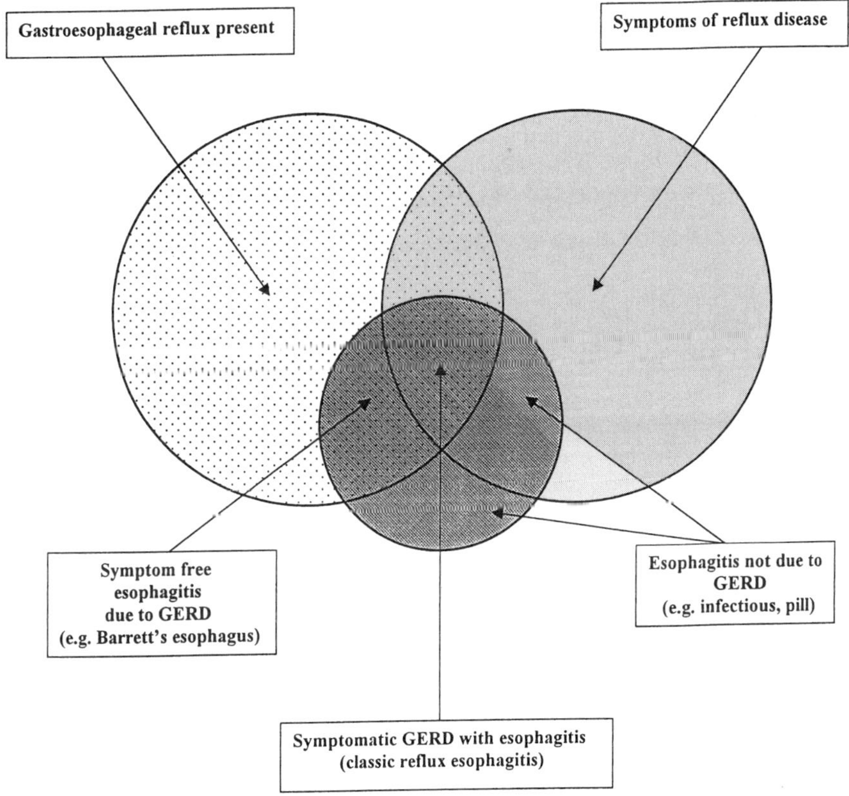

Figure 1 Relationship between GERD, symptoms, and esophagitis.

between symptom severity and mucosal damage makes the history alone an unreliable predictor of the presence of esophagitis or Barrett's esophagus, often necessitating further testing to address these issues.

In patients presenting with the classic symptoms of GERD, a presumptive diagnosis of reflux disease can be made without formal testing. This concept evolved from an important study by Klauser and associates, who evaluated over 300 patients with the chief complaint of heartburn and regurgitation (8). Heartburn was a major complaint in 68% of GERD patients confirmed by pH testing versus only 48% of patients without reflux ($p = 0.0009$). Complaints of acid regurgitation were present in 60% of patients with pathological pH tests compared to only 48% of normals ($p = 0.03$). Thus the sensitivity and specificity of heartburn for predicting GERD was 38% and 89%, respectively, whereas the sensitivity of acid regurgitation was only 6%, but its specificity 95%. Other symptoms were unable to predict GERD reliably (Table 1). Thus, the presence of heartburn and/or acid regurgitation allows the physician to confidently treat patients empirically for GERD without further testing; however, the absence of these complaints does not exclude the diagnosis (8). If patients describe less common complaints or symptoms suggestive of more aggressive reflux disease, such as dysphagia, odynophagia, or gastrointestinal bleeding, further investigation is warranted. Atypical complaints such as chest pain, hoarseness, sore throat, chronic cough, and asthma also deserve early exploration for esophageal reflux

Table 1 Prevalence of Symptoms in Patients with Normal and Abnormal Esophageal pH Monitoring

Symptom	Normal esophageal pH monitoring ($n = 138$) (%)	Abnormal esophageal pH monitoring ($n = 166$) (%)
Heartburn	48	68
Acid regurgitation	48	60
Odynophagia	8	10
Pharyngeal pain	15	19
Nausea	32	38
Belching	40	49
Epigastric pain	53	54
Retrosternal pain	61	57
Retrosternal burning	49	61

Derived from 304 patients with symptoms of reflux disease with an abnormal pH test consisting of esophageal pH < 4 for more than 8.2% of the upright or more than 3.0% of the supine recording time.
Percentage values are derived from the individual subgroups.

with diagnostic testing. Patients with symptoms refractory to treatment should undergo a thorough clinical investigation as well.

TESTS FOR REFLUX

Esophageal pH Monitoring

Continuous ambulatory pH monitoring of the distal esophagus is the most reliable test for determining quantitatively the amount of esophageal acid exposure (10). The test is performed by passing a thin pH probe transnasally to a level 5 cm above the manometrically defined lower esophageal sphincter (LES). Fluoroscopy, endoscopy, and the pH step-up technique have been tried to define eventual probe location, but are inaccurate compared to manometry (11,12). The pH probe is connected to a battery-powered data logger capable of recording pH values transmitted from the probe, typically at a rate of every 4–6 s. Patients can supplement this information by writing in a diary or pressing a manual event marker on the data logger indicating the appearance of symptoms, the timing of meals, periods of sleep, or other activities that may affect reflux. This method of recording data allows the physician to calculate a number of variables that attempt to identify the study as either normal (physiological) or abnormal (pathological). The current consensus is to measure the percentage of time that pH in the esophagus is <4 (13). If the esophageal acid exposure time is greater than an established threshold value, the test is considered positive. The most commonly cited normal value for percentage total time esophageal pH < 4 is 4.2% or less; however, different studies have defined various normals (Table 2). Other parameters that can be assessed with esophageal pH monitoring include: percentage of recumbent

Table 2 Esophageal Acid Exposure Values in Normal, Healthy Subjects

	% time esophageal pH < 4		
Ref.	Total	Upright	Supine
Kasapidas (n = 18)	1.9 ± 1	2.6 ± 1.6	0.5 ± 0.6
Matteoli (n = 20)	1.87 ± 1.56	2.78 ± 2.42	0.66 ± 0.81
Vitale (n = 22)	—	2.2 ± 0.4	1.0 ± 0.5
Masclee (n = 27)	1.7 (0.1–9.0)	2.6 (0.1–13.6)	0.0 (0.0–9.4)
Schindlbeck (n = 42)	2.6 (0–45.2)	3.8 (0–53.3)	0.5 (0–26.5)
Johnsson (n = 50)	3.4	4.6	3.2
DeMeester (n = 50)	4.5 ± 1.4	8.4 ± 2.3	3.5 ± 1.0
Richter (n = 110)	5.48	8.20	2.98

n = Number of subjects in study.

time pH < 4, percentage of time upright pH < 4, total number of reflux episodes, duration of longest reflux episode, and number of episodes greater than 5 min (14,15).

Prolonged esophageal pH monitoring for 16–24 h offers many advantages over other forms of reflux testing. Compared to scintigraphy and the older standard acid reflux test, pH monitoring is truly ambulatory. The patient can leave the testing facility to go home and conduct normal daily activities. Also, there is no limitation on diet and the patient is encouraged to eat regular meals. This is more comfortable for the patient and more likely to evoke GER than earlier approaches where diet was controlled (i.e., no food with pH < 4) and activities were limited (10). The probes are thin and well tolerated. Compared to radiographic testing, there is no radiation exposure. Testing allows different characteristics of reflux to be analyzed. The investigator can discern positional variations in reflux, upright versus supine events, meal- and sleep-related episodes, and even perform symptom correlation with reflux events (Fig. 2).

One important problem with continuous pH monitoring is that there exists no absolute threshold value that reliably identifies the presence of GERD. Validation studies comparing the presence of endoscopic esophagitis with pH measurements reveal a general difference between the pH exposures of patients with and without esophagitis (16–21). Reported sensitivities range from 77% to 100% with specificities from 85% to 100%. In the clinical setting, however, patients with endoscopic evidence of reflux esophagitis rarely need pH testing. Instead, patients with suspected reflux and no endoscopic evidence of esophagitis (i.e., nonerosive refluxers) should benefit most from ambulatory pH monitoring. However, the data are much less conclusive in this group. Studies reveal considerable overlap in esophageal acid exposure times between controls and nonerosive refluxers, thereby making interpretation of individual readings difficult (Table 3). Other drawbacks include possible equipment failure, the pH probe missing a reflux event because it is buried in a mucosal fold, and false-negative studies due to dietary or activity limitations resulting from irritation from the probe. Nevertheless, ambulatory 24-h pH monitoring is the best test available for diagnosing GERD.

The clinical indications for ambulatory pH monitoring are summarized in Table 4. Testing is valuable in the setting of antireflux surgery. Prior to fundoplication, pH testing is performed when endoscopy fails to identify reflux esophagitis (22). In this setting, pH monitoring can document the presence of GERD before committing to surgical intervention. If esophagitis is present, esophageal pH testing is not necessary because the disease has already been proven. When pH monitoring is performed prior to antireflux surgery, drugs (especially proton pump inhibitors, PPIs) are discontinued 1 week prior to esophageal testing to allow a washout period for the medications. Ambulatory pH testing also has a role after antireflux surgery. If the patient persists with symptoms or has evidence

Physiologic Reflux Pattern

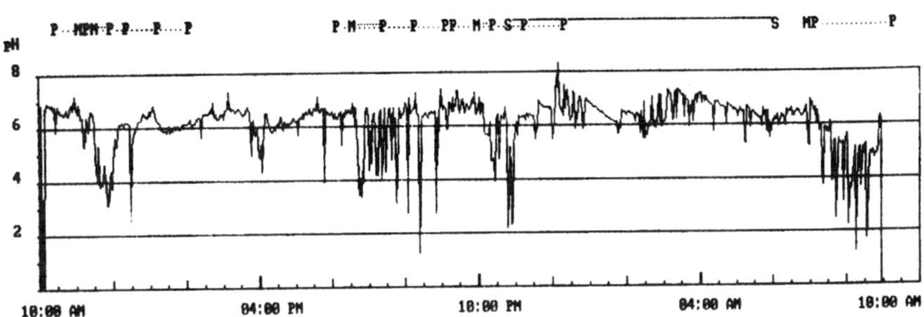

Upright Reflux Pattern

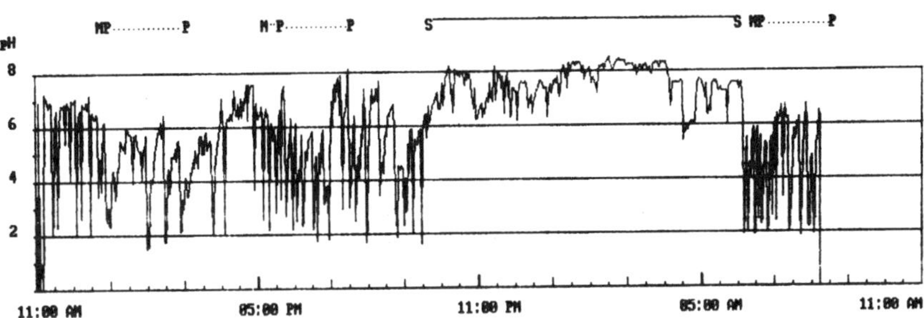

Combined Reflux Pattern

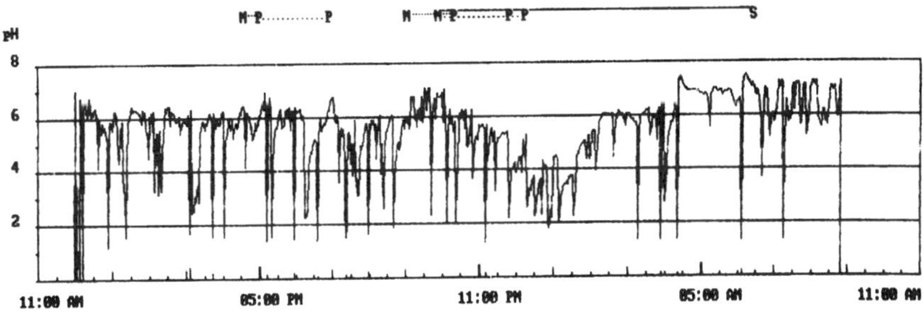

Figure 2 Common patterns of 24-h esophageal pH monitoring.

Table 3 Esophageal Acid Exposure Values in Controls vs. EGD-Negative Patients with GERD

Ref.	Controls % time esophageal pH < 4 (upper limit of normal)	EGD-negative patients % time esophageal pH < 4 (mean)
Kasapidas	3.9	11.6 ± 4.8
Matteoli	5.0	1.9 ± 1.6
Vitale	7.2	5.8 ± 1.1
Masclee	4	6.4 (0.3–18.7)
Schindlbeck	7.0	10.2 (1.3–78.7)

Means are provided with either ranges (in parentheses) or standard deviations (±).

of continued esophagitis on endoscopy, pH monitoring can confirm that the changes are indeed due to recurrent esophageal acid exposure (15).

Esophageal pH monitoring is indicated for evaluating patients who have symptoms suggestive of reflux disease that are resistant to treatment and in whom endoscopy is negative or equivocal (23). Two populations are defined by testing: those with and without continued esophageal acid exposure. The group with persistent acid reflux represents treatment nonresponders, and therapy should be advanced by either doubling the dose of PPIs or possibly adding H_2 blockers. The cohort of patients with normal reflux values denotes those with problems other

Table 4 Guidelines for the Clinical Use of Esophageal pH Monitoring

Definite indications
- To document abnormal esophageal acid exposure in an endoscopy-negative patient being considered for antireflux surgery
- To evaluate patients after antireflux surgery who are suspected by symptoms of persistent esophagitis to still have ongoing abnormal reflux
- To evaluate patients with either normal or equivocal endoscopic findings and reflux symptoms that are refractory to PPIs

Possible indications
- To evaluate patients for suspected atypical or extraesophageal presentations of GERD

Not indicated
- To detect or verify reflux esophagitis, which is best done by endoscopy with biopsies

than acid reflux such as bile reflux, aerophagia, dyspepsia, or psychological problems.

Ambulatory pH testing also helps further define the patients with extraesophageal manifestations of GERD. In this group, pH testing can be done initially to confirm the coexistence of GERD; however, this does not guarantee the causality of symptoms. Therefore, an alternative approach is to treat the patient first aggressively with PPIs if acid reflux is suspected, reserving pH testing only for those patients not responding after 4–8 weeks of therapy (15).

Technetium 99 Scintiscanning

The technique of ingesting a radionuclide colloid to quantitate gastroesophageal reflux is known as gastroesophageal scintigraphy. It is performed by having a supine patient ingest a set volume of water containing a radionuclide-labeled colloid, usually ^{99m}technetium, that is routinely used in liver-spleen scans. Subsequently, serial images of the chest are obtained with a gamma camera to observe both the esophagus and stomach. These baseline measurements are followed by provocative maneuvers to induce reflux, such as Valsalva or application of an abdominal binder. The presence of reflux is determined by gross visual review of the serial images and by assessing the amount of radioisotope in the stomach compared to that in the esophagus. Analysis is generally done by computer measurements (24).

Advantages of this test are that it is noninvasive and exposes the patient to minimal amounts of radiation. It does not require prolonged monitoring and can be conducted quickly. Because it measures mechanical function and volume of the refluxate, it is an "acid independent" test. Indeed, Shay and associates demonstrated that scintigraphy identified 61% of postprandial reflux events as opposed to 16% for pH monitoring (25). The greater sensitivity of scintigraphy was primarily due to its ability to identify reflux occurring immediately after a meal when the food buffers the gastric acid, raising the pH to a level greater than 4, or when the pH was already less than 4 in the esophagus. During these periods, pH monitoring cannot detect most reflux events because the intraesophageal pH does not change significantly.

Disadvantages to scintigraphy are primarily related to its poor sensitivity and specificity for detecting GERD. The reported sensitivity of scintigraphy in adults ranges widely from 14% to 90% with an average of 65%. Specificity is only slightly better, ranging from 60% to 90% (26–29). Additionally, this test suffers from its relatively short monitoring period and the fact that reflux by nature occurs intermittently and frequently after meals, even in healthy subjects. Use of the abdominal binder increases the sensitivity of scintigraphy but does so at the expense of specificity, thereby decreasing the positive predictive value of the test (30). Specificity is also diminished when false-positive results are due to double swallows and hiatal hernias. Finally, the cost of scintigraphy can be a drawback, approaching the cost of endoscopy in some centers. In clinical practice, pH monitoring has replaced esophageal scintigraphy, except in the situation where nonacid reflux is suspected.

Barium Esophagram

The barium esophagram is the cheapest and most readily available test for assessing gastroesophageal reflux. Technique varies according to the question being asked and the suspected underlying pathology, yet all phases of testing involve the patient ingesting a quantity of barium contrast followed by radiographic monitoring. The double-contrast method displays the esophagus by having the upright patient swallow high-density barium as well as a gas-forming agent. Initially, double-contrast views of the esophagus are obtained that detail the esophageal mucosa, attempting to highlight mucosal lesions. Next, double-contrast views of the gastric cardia are gathered to check for possible causes of dysphagia. Next, the patient is placed in the prone position and esophageal motility assessed fluoroscopically by observing multiple swallows of barium separated by 20 s to allow for esophageal recovery. In the same position, single-contrast views of the esophagus are also obtained while the patient quickly ingests a thin barium solution. This act maximally distends the esophagus and esophagogastric junction revealing small strictures, rings, and hiatal hernias. Finally, various maneuvers are performed to provoke reflux, including coughing, rolling side to side, leg lifting, and the water-siphon test (2).

Barium studies identify gastroesophageal reflux when contrast moves in a retrograde fashion from the stomach into the esophagus. If this occurs repeatedly or to a significant degree well into the mid- or proximal esophagus, the test is positive. ''Free reflux'' occurs when spontaneous retrograde movement of barium is present. Sensitivities reported in the literature range from 20% to 73% with an average of 39% for detecting free reflux. ''Stress reflux'' occurs if a provocative maneuver, such as the water-siphon test, is used to induce these episodes (30).

Major advantages to barium testing are its availability, noninvasive nature, and relatively inexpensive cost. With fluoroscopy, the extent and frequency of reflux can be addressed as well as the effectiveness of esophageal clearance. Some have suggested that provocative maneuvers decrease the specificity of identifying GER. However, we found that provocative tests increased the sensitivity of the barium esophagram to 70% compared to pH testing with a concomitant specificity of 74%, yielding a positive predictive value of 80% (31). Perhaps the greatest advantage of barium testing, though, is its ability to demonstrate structural narrowing of the esophagus. Subtle findings such as Schatzki's rings, webs, or small peptic strictures are often seen only with an esophagram, being missed

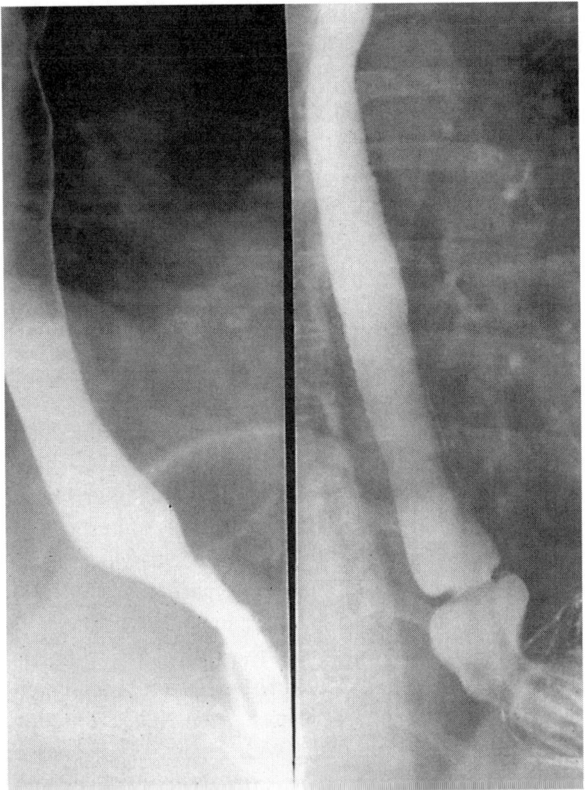

Figure 3 (Left) Barium esophagram suggesting a subtle stricture. (Right) Same patient with ring well defined with hiatal hernia after Valsalva maneuver.

by endoscopy, which may not adequately distend the esophagus (Fig. 3). When a 13-mm radioopaque pill or marshmallow is consumed along with the barium liquid, this method is the most sensitive test for detecting esophageal narrowing, with values reported between 95% and 100%. Hiatal hernias also are best diagnosed with the barium esophagram (30).

Disadvantages of the barium esophagram rest on the test's poor ability to demonstrate fine mucosal detail. While sensitivities of 79–93% have been reported for detecting moderate esophagitis and 95–100% for severe esophagitis, mild esophagitis with lesser mucosal alterations is frequently missed. In patients with mild reflux disease, radiographic detection varies from 0% to 53%, depending on the definition used in grading the esophagitis endoscopically (30). Barium testing also falls short when addressing the presence of Barrett's esophagus. Although its presence is suggested by seeing an area of focal esophagitis, ulcer, or stricture separated by normal mucosa from a hiatal hernia, biopsies are necessary to make the diagnosis of Barrett's esophagus.

The barium esophagram is primarily used in the evaluation of the GERD patient complaining of dysphagia. It should be the first diagnostic study in the patient with new-onset dysphagia because of its ability to define subtle strictures and rings as well as assess motility. On the other hand, endoscopy is the diagnostic test of choice in the patient with recurrent dysphagia known to have a stricture or when the suspicion of cancer is high.

Bilirubin (Bile) Monitoring

Recently, the concept that symptoms and/or complications of GERD may be related to reflux of duodenal contents has received attention. Known as duodenogastroesophageal reflux (DGR), duodenal constituents such as trypsin, lysolecithin, and bile acids are postulated to initiate esophageal mucosal injury when mixed with the gastric contents, pepsin, and hydrochloric acid. Animal studies and human investigations have demonstrated that esophagitis occurs when conjugated bile acids persist in the esophagus within an acidic environment (32–34). Studies identifying mucosal damage from bile salts or trypsin in an alkaline environment are less conclusive and more controversial (35–37).

One of the major problems in studying DGR is the lack of a tool accurately identifying its presence. Methods attempted in the past, including endoscopy, scintigraphy, aspiration studies, and pH monitoring with a pH > 7 defined as "alkaline" reflux, either yielded marginal results or were difficult to perform. Initially, pH was thought to be an ideal marker of DGR because duodenal contents usually have a pH greater than or equal to 7. To be confident of this assumption, however, other possible causes of pH > 7 have to be excluded, such as equipment error, dietary considerations, dental infections raising salivary pH, pooling of saliva in the esophagus, and increased salivation secondary to irritation from the pH probe or acid reflux (38). Recent studies suggest these latter factors, especially increased salivation, are the most common causes of an esophageal pH > 7 (39,40).

The most sensitive method for detecting DGR is bilirubin monitoring. This technique utilizes the spectrophotometric property of bilirubin, the most common pigment in bile (Fig. 4). Using a fiberoptic probe, a light source is introduced into the esophagus with a data collection system worn on a waist belt, similar to esophageal pH monitoring. A spectrophotometer measures the absorption of wavelengths at 450 nm (bilirubin) and 490 nm or 565 nm (reference) every 8 s. An integrated microcomputer calculates the differences of the absorbances, which is directly proportional to the bilirubin concentration in the sample. The presence of bilirubin as a surrogate marker of bile suggests the presence of DGR. Normal

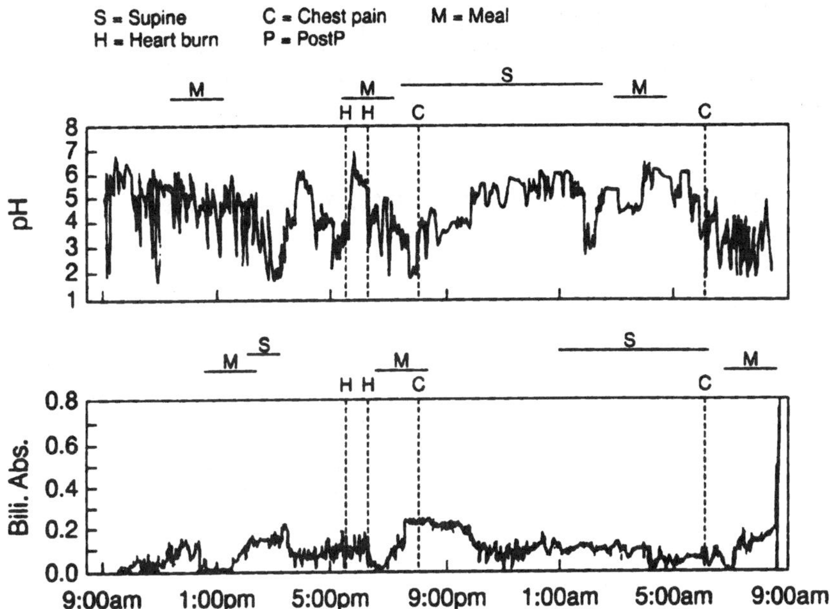

Tracings representing simultaneous 24-hour pH and bilirubin monitoring in a patient with Barrett's esophagus.

Figure 4 Tracings representing simultaneous 24-h pH and bilirubin monitoring in patient with Barrett's esophagus. Note rise in bilirubin absorption associated with fall in pH < 4 confirming that acid and bilirubin (bile) reflux occur simultaneously.

values have been established for total, upright, and supine exposure times to bilirubin. Abnormal DGR exists if bilirubin absorbance is detected ≥1.8% of the total monitoring time (32).

Advantages of bilirubin monitoring for defining DGR are its ambulatory nature, ease of performance, and relative independence of pH. Disadvantages also exist. Bilirubin undergoes a transformation from a monomer to dimer at pH < 3.5, and the absorption band of the dimeric form shifts to 400 nm. Therefore, at low pH, the degree of DGR may be underestimated. Also, other substances may have an absorption characteristic similar to bilirubin; hence patients must remain on a standardized diet to ensure there is not an overestimation of DGR. Even with these limitations, bilirubin monitoring has yielded good correlation with aspiration studies confirming DGR with *r*-values of 0.71 and 0.82 (38,41,42).

Bilirubin monitoring has limited clinical utility and is primarily a research tool. We use it combined with pH monitoring in evaluating patients with reflux-like symptoms who are post gastric surgery or gastrectomy where alkaline reflux is problematic. We have not found it useful in patients with intact stomachs as bilirubin reflux always parallels acid reflux (43).

TESTS FOR SYMPTOM CORRELATION WITH REFLUX

Esophageal pH Monitoring

One of the values of 24-h esophageal pH monitoring is its ability to associate symptoms with acid reflux into the esophagus. During testing, the patient is encouraged to push an event marker on the data logger when symptoms are noted as well as recording them in a diary. When the study is complete, the data are downloaded and analyzed permitting an evaluation of the relationship between reflux episodes and symptoms. The key to successful testing is ensuring that the patient has a typical day, thereby providing the best opportunity to evoke a number of symptom episodes.

Reflux episodes are not always associated with symptoms. In patients with well-established GERD, from either a positive endoscopy or pH study, the symptom of heartburn correlates with a pH < 4 80–90% of the time. Overall, however, only 10–20% of reflux episodes are associated with the symptom of heartburn or acid regurgitation (44). The relationship of symptoms to acid reflux is also important in patients with atypical presentations of reflux disease. For example, in a study evaluating the etiology of chest pain, 50 of 100 patients with chest pain and normal coronary arteries experienced the onset of pain with the occurrence of esophageal acid reflux (45). Additionally, an investigation in 48 patients examining the temporal relationship between asthma and esophageal reflux identified that 45% of wheezing episodes happened either just before, during, or just after a reflux event in 48 patients (46).

Since it is rare for all reflux episodes to produce symptoms, different statistical analyses have evolved attempting to define a significant association between these two variables (Table 5). Initially the "symptom index" was devised. This is defined as the percentage of symptom episodes associated with acid reflux divided by the total symptom episodes (47). This was modified to produce the "symptom sensitivity index," or the percentage of reflux-associated symptom episodes per total number of reflux episodes (48). Most recently, the "symptom-association probability" (SAP) was developed. This scheme evaluates the four possible associations between reflux events and symptoms: reflux with symptoms, reflux without symptoms, symptoms without reflux, and no reflux without symptoms (49). The advantage of the SAP is that all the relevant data are taken into account. By breaking the 24-h study period into 720 2-min blocks, one can establish a 2×2 contingency table comparing symptoms to reflux events. A *p*-

Table 5 Endoscopic Grading Systems for Degrees of Esophagitis

	Savary-Miller classification	Hetzel classification
Grade 0	NA	Normal-appearing mucosa
Grade I	Single, erosive or exudative lesion, oval or linear, taking only one longitudinal fold	Mucosal edema, hyperemia, and/or friability of mucosa
Grade II	Noncircular multiple erosions or exudative lesions taking more than one longitudinal fold with or without confluence	Superficial erosions involving <10% of mucosal surface of last 5 cm of esophageal squamous mucosa
Grade III	Circular erosive or exudative lesion	Superficial erosions/ulcerations involving 10–50% of distal esophagus
Grade IV	Chronic lesions: ulcers, strictures, or short esophagus, isolated or associated with lesions grade I–III	Deep peptic ulceration anywhere in the esophagus or confluent erosion of >50% of the distal esophageal squamous mucosa
Grade V	Barrett's epithelium isolated or associated with lesions grade I–III	NA

	Los Angeles classification
Grade A	One or more mucosal breaks confined to the folds, each no longer than 5 mm
Grade B	At least one mucosal break more than 5 mm long confined to the mucosal folds but not continuous between the tops of the mucosal folds
Grade C	At least one mucosal break continuous between the tops of two or more mucosal folds but not circumferential
Grade D	Circumferential mucosal break

value can be computed, and if it is less than 0.05, then the probability that the symptom-reflux association is not caused by chance is at least 95%.

Another important factor in determining symptom correlation is the definition of the time interval around a pain episode where a reflux episode is deemed causative. Different studies have used time windows ranging from 10 min before or after pain to 2–5 min before pain ensues (50). Lam et al. investigated a group of patients with noncardiac chest pain using times up to 6 min before and 6 min after a pain episode to define a time window (51). With the use of mathematical modeling, they concluded that the time window ranging from 2 min before a pain episode until the onset of the symptom was optimal.

Unfortunately, despite the eloquence of these analyses, no studies to date have defined the accuracy of any of the symptom scores in predicting response to therapy. Therefore, although pH testing and symptom correlation defines an association between these two processes, only treatment trials address the true definition of a causal relationship.

Bilirubin Monitoring

The same techniques utilized by patients undergoing 24-h pH testing can be used by patients being monitored for the presence of DGR. Again, an event recorder identifies the appearance of symptoms with a mark on the data strip while recording bilirubin absorbance and pH in the esophagus. After testing is complete, an assessment of DGR events and symptoms can be conducted.

Using this technique, Vaezi and Richter studied 32 patients with partial gastrectomies and upper gastrointestinal (GI) complaints, assessing the role of acid and DGR in symptom production (43). A total of 133 symptoms were reported during the 24-h monitoring periods. Simultaneous reflux of both DGR and acid was recorded in 92% of heartburn episodes, 70% of abdominal pain events, and 89% of regurgitation symptoms. The vast minority of symptoms were associated with DGR only: 6% of heartburn episodes, 30% of abdominal pain events, and 11% of regurgitation symptoms. Most interestingly, esophagitis occurred only in the patients with both abnormal amounts of DGR and acid and not in the DGR-alone group. This suggests that symptoms may be caused by DGR alone, but acid is required for the development of mucosal injury.

Bernstein Test

The Bernstein test helps address whether a patient's symptoms are due to acid in the esophagus (52). With the patient seated or supine, normal saline is infused through a nasogastric tube located in the middle third of the esophagus (Fig. 5). This is followed by the introduction of 0.1 N HCl at the rate of 6–8 mL/min. If typical symptoms arise (i.e., heartburn or chest pain) in the following 15–30 min, the acid drip is halted and saline again infused. If this eases or relieves the symptoms, the patient is exposed to acid again and the sequence repeated. A positive test is defined as symptom production with acid, which is then relieved with saline. To accurately reflect an esophageal origin of pain, the sensation of chest discomfort provoked by testing must be similar to the spontaneous pain episodes. If not, the test is considered indeterminate.

Multiple studies have evaluated the value of the Bernstein acid perfusion test. When the production of heartburn is the endpoint for GERD, sensitivities of 42–100% have been published with specificities ranging from 50% to 100% (2). If studying atypical chest pain and GERD, the sensitivity of the Bernstein test is poor, only 7–36%, yet the specificity is better, ranging from 83% to 94% (53–55). Thus, a positive test reliably attributes a patient's complaint of chest

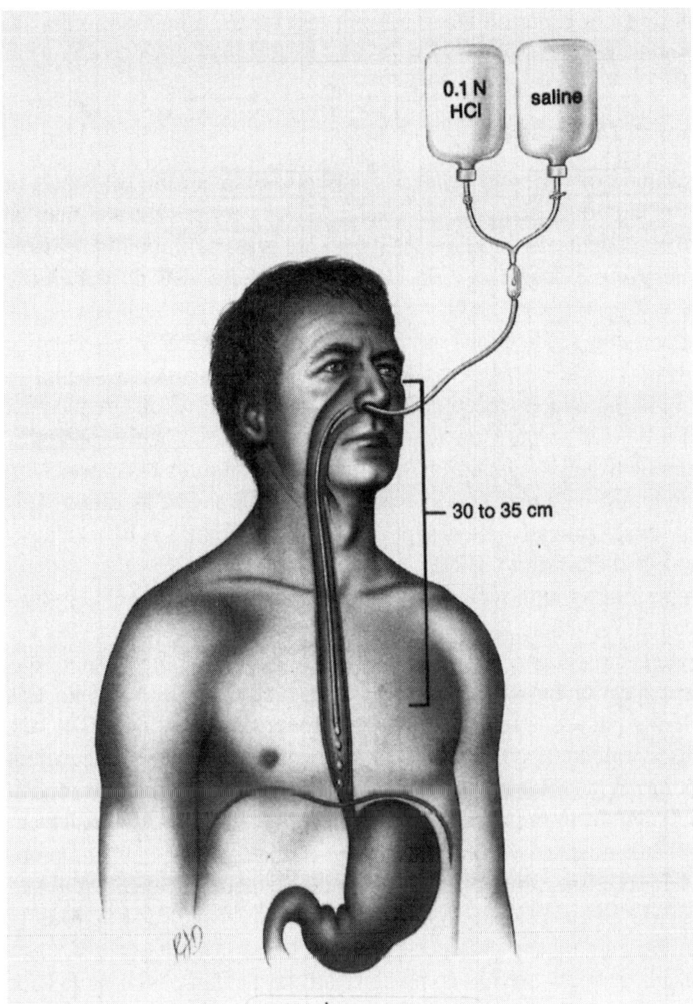

Figure 5 Acid perfusion (Bernstein) test.

pain to esophageal acid exposure, whereas a negative study has little clinical importance.

These studies highlight the limitations of the Bernstein test. Furthermore, the Bernstein test is found lacking when compared to 24-h esophageal pH monitoring. The latter test is not dependent on exogenous acid and can monitor multiple episodes of pain and relate them to position, meals, and activity. Therefore,

24-h pH monitoring has replaced the Bernstein test for ascribing symptoms to acid reflux episodes.

Empirical Trial of Medication

Although a multitude of different tests exist to help establish the diagnosis of GERD, no tool is yet 100% sensitive or specific. Tests vary in cost and may be poorly tolerated by patients. In addition, most tests are at least minimally invasive and therefore carry some degree of risk. Furthermore, these tests do not ensure that acid reflux is causing the patient's symptoms. Because of these issues, the use of acid-suppressing medications as a tool to diagnose GERD has become more accepted (56,57). The decision to take this approach was aided by the introduction of the PPIs. Unlike H_2-receptor antagonists, PPIs drastically reduce the amount of acid produced in the stomach as well as the time to heal esophagitis (58–61). Symptoms usually respond in 7–14 days. If symptoms disappear with therapy and then return with medication cessation, GERD may be assumed. This approach makes sense clinically and is supported by the literature as being a cost-effective method of diagnosing GERD.

A patient presenting with typical complaints of heartburn and acid regurgitation is an excellent candidate for empirical therapy with a PPI (1,62). After the history is obtained, the patient is given a high dose of either omeprazole (40–80 mg orally per day) or lansoprazole (60–90 mg orally per day) for not less than 14 days. If the patient reports symptom improvement of at least 50%, the medication is discontinued. If symptoms recur within the next 2 weeks, the patient is diagnosed as having GERD and therapy is reinstituted. If the patient reports minimal or no symptom improvement, the medication can be increased for another 2 weeks. If still no improvement, the patient is diagnosed as having a problem other than GERD. Using this approach, Schindlbeck and colleagues observed that an empirical trial of omeprazole 40 mg orally twice daily showed a sensitivity above 83% for determining the presence of GERD (63).

Patients with atypical GERD complaints are particularly well suited for empirical therapy. Fass and colleagues demonstrated the benefits of this treatment approach, which they called the ''omeprazole test,'' in a cohort of patients with noncardiac chest pain (64). Participants were initially evaluated by endoscopy and 24-h esophageal pH monitoring. Treatment was initiated with omeprazole 40 mg po orally every morning and 20 mg orally every evening or placebo for 7 days. The study incorporated a washout period and patient crossover. Empirical therapy was found to have a sensitivity of 78% and specificity of 86% in detecting GERD, when compared to traditional testing.

An empirical trial of PPI for diagnosing GERD has many advantages. The test is office based, easily performed, relatively inexpensive, available to all physicians in the community, and avoids many needless procedures. Fass and colleagues highlighted the economic benefits of empirical testing (64). They showed a savings of greater than $570 per average patient due to a 59% reduction in the number of diagnostic tests performed when evaluating patients with noncardiac chest pain. Similarly, a cost analysis performed on patients with chronic cough by Ours and colleagues demonstrated the cost benefits of empirical testing over manometry and pH testing, showing savings of almost $1000 per patient (65).

Disadvantages are few but include false-positive results secondary to a placebo effect from the medication. Furthermore, no assessment is made of the esophageal mucosa, nor is any attempt made to quantitate the amount of reflux. These issues aside, empirical therapy with the acid-suppressing PPIs has become the preferred method of initially diagnosing and managing patients suspected of having both typical and atypical presentations of GERD.

Who does not fit the criteria for an empirical therapy trial? Any patient with ''alarm'' symptoms suggesting progressive or complicated disease needs more conclusive testing. Complaints of dysphagia, odynophagia, GI bleeding, or long-standing symptoms of at least 5 years warrant initial testing with endoscopy to assess the esophageal mucosa for strictures, cancers, and Barrett's esophagus as well as exclude other gastroduodenal pathology (66).

TESTS FOR TYPE/SEVERITY OF ESOPHAGEAL INJURY

Endoscopy

When the diagnosis of GERD is suspected, endoscopy is usually the first test pursued to identify the presence of esophagitis and exclude other etiologies for the patient's complaints (67). The advancements in the optical capabilities of endoscopy provide the physician an excellent opportunity to visualize directly the esophageal mucosa and assess tissue injury. A number of endoscopic criteria have evolved helping to diagnose reflux esophagitis; unfortunately, the interpretation of some of these signs is subject to interobserver and even intraobserver variability (68–70). This problem is less a factor when dealing with mucosal erosions and ulcerations, but is more apparent when attempting to diagnose esophagitis when minimal inflammation exists. Furthermore, only 40–60% of patients with abnormal esophageal reflux by pH testing have endoscopic evidence of esophagitis. Thus the sensitivity of endoscopy for GERD is 60–70% at best, but it has excellent specificity at 90–95% (70,71).

Mucosal abnormalities associated with GERD include erythema, edema, friability, and granularity. Complications of reflux recognized by endoscopy include erosions, ulcers, exudate, stricture, and Barrett's esophagus. The earliest-encountered endoscopic abnormalities of GERD include edema and erythema. Edema is noted when there is loss of the fine vascular pattern just above the squamocolumnar junction. Erythema (i.e., redness) reflects a further degree of inflammation. Neither of these findings is specific for GERD as some degree of edema can be seen in up to 60% of healthy subjects and both are very dependent upon the quality of endoscopic visual images (70). More reliable are the findings of friability, granularity, and red streaks. Friability, or the easy bleeding that occurs with gentle pressure on the mucosa, results from the development of enlarged capillaries near the mucosal surface in response to acid. Red streaks may extend upward from the esophagogastric (EG) junction along the ridges of esophageal folds. In studies evaluating these stigmata, nearly all patients were found to have GERD (72). When acid injury progresses, erosions develop (Fig. 6). These are characterized by shallow thinning of the mucosa associated with a white or yellow exudate surrounded by erythema. They are most commonly located just above the EG junction and may be either single lesions or coalesced regions. Typically, they occur along the tops of mucosal folds, areas most prone to acid exposure (73). Erosions may also be caused by NSAID use, heavy smoking, and infectious esophagitis (e.g., *Candida*, herpes); therefore, they are not 100% specific for the diagnosis of GERD (72). Ulcers reflect more severe damage to the esophagus. These have depth into the mucosa, tend to have either a white or yellow discolored base, and may be seen either isolated along a fold or surrounding the EG junction (Fig. 7).

Beyond these mucosal findings, other complications of acid reflux disease often are noted at endoscopy including rings, strictures, or Barrett's mucosa. The Schatzki's ring is a thin, pearly white tissue structure located at the squamoco-

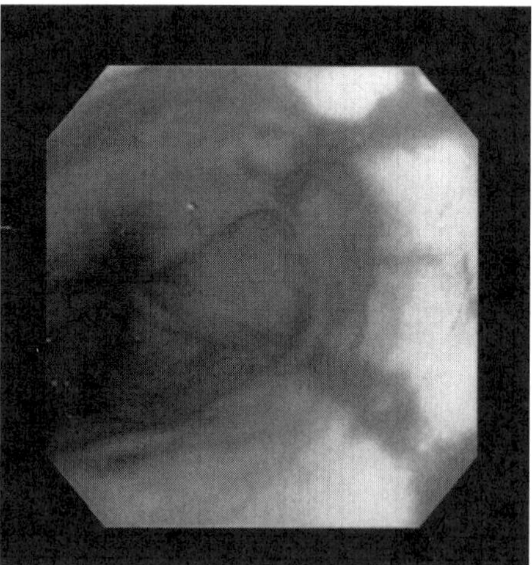

Figure 6 Two linear erosions extending proximally from squamocolumnar junction at the proximal border of a hiatal hernia.

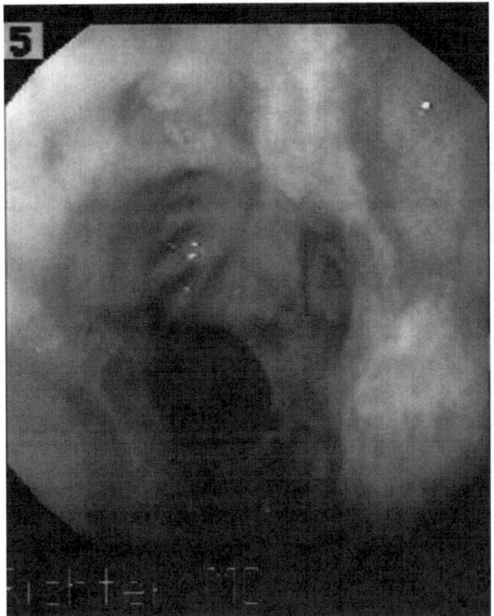

Figure 7 Circumferential ulcer with stricture of esophagus.

lumnar junction. Its etiology is controversial but recent debate suggests it is a complication of GERD for several reasons: (1) the mucosa above the ring resembles the mucosa of chronic reflux, devoid of submucosal vessels; (2) the ring may be associated with other evidence of endoscopic esophagitis; and (3) some rings progress to strictures. Peptic strictures cause narrowing of the distal esophagus because of chronic acid-induced inflammation, which eventually stimulates collagen formation and the creation of a shortened, thick, noncompliant region of scarring. Like rings, peptic strictures tend to occur distally at the EG junction. They are typically short and less than 1 cm in length. If they are longer, other etiologies such as Zollinger-Ellison syndrome, pill esophagitis, or mechanical trauma from a long-term indwelling nasogastric tube should be sought (70). Further evidence of esophagitis is often seen proximal to the stricture. Barrett's esophagus, which appears as a salmon- or pink-colored mucosa in the tubular esophagus, is another complication of GERD (Fig. 8). Although the diagnosis can be suggested at endoscopy, mucosal biopsies are always necessary to confirm the presence of specialized intestinal metaplasia (67).

Endoscopic grading of GERD depends upon the endoscopist's interpretation of these visual images. Unfortunately, there exists no standard classification

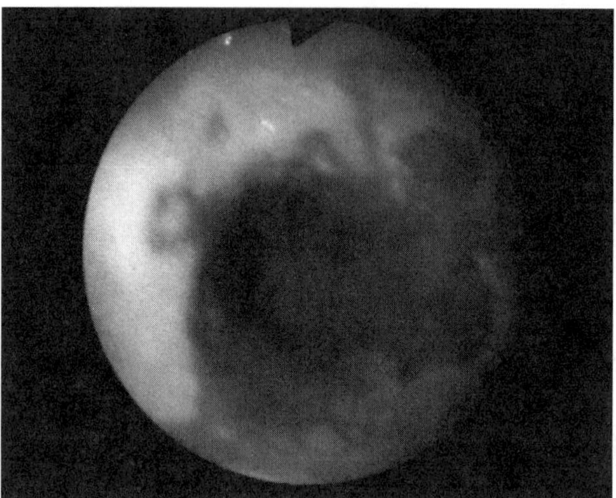

Figure 8 Barrett's esophagus.

scheme for endoscopic findings. Instead, several grading systems are available but none are completely satisfactory (Table 6). The most commonly employed scheme is the Savary-Miller classification (74). A score of 0 reflects normal-appearing mucosa while a value from I to III is assigned depending upon the degree of mucosal erosions. Grade IV is reserved for any complication of GERD such as ulceration, stricture, or Barrett's esophagus. The MUSE system stands for metaplasia, ulceration, stricture, and esophagitis (9). It calls for the individual grading of these findings on a scale from 0 to 3. Unfortunately, this scheme is cumbersome and difficult to use routinely. The Hetzel system grades severity not by the number of erosions but instead by the area of injury to the esophageal mucosal surface (75). The Los Angeles system uses a grading scale from A to D. The number, length, and location of mucosal breaks determine the degree of esophagitis (69). These different classification systems diverge the most when defining the subtlest degree of injury. When erythema, edema, and indistinct Z-line are included, the sensitivity of diagnosing GERD rises at the expense of specificity.

Even though endoscopy offers many advantages in diagnosing GERD and defining the extent of disease, most patients with reflux disease are treated initially without endoscopy. The important exception to this rule is the patient experiencing "alarm" symptoms. These are defined as dysphagia, odynophagia, weight loss, and gastrointestinal bleeding. Here, endoscopy should be performed early to rule out the presence of other entities such as infections, ulcers, cancer, or varices.

Table 6 Indices Relating Reflux Events and Symptoms

Symptom index (SI):

$$SI = \frac{\text{(number of reflux episodes} - \text{related symptom episodes)}}{\text{total number of symptom episodes}} \times 100\%$$

Symptom sensitivity index (SSI):

$$SSI = \frac{\text{number of symptomatic reflux episodes}}{\text{total number of reflux episodes}} \times 100\%$$

Symptom association probability (SAP):

Symptoms (S)

Reflux (R)		+	−	
	+	S+R+	−R+	R+
	−	S+R−	S−R−	R−
		S+	S−	Total

Calculate *p*-value using Fisher Exact test:

$$p = \frac{(R + !)\ (R - !)\ (S + !)\ (S - !)}{(Total!)\ (S + R + !)\ (S - R + !)\ (S + R - !)\ (S - R - !)}$$

$$SAP = (1 - p) \times 100\%$$

The role of endoscopy in GERD patients without alarm symptoms is more controversial. Initially, it was felt that endoscopy could dichotomize patients into two groups, nonerosive or mild disease and severe erosive disease, and better direct their management. Since the former population rarely develops complications, they could be treated less aggressively with H_2-receptor antagonists or promotility agents. The latter group, being more prone to complications and requiring maintenance therapy, needed more aggressive treatment with PPIs or surgery. Endoscopy was performed to assess disease severity either before initiating treatment or when symptoms relapsed after medications were discontinued. This practice is now less popular with the use of PPIs as first-line therapy for GERD. Since this drug class treats both groups of patients equally well, early endoscopy has less impact in influencing the choice of therapy. Currently, the most important reason to perform endoscopy in GERD patients is to identify peptic strictures or Barrett's esophagus. The latter is diagnosed most reliably on biopsy, and the presence of dysplasia can be affected adversely by active inflammation (76). Therefore, biopsies are usually not taken to exclude Barrett's mucosa if acute inflammation is present, but rather the patient is treated aggressively with PPIs for 8 weeks, and then endoscopy is repeated with biopsies. This allows better definition of the classic finding of Barrett's epithelium and prevents false-positive grading of low- or high-grade dysplasia due to inflammation. Using this rationale, the vast majority of patients with chronic GERD need only one endoscopy while on therapy. If Barrett's esophagus is identified, enrollment into an endoscopic surveillance program is appropriate (66).

Even though endoscopy is a vital tool in the diagnosis and surveillance of GERD, it should be used prudently. The test adds cost to the medical care of the patient, has a small but real potential for complications, and may prolong the length of time between the patient's presentation to the physician and initiation of therapy.

Esophageal Biopsy

The ability to obtain tissue during endoscopy is very important. Biopsies of the esophagus are warranted to identify the presence of reflux injury, exclude other esophageal diseases and confirm the presence of complications, especially Barrett's esophagus. Microscopic changes indicative of reflux may occur even when the mucosa appears normal endoscopically (77). In the presence of macroscopic abnormalities, such as a stricture or ulceration, biopsy provides tissue to exclude other possible diagnoses such as neoplasm, infection, pill injury, or bullous disease. Often, the presence of intestinal metaplasia is in question. What appears to be Barrett's esophagus due to the classic endoscopic salmon-colored mucosal appearance may actually represent gastric mucosa. Biopsy evidence of goblet cells suggests intestinal metaplasia while their absence confirms the presence of gastric cardia–type mucosa (76).

The most sensitive histological markers of reflux disease are reactive epithelial changes characterized by an increase in the basal cell layer greater than 15% of the epithelium thickness or papillae elongation into the upper third of the epithelium (Fig. 9). These changes represent increased epithelial turnover of the squamous mucosa. Papillae, or rete peg, height increases due to loss of surface cells from acid injury, while basal cell hyperplasia is indicative of mucosal repair. Unfortunately, these changes are also noted in up to 50% of normal individuals when biopsies are taken from the distal 2–3 cm of the esophagus and in up to 20% of normal individuals with biopsies from the more proximal esophagus (76). Hence, these changes are sensitive markers for GERD but have poor specificity.

More severe esophageal inflammation is characterized by cellular infiltration. Neutrophils and eosinophils are not usually present in the esophageal mucosa; therefore, their appearance in biopsy tissue is highly suggestive of GERD

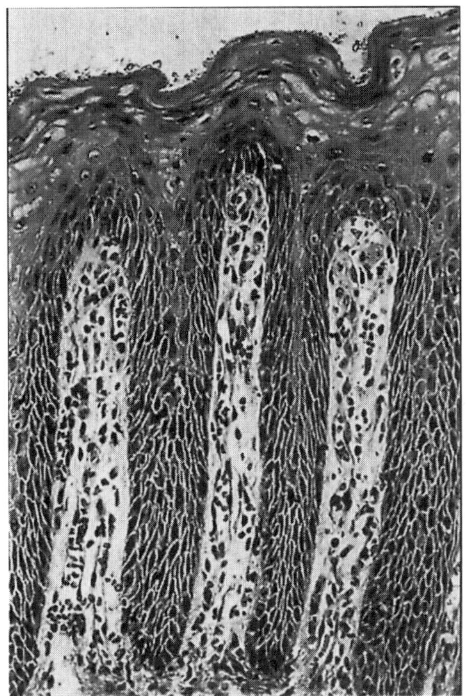

Figure 9 Reparative changes secondary to reflux disease characterized by basal cell hyperplasia and marked elongation of the rete pegs.

(76). Current theory suggests that reflux causes an acute injury to the vascular bed of the esophagus, leading to the release of vasoactive substances, which promotes edema and stimulates the migration of neutrophils and eosinophils into the area. Unfortunately, the detection of neutrophils is an insensitive marker for reflux disease, being present in no more than 40% of GERD patients (78). The sensitivity of eosinophils for GERD is better, reported as high as 69%; however, specificity may be lacking. In one study, 4 of 12 (33%) normal individuals were noted to have rare eosinophils present on biopsy (79). It is hypothesized that this decline in specificity reflects an association of eosinophilia with other diseases such as asthma or eosinophilic gastroenteritis. Interestingly, the sensitivity and specificity in children is much stronger reflecting the lack of eosinophils in the juvenile inflammatory response (76,80).

Further evaluation of microscopic changes associated with reflux disease can be assessed with electron microscopy. Studies with transmission electron microscopy performed on human esophageal biopsies demonstrate the presence of dilated intercellular spaces in patients with both erosive and nonerosive reflux diseases (81). This finding precedes the onset of gross morphological damage, thus representing one of the earlier alterations in GERD. Scanning electron microscopy also has been used to study the pathological changes associated with reflux. Initially, studies identified a decrease in the number of microridges, infoldings of the plasmalemma on the luminal surface of the squamous epithelium, in patients with heartburn or reflux esophagitis (82,83). Further studies, however, failed to confirm an association between microridge loss and the presence of GERD (84).

Unfortunately, performing esophageal mucosal biopsies is not without its problems. The diagnostic yield is dependent upon the sample size, biopsy location, and tissue orientation. Initial studies were performed with pinch biopsies taken tangentially to the esophageal surface. This practice yielded small amounts of tissue, which were challenging to interpret because of difficulty in proper tissue orientation. To improve upon the pinch biopsy method, the suction biopsy and the jumbo biopsy techniques were developed. These allow a greater sampling volume per biopsy and therefore provide tissue that is easier to study. If lesions associated with GERD are present, such as ulcers or erosions, biopsies are obtained from the base of the lesion to demonstrate the depth of tissue injury as well as the reparative process. Biopsy of the surrounding area discloses the local cell infiltration. In contrast, if no lesions are noted at the time of endoscopy, biopsies are performed at least 3 cm above the EG junction (Z-line) to look for reactive changes due to reflux. Multiple biopsies are gathered because of the sporadic nature of the histological changes. Tissue closer to the Z-line is not sampled because of the decreased specificity for diagnosing GERD (76,85).

Esophageal Manometry

Esophageal manometry provides information on the functional ability of the esophageal muscles by quantifying the contractile activities of the esophageal sphincters and body during swallowing. The equipment necessary to perform manometric testing includes a catheter, pressure transducers, and a recorder. Testing is performed by first passing the catheter apparatus into the esophagus. The assembly is capable of recording multiple pressure readings simultaneously from within the esophagus. The number of readings is dependent upon the number of sensors, typically spaced 3–5 cm apart along the catheter. From three to eight sensors are connected to transducers that convert the physical changes of pressure to electrical signals. These signals are transmitted to a recorder that transforms the information to a visual display by way of a polygraph. Either a water-perfused catheter system or one based on solid-state circuitry is typically employed. The solid-state systems are more expensive and fragile; however, they are better able to accurately record pressures in both the esophagus and pharynx, and testing can be performed with solid and semisolid boluses in addition to water. With this technique of resting pressures of the lower and upper esophageal sphincters as well as the timing and completeness of their relaxations are recorded. In the esophageal body, peristalsis is evaluated by assessing the presence, propagation, velocity, amplitude, and duration of contraction waves (2,15).

The measurement of lower esophageal sphincter (LES) pressure logically should be associated with the severity of GERD because of its importance as a major barrier to reflux. In fact, the majority of patients investigated in early studies, usually those with severe esophagitis prior to surgery, had LES pressures < 10 mmHg. However, recent studies find that over 60% of patients with GERD have a normal resting LES pressure of 10–30 mmHg, while an occasional asymptomatic subject has pressures below this value (86). This observation is not surprising since current studies find that transient relaxations of the LES are the primary mechanisms by which reflux occurs. In between these episodes, the basal LES pressure, which is traditionally measured by stationary manometry, is normal. Consequently, LES pressure in a given patient is too imprecise for identifying the potential for reflux (70).

Quantitative assessment of peristaltic activity in the esophageal body is also an important test in assessing the severity of reflux disease (20). As the degree of GERD worsens, increasing dysmotility is noted characterized by frequent simultaneous or nonconducted contractions and low-amplitude (<35 mmHg) peristaltic contraction (Fig. 10). These changes are termed ''ineffective peristalsis'' as they do not predictably clear the esophagus of refluxed acid. In our experience, ineffective peristalsis in the distal esophagus is much more common (30–40%) than low LES pressure (approximately 10%). Manometry is crucial for identifying these abnormalities in esophageal function (71).

In clinical practice, esophageal manometry has no role in the evaluation of uncomplicated GERD. Manometry serves as an integral component of pH monitoring by accurately defining the location of the LES, a task poorly performed by endoscopy, fluoroscopy, or the pH pull-through technique. However, it is an essential test in the preoperative evaluation of patients prior to antireflux surgery (22,87). A normal LES pressure does not preclude surgery for the reasons previously discussed, yet occasionally a diagnosis of achalasia or scleroderma is made, changing the clinical approach. Most importantly, the presence of ineffective peristalsis suggests a weak esophageal pump and helps tailor the antireflux surgery. In these patients, adapting the surgical approach to incorporate an incomplete Toupet procedure rather than a Nissen fundoplication minimizes the risk of postoperative dysphagia (15,88).

Esophageal Potential Difference Measurement

The potential difference across the esophageal epithelium is due to the transport of ions, principally sodium, across the cell's basolateral membrane in conjunction with the resistance to passive ion movement across tight junctions and cellular

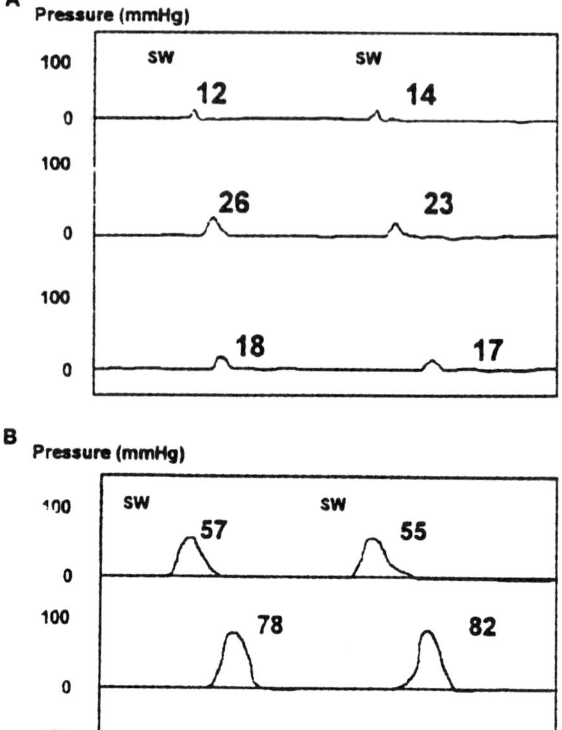

Figure 10 Examples of ineffective peristalsis by esophageal manometry. (A) Low-amplitude peristalsis (normal > 35 mmHg). (B) Frequent nontransmitted contractions (NT) in the distal esophagus.

membranes. This active process (requiring ATP) sets up concentration gradients of ions between the intracellular and extracellular spaces. Using Ohm's law:

$$PD \text{ (millivolts)} = I \text{ (microamps)} \times R \text{ (ohms·cm}^2\text{)}$$

where *PD* is potential difference, *I* is current, and *R* is electrical resistance, a voltage potential can be calculated for normal esophageal tissue. If this tissue is damaged structurally or functionally, the potential difference changes. With acid exposure, there is a brief rise in the measured voltage that is followed by a gradual decrease. The fall in voltage reflects the movement of ions back along the concentration gradient toward a state of equilibrium. Initially, this is due to increased permeability of the intercellular tight junctions secondary to acid-related injury. As acid exposure continues, the active transport of Na is disturbed and eventually disrupted completely. When the potential difference is zero, normal epithelial function is absent. This reflects either complete necrosis or scar formation of the tissue. A potential difference other than normal or zero reflects the degree of tissue injury or possibly the transition to an alternate epithelium such as Barrett's esophagus (89,90).

The measurement of the resting electrical potential difference across the epithelium is primarily a research technique used to assess the integrity of the esophageal epithelium. Currently, it has no use in the clinical diagnosis of GERD.

TESTS FOR MECHANISMS OF ESOPHAGEAL INJURY

Esophageal Manometry/pH Monitoring

As discussed earlier, manometry has limited ability to distinguish the severity of GERD. It does, however, have a role in determining the mechanism of esophageal injury. By assessing the character of esophageal peristalsis along with the function of the esophageal sphincters, manometry can identify functional abnormalities promoting the development of reflux. More importantly, manometry may identify specific problems, which helps tailor possible surgical therapy for GERD. Support for this rationale comes from retrospective studies. In one review, preoperative manometry influenced surgical technique in 10% of patients undergoing laparoscopic fundoplication. Results of surgery demonstrated a 96% success rate (22). In another study, patients with impaired esophageal motility underwent laparoscopic antireflux surgery. More severe dysphagia was reported in the Nissen fundoplication group (57%) versus the Toupet group (9%) (91). These findings demonstrate that manometry is an important preoperative test to customize antireflux surgery.

Esophageal pH monitoring also helps in understanding the mechanisms of acid reflux injury. Johnson and DeMeester found that the circadian pattern of GER helps to predict the degree of acid injury and esophagitis (92,93). Patients with reflux only during the day have frequent symptoms but minimal esophagitis due to rapid acid clearance. In contrast, nocturnal reflux is frequently associated with esophagitis and the complications of GERD. At night in the supine position, poor acid clearance occurs because of the lack of gravity, peristalsis, and saliva production while asleep. Nevertheless, acid reflux patterns and total acid exposure times overlap considerably in individual patients with GERD suggesting that other factors such as mucosal resistance are important in protecting esophageal integrity.

Barium Esophagram

Direct visualization of the esophagus with fluoroscopy is another method for determining the mechanism of esophageal injury. With this technique, abnormalities such as nonperistaltic contractions, incomplete primary peristalsis, and aperistalsis may be observed. These findings typically occur in the lower half of the esophagus. Observing barium swallows compares favorably to manometry in evaluating primary esophageal motility. Barium can also estimate esophageal clearance. Normal individuals in a recumbent position should remove all barium swallowed with one peristaltic sequence. Finally, barium may disclose the presence of a hiatal hernia, which acts to decrease the integrity of the LES by altering the anatomical relationships between the gastroesophageal junction, diaphragm, and associated ligaments (30).

CONCLUSION

The diagnosis of GERD at times poses a challenge for even the most skilled clinician. Without a test that is 100% sensitive and specific for disease, the physician must assimilate the patient's presentation and adopt an individualized strategy that will best arrive at a diagnosis. This demands a fundamental understanding of the many tests available for detecting GERD, the strengths and weaknesses of each test, and the indications for their use. By employing this approach, the physician optimizes his or her opportunity to correctly identify GERD and its relationship to the patient's complaints.

REFERENCES

1. Richter JE. Typical and atypical presentations of gastroesophageal reflux disease. The role of esophageal testing in diagnosis and management. Gastroenterol Clin North Am 1996; 25:75–102.
2. Richter JE. Disorders of esophageal function. In: McCallum RW, Phillips SF, Reynolds JC, eds. Gastrointestinal Motility Disorders for the Clinician: Practical Guidelines for Patient Care. New York: Academy Professional Information Services, 1998: 5.1–5.28.
3. Koufman JA. The otolaryngologic manifestations of gastroesophageal reflux disease: a clinical investigation of 225 patients using ambulatory 24-hour pH monitoring and an experimental investigation of the role of acid and pepsin in the development of laryngeal injury. Laryngoscope 1991; 101:1–65.
4. Hewson EG, Sinclair JW, Dalton CB, Richter JE. 24-hour esophageal pH monitoring: the most useful test for evaluating non-cardiac chest pain. Am J Med 1991; 90: 576–583.

5. Castell DO. Esophageal disorders in the elderly. Gastroenterol Clin North Am 1990; 19:235–254.
6. Knill-Jones RP, Card WI, Crean GP, James WB, Spiegelhalter DJ. The symptoms of gastro-oesophageal reflux and of oesophagitis. Scand J Gastroenterol 1984; 19: 72–76.
7. Spechler SJ. Barrett's esophagus: what's new and what to do. Am J Gastroenterol 1989; 84:220–223.
8. Klauser AG, Schindlbeck NE, Muller-Lissner SA. Symptoms in gastro-oesophageal reflux disease. Lancet 1990; 335:205–208.
9. Armstrong D, Emde C, Inauen W, Blum AL. Diagnostic assessment of gastroesophageal reflux disease: what is possible vs. what is practical? Hepato-Gastroenterol 1992; 39:3–13.
10. Kahrilas PJ, Quigley EMM. Clinical esophageal pH recording: a technical review for practice guideline development. Gastroenterology 1996; 110:1982–1996.
11. Klauser AG, Schindlbeck N, Muller-Lissner SA. Esophageal 24-hour pH monitoring: is prior manometry necessary for correct positioning of the electrode? Am J Gastroenterol 1990; 85:1463–1467.
12. Mattox HE, Richter JE, Sinclair JW. Gastroesophageal pH step-up inaccurately locates the proximal border of the lower esophageal sphincter. Dig Dis Sci 1992; 37: 1185–1191.
13. Schindlbeck NE, Ippisch H, Klauser AG, Muller-Lissner SA. Which pH threshold is best in esophageal pH monitoring? Am J Gastroenterol 1991; 86:1138–1141.
14. Jamieson JR, Stein HJ, DeMeester TR, Bonavina L, Schwizer W, Hinder RA, Albertucci M. Ambulatory 24-H esophageal pH monitoring: normal values, optimal thresholds, specificity, sensitivity, and reproducibility. Am J Gastroenterol 1992; 87: 1102–1111.
15. Ergun GA, Kahrilas PJ. Clinical applications of esophageal manometry and pH monitoring. Am J Gastroenterol 1996; 91:1077–1089.
16. Vitale GC, Cheadle WG, Sadek S, Michel ME, Cuschieri A. Computerized 24-hour ambulatory esophageal pH monitoring and esophagogastroduodenoscopy in the reflux patient. Ann Surg 1984; 20:724–728.
17. Schindlbeck NE, Heinrich C, Konig A, Dendorfer A, Pace F, Muller-Lissner SA. Optimal thresholds, sensitivity, and specificity of long-term pH-metry for the detection of gastroesophageal reflux disease. Gastroenterology 1987; 93:85–90.
18. Masclee AAM, De Best ACAM, De Graaf R, Cluysenaer OJJ, Jansen JBMJ. Ambulatory 24-hour pH-metry in the diagnosis of gastroesophageal reflux disease. Scand J Gastroenterol 1990; 25:225–230.
19. Mattioli S, Pilotti V, Spangaro M, Grigioni WF, Zannoli R, Felice V, Conci A, Gozzetti G. Reliability of 24-hour home esophageal pH monitoring in diagnosis of gastroesophageal reflux. Dig Dis Sci 1989; 34:71–78.
20. Kasapidis P, Xynos E, Mantides A, Chrysos E, Demonakou M, Nikolopoulos N, Vassilakis JS. Differences in manometry and 24-hour ambulatory pH-metry between patients with and without endoscopic or histologic esophagitis in gastroesophageal reflux disease. Am J Gastroenterol 1993; 88:1893–1899.
21. Johnsson F, Joelsson B, Isberg P. Ambulatory 24 hour intraesophageal pH-monitoring in the diagnosis of gastroesophageal reflux disease. Gut 1987; 28:1145–1150.

22. Waring JP, Hunter JG, Oddsdottir M. The preoperative evaluation of patients considered for laparoscopic antireflux surgery. Am J Gastroenterol 1995; 90:35–38.
23. Katzka DA, Paoletti V, Leite L, Castell DO. Prolonged ambulatory pH monitoring in patients with persistent gastroesophageal reflux disease symptoms: testing while on therapy identifies the need for more aggressive anti-reflux therapy. Am J Gastroenterol 1996; 91:2110–2113.
24. Shay SS, Abreu SH, Tsuchida A. Scintigraphy in gastroesophageal reflux disease: a comparison to endoscopy, LESp, and 24-hour pH score, as well as to simultaneous pH monitoring. Am J Gastroenterol 1992; 87:1094–1101.
25. Shay SS, Eggli D, Johnson LF. Simultaneous esophageal pH monitoring and scintigraphy during the postprandial period in patients with severe reflux esophagitis. Dig Dis Sci 1991; 36:558–564.
26. Petersen KH, Erichsen GH, Myrvold HE. Scintigraphy, pH measurement, and radiography in the evaluation of gastroesophageal reflux. Scand J Gastroenterol 1985; 20:289–294.
27. Fung W, Van der Schaaf A, Grieve JC. Gastroesophageal scintigraphy and endoscopy in the diagnosis of esophageal reflux and esophagitis. Am J Gastroenterol 1985; 80:245–247.
28. Jenkins AF, Cowan RJ, Richter JE. Gastroesophageal scintigraphy: is it a sensitive screening test for gastroesophageal reflux disease? J Clin Gastroenterol 1985; 7: 127–131.
29. Kjellen G, Brudin L, Hakansson HO. Is scintigraphy of value in the diagnosis of gastro-oesophageal reflux disease? Scand J Gastroenterol 1991; 26:425–430.
30. Ott DJ. Gastroesophageal reflux disease. Radiol Clin North Am 1994; 32:1147–1166.
31. Thompson JK, Koehler RE, Richter JE. Detection of gastroesophageal reflux: value of barium studies compared with 24 hour pH monitoring. Am J Radiol 1994; 162: 621–626.
32. Vaezi MF, Richter JE. Role of acid and duodenogastroesophageal reflux in gastroesophageal reflux disease. Gastroenterology 1996; 111:1192–1199.
33. Vaezi MF, Richter JE. Synergism of acid and duodenogastroesophageal reflux in complicated Barrett's esophagus. Surgery 1995; 117:699–704.
34. Vaezi MF, Singh S, Richter JE. Role of acid and duodenogastric reflux in esophageal mucosal injury: a review of animal and human studies. Gastroenterology 1995; 108: 1897–1907.
35. Attwood SEA, DeMeester TR, Bremner CG, Barlow AP, Hinder RA. Alkaline gastroesophageal reflux: implications in the development of complications in Barrett's columnar-lined lower esophagus. Surgery 1989; 106:764–776.
36. Attwood SEA, Ball CS, Barlow AP, Jenkinson L, Norris TL, Watson A. Role of intragastric and intraoesophageal alkalinization in the genesis of complications in Barrett's columnar lined lower esophagus. Gut 1993; 34:11–15.
37. Bremner RM, Crookes PF, DeMeester TR. Concentration of refluxed acid and esophageal mucosal injury. Am J Surg 1992; 164:522–527.
38. Champion G, Richter JE, Vaezi MF, Singh S, Alexander R. Duodenogastroesophageal reflux: relationship to pH and importance in Barrett's esophagus. Gastroenterology 1994; 107:747–754.

39. Devault KR, Georgeson S, Castell DO. Salivary stimulation mimics esophageal exposure to refluxed duodenal contents. Am J Gastroenterol 1993; 88:1040–1043.
40. Singh S, Bradley LA, Richter JE. Determinants of oesophageal ''alkaline'' pH environment in controls and patients with gastro-oesophageal reflux disease. Gut 1993; 34:309–316.
41. Bechi P, Pucciani F, Baldini F, Cosi F, Falciai R, Mazzanti R, Castagnoli A, Pesseri A, Boscherini S. Long-term ambulatory enterogastric reflux monitoring. Validation of a new fiberoptic technique. Dig Dis Sci 1993; 38:1297–1306.
42. Vaezi MF, LaCamera RG, Richter JE. Bilitec 2000 ambulatory duodenogastric reflux monitoring system. Studies on its validation and limitations. Am J Physiol 1994; 30:1050–1056.
43. Vaezi MF, Richter JE. Contribution of acid and duodenogastroesophageal reflux to oesophageal mucosal injury and symptoms in partial gastrectomy patients. Gut 1997; 41:297–302.
44. Baldi F, Ferrarini F, Longanesi A, Ragazzini M, Barbara L. Acid gastroesophageal reflux and symptom occurrence. Analysis of some factors influencing their association. Dig Dis Sci 1989; 34:1890–1893.
45. Hewson RA. 24-hour esophageal pH monitoring: the most useful test for evaluating non-cardiac chest pain. Am J Med 1991; 90:576.
46. Sontag S, O'Connell S, Khandelwal S. Does wheezing occur in association with an episode of gastroesophageal reflux? (abstr). Gastroenterology 1989; 96:482.
47. Wiener GJ, Richter JE, Cooper JB, Wu WC, Castell DO. The symptom index: a clinically important parameter of ambulatory 24-hour esophageal pH monitoring. Am J Gastroenterol 1988; 83:358–361.
48. Brumelhof R, Smout AJPM. The symptom sensitivity index: a valuable additional parameter in 24-hour esophageal pH recording. Am J Gastroenterol 1991; 86:160–164.
49. Weusten BLAM, Roelofs JMM, Akkermans LMA, vanBerge-Henegouwen GP, Smout AJPM. The symptom association probability: an improved method for symptom analysis of 24-hour esophageal pH data. Gastroenterology 1994; 107:1741–1745.
50. Weusten BLAM, Smout AJPM. Symptom analysis in 24-hour esophageal pH monitoring. In: Richter JE, ed. Ambulatory Esophageal pH Monitoring: Practical Approach and Clinical Applications, 2nd ed. Baltimore: Williams & Wilkins, 1997: 97–105.
51. Lam HGT, Breumelhof R, Roelofs JMM, vanBerge-Henegouwen GP, Smout AJPM. What is the optimal time window in symptom analysis of 24-hour esophageal pressure and pH data? Dig Dis Sci 1994; 89:402–409.
52. Bernstein LM, Baker LA. A clinical test for esophagitis. Gastroenterology 1958; 34:760–781.
53. Katz PO, Dalton CB, Richter JE, Wu WC, Castell DO. Esophageal testing in patients with noncardiac chest pain and/or dysphagia. Results of three years' experience with 1161 patients. Ann Intern Med 1987; 106:593–597.
54. Richter JE, Hewson EG, Sinclair JW, Dalton CB. Acid perfusion test and 24-hour esophageal pH monitoring with symptom index: comparison of tests for esophageal acid sensitivity. Dig Dis Sci 1991; 36:565–571.

55. Richter JE, Hewson EG, Sinclair J, Dalton CB. Acid perfusion test: an obsolete screening test for acid induced non-cardiac chest pain (abstr). Gastroenterology 1990; 98:A112.
56. Schenk BE, Kuipers EJ, Klinkenberg-Knol EC, Festen HPM, Jansen EH, Tunyman HARE, Schrijver M, Dieleman LA, Meuwissen SGM. Omeprazole as a diagnostic tool in gastroesophageal reflux disease. Am J Gastroenterol 1997; 92:1997–2000.
57. Sonnenberg A, Fabiola D, El-Serag HB. Empirical therapy versus diagnostic tests in gastroesophageal reflux disease. A medical decision analysis. Dig Dis Sci 1998; 43:1001–1008.
58. Feldman M, Harford WV, Fisher RS, Sampliner RE, Murray SB, Greski-Rose PA. Treatment of reflux esophagitis resistant to H2-receptor antagonists with lansoprazole, a new H+/K+-ATPase inhibitor: a controlled, double-blind study. Am J Gastroenterol 1993; 88:1212–1217.
59. Marks RD, Richter JE, Rizzo J, Koehler RE, Spenney JG, Mills TP, Champion G. Omeprazole versus H2-receptor antagonists in treating patients with peptic stricture and esophagitis. Gastroenterology 1994; 106:907–915.
60. Dent J, Yeomans ND, Mackinnon M, Reed W, Narielvala FM, Hetzel DJ, Solcia E, Shearman DJC. Omeprazole versus ranitidine for prevention of relapse in reflux oesophagitis. A controlled double blind trial of their efficacy and safety. Gut 1994; 35:590–598.
61. Robinson M, Lanza F, Avner D, Haber M. Effective maintenance treatment of reflux esophagitis with low-dose lansoprazole. A randomized, double-blind, placebo-controlled trial. Ann Intern Med 1996; 124:859–867.
62. DeVault KR, Castell DO. Guidelines for the diagnosis and treatment of gastroesophageal reflux disease. Ann Intern Med 1995; 155:2165–2173.
63. Schindlbeck NE, Klauser AG, Voderholzer WA, Muller-Lissner S. Empiric therapy for gastroesophageal reflux disease. Arch Intern Med 1995; 155:1808–1812.
64. Fass R, Fennerty MB, Ofman JJ, Gralnek IM, Johnson C, Camargo E, Sampliner RE. The clinical and economic value of a short course of omeprazole in patients with noncardiac chest pain. Gastroenterology 1998; 115:42–49.
65. Ours TM, Kavuru MS, Schilz RJ, Richter JE. A prospective evaluation of esophageal testing and a double blind, randomized study of omeprazole in a diagnostic and therapeutic algorithm for chronic cough. In press.
66. Kahrilas PJ. Gastroesophageal reflux disease. JAMA 1996; 276:983–988.
67. Weinberg DS, Kadish SL. The diagnosis and management of gastroesophageal reflux disease. Med Clin North Am 1996; 80:411–429.
68. Bytzer P, Havelund T, Moller Hansen J. Interobserver variation in the endoscopic diagnosis of reflux esophagitis. Scand J Gastroenterol 1993; 28:119–125.
69. Armstrong D, Bennett JR, Blum AL, Dent J, De Dombal FT, Galmiche J-P, Lundell L, Margulies M, Richter JE, Spechler SJ, Tytgat GNJ, Wallin L. The endoscopic assessment of esophagitis: a progress report on observer agreement. Gastroenterology 1996; 111:85–92.
70. Richter JE. Severe reflux esophagitis. Gastrointest Endosc Clin North Am 1994; 4: 677–697.
71. Richter JE, Castell DO. GE reflux: pathogenesis, diagnosis and therapy. Ann Intern Med 1982; 97:93–103.

72. Johnson LF, DeMeester TR, Haggitt RC. Endoscopic signs of gastroesophageal reflux objectively evaluated. Gastrointest Endosc 1976; 22:151–155.
73. Hatlebakk JG, Berstad A. Endoscopic grading of reflux esophagitis: what observations correlate with gastro-oesophageal reflux? Scand J Gastroenterol 1997; 32:760–765.
74. Ollyo JB, Lang F, Fontolliet C, Monnier P. Savary-Miller's new endoscopic grading of reflux-oesophagitis: a simple, reproducible, logical, complete and useful classification. Gastroenterology 1990; 98:A100.
75. Hetzel DJ, Dent J, Reed WD, Narielva FM, Machinnon M, McCarthy JH, Mitchell B, Beveridge BR, Laurence BH, Gibson GG, Grant AK, Shearman DJC, Whitehead R, Buckle PJ. Healing and relapse of severe peptic esophagitis after treatment with omeprazole. Gastroenterology 1988; 95:903–912.
76. Riddell RH. The biopsy diagnosis of gastroesophageal reflux disease, "carditis," and Barrett's esophagus, and sequelae of therapy. Am J Surg Pathol 1996; 20:31–50.
77. Funch-Jensen P, Kock K, Christensen LA, Fallingborg J, Kjaergaard JJ, Paulin Anderson S, Stubbe Teglbjaerg P. Microscopic appearance of the esophageal mucosa in a consecutive series of patients submitted to upper endoscopy. Correlation with gastroesophageal reflux symptoms and macroscopic findings. Scand J Gastroenterol 1986; 21:65–69.
78. Seefeld U, Krejs GJ, Siebenmann RE, Blum AL. Esophageal histology in gastroesophageal reflux. Morphometric findings in suction biopsies. Dig Dis Sci 1977; 22:956–964.
79. Tummala V, Barwick KW, Sontag SJ, Vlahcevic RZ, McCallum RW. The significance of intraepithelial eosinophils in the histologic diagnosis of gastroesophageal reflux. Am J Clin Pathol 1987; 87:43–48.
80. Winter HS, Madara JL, Stafford RJ, Grand RJ, Quinlan JE, Goldman H. Intraepithelial eosinophils: a new diagnostic criterion for reflux esophagitis. Gastroenterology 1982; 83:818–823.
81. Tobey NA, Carson JL, Alkiek RA, Orlando RC. Dilated intercellular spaces: a morphological feature of acid reflux-damaged human esophageal epithelium. Gastroenterology 1996; 111:1200–1205.
82. Goran DA, Shields HM, Bates ML, Zuckerman GR, DeSchryver-Kecskemeti K. Esophageal dysplasia. Assessment by light microscopy and scanning electron microscopy. Gastroenterology 1984; 86:39–50.
83. Danton MHD, Nunn S, Dolan S, Collins BJ, Sloan JM, Carr KE. A scanning electron microscope study of reflux oesophagitis. J Anat 1991; 176:247.
84. Johnston BT, Nunn S, Sloan JM, Collins JSA, McFarland RJ, Parkin S, Carr KE, Collins BJ. The application of microridge analysis in the diagnosis of gastro-oesophageal reflux disease. Scand J Gastroenterol 1996; 31:97–102.
85. Kaul B, Halvorsen T, Peterson H, Grette K, Myrvold HE. Gastroesophageal reflux disease. Scintigraphic, endoscopic, and histologic considerations. Scand J Gastroenterol 1986; 21:134–138.
86. Behar J, Biancani P, Sheahan DG. Evaluation of esophageal tests in the diagnosis of reflux esophagitis. Gastroenterology 1976; 71:9–15.
87. Spechler SJ. Comparison of medical and surgical therapy for complicated gastroesophageal reflux disease in veterans. N Engl J Med 1992; 326:786–792.

88. Falk GW. GERD diagnostic tests: manometry and pH monitoring (personal communication), 1998.
89. Vidins EI, Fox JA, Beck IT. Transmural potential difference (PD) in the body of the esophagus in patients with esophagitis, Barrett's epithelium, and carcinoma of the esophagus. Am J Dig Dis 1971; 16:991–999.
90. Herlihy KJ, Orlando RC, Bryson JC, Bozymski EM, Carney CN, Powell DW. Barrett's esophagus: clinical, endoscopic, histologic, manometric and electrical potential difference characteristics. Gastroenterology 1984; 86:436–443.
91. Lund RJ, Wetscher GJ, Raiser F, Glaser K, Perdikis G, Gadenstatter M, Katada N, Hinder RA. Laparoscopic Toupet fundoplication for gastroesophageal reflux disease with poor esophageal body motility. Gastroenterology 1996; 110:PA 1401.
92. Johnson LF, DeMeester TR, Haggitt RC. Esophageal epithelial response to gastroesophageal reflux, a quantitative study. Am J Dig Dis 1978; 23:498–509.
93. Johnson LF, DeMeester TR. Evaluation of elevation of the head of the bed, bethanechol, and antacid foam tablets on gastroesophageal reflux. Dig Dis Sci 1981; 26:673–680.

5

Pathophysiology of Gastroesophageal Reflux Disease

The Antireflux Barrier and Luminal Clearance Mechanisms

Peter J. Kahrilas and Guoxiang Shi
Northwestern University Medical School, Chicago, Illinois

Gastroesophageal reflux disease (GERD) encompasses a spectrum of disorders inclusive of both symptomatic conditions related to the reflux of gastric juice across the esophagogastric junction (EGJ) and potential damage to the esophageal or supraesophageal epithelium related to that reflux. In either case, the fundamental aberration is excessive esophageal or supraesophageal epithelial exposure to gastric refluxate. However, it is important to note that no absolute cutoff values exist for what constitutes pathological reflux. A minority of individuals with GERD will have visually evident erosion, ulceration, stricture formation, or metaplasia, in which cases it is clear that the caustic exposure sustained exceeded the defensive ability of the involved epithelium. On the other hand, in the majority of individuals without visual evidence of the disease, symptoms emanate from reflux either because of changes in the fine structure of the epithelium not evident endoscopically, or because the epithelium is excessively sensitive to what would be a tolerable exposure to refluxate for another individual. Thus, a comprehensive understanding of the pathogenesis of GERD must consider both the determinants of epithelial acid exposure and the defensive mechanisms of the epithelium. Significant aberration in either of these pathophysiological influences can tip the balance from a compensated condition toward a decompensated condition, be that heartburn, chest pain, laryngitis, or esophagitis. The intermittent nature of symptoms in many individuals with GERD suggests that the aggressive and defensive forces are part of a delicately balanced system susceptible to perturbation not only by the quantitative attributes of reflux, but also by cofactors related to diet, concurrent medications, voice use, cigarette smoking, or emotional stress. This chapter will focus on the determinants of esophageal acid exposure, specifically, gastroesophageal reflux and mechanisms of acid clearance. A subsequent chapter will review our current understanding of epithelial defense mechanisms.

MECHANISMS OF ACID REFLUX

The prerequisite for the development of GERD is movement of gastric juice from the stomach into the esophagus. Under normal circumstances, reflux is prevented as a function of the EGJ. The antireflux barrier at the EGJ is an anatomically complex zone whose functional integrity has been variably attributed to intrinsic lower esophageal sphincter (LES) pressure, extrinsic compression of the LES by the crural diaphragm, the intra-abdominal location of the LES, integrity of the phrenoesophageal ligament, and maintenance of an acute angle of His (the angle of entry of the esophagus into the stomach). Although there is probably some merit to each of these possibilities, supporting evidence is more compelling in some cases than in others. Quite possibly, competence of the antireflux barrier is attributable to more than one factor and incompetence becomes increasingly severe as more antireflux mechanisms are disabled. The antireflux barrier needs to be dynamic because it must guard against reflux in a variety of circumstances. Furthermore, the dominant mechanism protecting against reflux may vary with circumstance. For example, the intra-abdominal segment of the LES may be important in preventing reflux during swallowing, the diaphragmatic crus may be of cardinal importance during abdominal straining, and basal LES pressure may be of primary importance during restful recumbency. The total number of reflux events sustained would then increase progressively as each of these protective mechanisms is compromised.

The complexity of the antireflux barrier has led investigators to focus on several different potential mechanisms of reflux. Three dominant theories of pathogenesis attribute EGJ incompetence to: (1) transient lower esophageal sphincter relaxations (tLESRs) without any necessary accompanying anatomical abnormality, (2) simply a result of a hypotensive LES, again, without any accompanying anatomical abnormality, or (3) anatomical disruption of the EGJ inclusive of, but not limited to, hiatal hernia. Individuals can be found exemplifying each of these mechanisms; however, what proportion of the entire GERD population can be attributed to each mechanism remains a hotly debated issue. Recent evidence also suggests that the dominant mechanism may vary as a function of disease severity with tLESRs dominating with mild disease and mechanisms associated with a hiatus hernia and/or weak sphincter dominating with more severe disease (1).

Transient Lower Esophageal Sphincter Relaxations

There is compelling evidence that tLESRs account for the overwhelming majority of reflux events in healthy individuals and in GERD patients with normal LES pressure (>10 mmHg) at the time of reflux (2–4). Figure 1 highlights differences between tLESRs and swallow-induced LES relaxation: tLESRs occur without an associated pharyngeal contraction, are unaccompanied by esophageal peristalsis, and persist longer (>10 s) than do swallow-induced LES relaxations (6). However, not all tLESRs are accompanied by reflux, with different investigators reporting reflux during as many as 93% or as few as 9–15% (4,5). What has become clear is the role of tLESRs in belching (7,8). The frequency of tLESRs is greatly increased by distension of the stomach by gas as it is by an upright as opposed to the supine posture. It seems likely that some of the confusion surrounding tLESRs stems from lack of a consistent definition; some investigators invoke the phenomenon with any nonswallow LES relaxation and others require more precise characteristics of the relaxations. Furthermore, it is increasingly appreciated that tLESRs are integrated motor responses involving not only LES relaxation, but also inhibition of the crural diaphragm and contraction of the costal diaphragm (9). In view of the circumstances in which they appear, it seems most likely that tLESRs are a physiological response to gastric distension by food or gas and are the mechanism responsible for gas venting of the stomach; acid reflux is an inconstant associated phenomenon.

Some investigators have suggested that tLESRs are manifestations of "subthreshold swallows" in response to pharyngeal stimulation (4). Supportive evidence of this includes the demonstration of isolated LES relaxation in response to pharyngeal stimulation with water (10,11) and from the observation made on a small number of gastrostomy patients (in whom LES recordings could be made through their gastrostomy site) that tLESR frequency was greatly enhanced during periods in which the free end of a second catheter was left dangling in the hypopharynx (12). However, it is clear that in at least some of these circumstances, investigators are invoking the phenomenon of tLESR with any nonswallow LES relaxation, ignoring the other components of the integrated response (crural diaphragm inhibition, costal diaphragm contraction, relaxation in excess of 10 s, esophageal aftercontraction) (9). It is also *unclear* to this investigator (PJK) what the relevant proposed *indigenous* stimulus would be to argue the importance of the pharyngeal stimulation mechanism. Thus, while there is convincing evidence that a variety of pharyngeal stimuli can elicit partial or complete LES relaxation, it remains disputable as to whether such relaxations have a clinically relevant relationship to tLESRs.

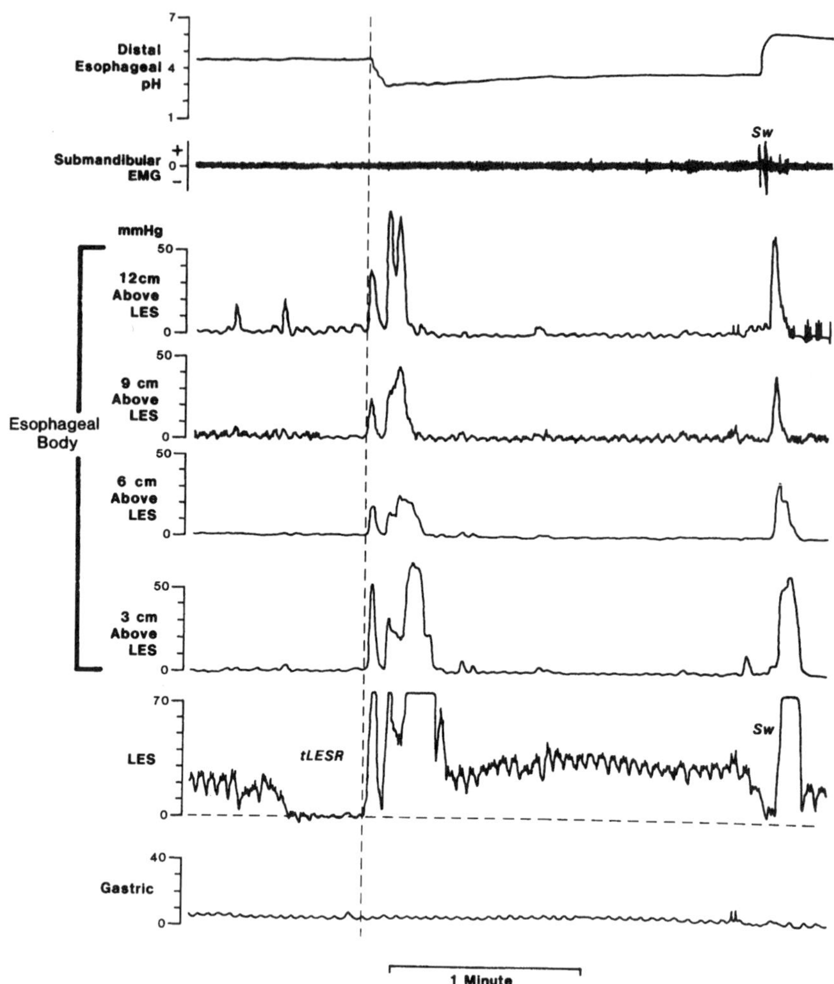

Figure 1 Example of a tLESR. Lower-esophageal-sphincter pressure is referenced to gastric pressure by the horizontal dotted line on the LES tracing (0 mmHg) representing mean intragastric pressure. Note that the tLESR persisted for 30 s while the swallow-induced LES relaxation to the right (Sw) persisted for only 5 s. Also note the absence of a submental EMG signal during the tLESR indicating the absence of a swallow. Finally, the associated esophageal motor activity is different in the two types of LES relaxation: the swallow is associated with primary peristalsis while the tLESR is associated with a vigorous, repetitive ''off-contraction'' throughout the esophageal body. (From Ref. 5, with permission.)

Recognizing the importance of tLESRs in promoting reflux, several groups of investigators are exploring the pharmacological manipulation of tLESRs as a potential therapy for GERD. Cholecystokinin (CCK) is one of the most extensively studied. Cholecystokinin-8 infused intravenously increased the occurrence of tLESRs in a dose-dependent fashion in both dogs and human subjects and this effect was blocked by CCK-A antagonists (13,14). Endogenous CCK was also demonstrated to play a role in the occurrence of tLESRs triggered by gastric distension with a barostat (14), gastric air distension (15), cholestyramine administration (16), oral administration of a liquid meal (17) or duodenal infusion of a liquid meal (18). These effects could not be demonstrated with infusion of CCK-33 (19), the hormonally acting form, suggesting that the effects are attributable to CCK acting as a neurotransmitter (20). Other interesting data pertain to morphine and atropine. Morphine decreased the number of tLESRs triggered by dextrose infusion into the stomach of GERD patients and this effect was blocked by nalaxone (21). Atropine potently inhibited tLESRs triggered by gastric distension or a meal in healthy subjects (22,23) or by a meal in GERD patients (24). Atropine, however, also reduces basal LES pressure and peristaltic efficacy (25), effects generally viewed as deleterious in GERD patients.

Hypotensive Lower Esophageal Sphincter

Physiologically, the LES is a 3–4-cm segment of tonically contracted smooth muscle at the distal end of the esophagus. Resting tone of the LES varies among normal individuals from 10 to 30 mmHg relative to intragastric pressure. Lower esophageal sphincter pressure is least in the postprandial period and greatest at night (2). Intra-abdominal pressure, gastric distension, peptides, hormones, various foods, and many drugs affect the LES pressure (Table 1). The mechanism of LES tonic contraction is not fully understood but seems to be a property of the muscle itself rather than of nerves affecting the sphincter. This conclusion is supported by the observation that pressure within the sphincter is minimally affected following the elimination of neural activity by close intra-arterial injection of tetrodotoxin (27). Furthermore, biochemical evidence suggests that the properties of the sphincter are defined by properties of the circular muscle. Specifically, the tonic contraction of the sphincter is not wholly associated with electrical transients (28,29), it has a lower resting membrane potential than the adjacent circular muscle (30,31), it exhibits increased passive permeability to potassium (32), and it seems to have a higher intracytosolic concentration of calcium (33). Sphincter tone may be maintained by the inositol phosphate–mediated continuous release of intracellular calcium. Although, inositol phosphates are found in higher concentrations in the LES than in adjacent circular muscle, resting sphincter tone is readily altered by exogenous agents such as hormones and a multitude of nerves as shown in Table 1. Further, 50–70% of LES tone of humans can be inhibited

Table 1 Substances Influencing LES Pressure

	Increase LES pressure	Decrease LES pressure
Hormones	Gastrin	Secretin
	Motilin	Cholecystokinin
	Substance P	Glucagon
		Somatostatin
		Gastric inhibitory polypeptide (GIP)
		Vasoactive intestinal polypeptide (VIP)
		Progesterone
Neural agents	α-Adrenergic agonists	α-Adrenergic antagonists
	β-Adrenergic antagonists	β-Adrenergic agonists
	Cholinergic agonists	Cholinergic antagonists
		Botulinum toxin
Foods	Protein	Fat
		Chocolate
		Ethanol
		Peppermint
Miscellaneous	Histamine	Theophylline
	Antacids	Prostaglandins E2 and I2
	Metoclopramide	Serotonin
	Domperidone	Meperidine
	Prostaglandin F2α	Morphine
	Cisapride	Dopamine
	Vecuronium	Calcium channel blockers
		Diazepam
		Barbiturates
		Nicotine
		Halothane
		Isoflurane
		Suxamethonium

Source: Modified from Ref. 26.

by atropine (25). Such influences may be especially important in modification of closure force in response to stimuli such as feeding and fasting.

Gastroesophageal reflux can occur with a diminished LES pressure by either strain-induced reflux or free reflux. Strain-induced reflux results when a hypotensive LES is overcome and ''blown open'' by an abrupt increase of intra-abdominal pressure (Fig. 2). Free reflux is characterized by a fall in intraesophageal pH without an identifiable change in either intragastric or LES pressure. Manometric data suggest that stress reflux or free reflux is relatively unusual, operant mainly when the LES pressure is less than 10 mmHg and 4 mmHg,

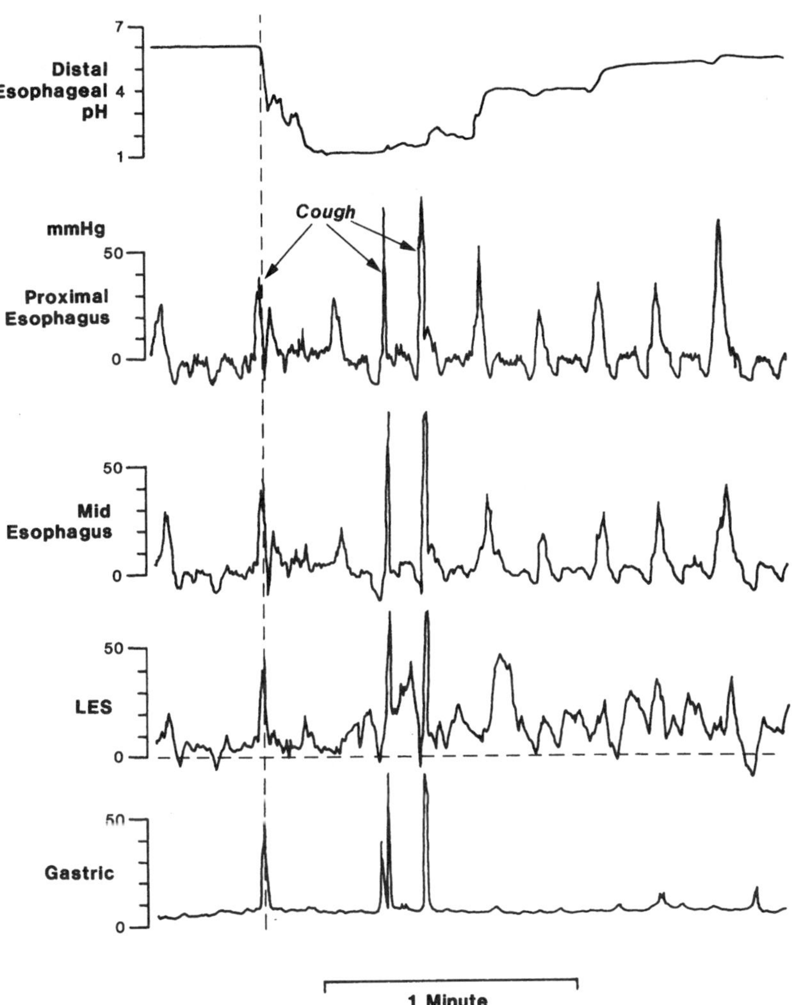

Figure 2 Example of stress reflux induced by coughing in an individual with a hypotensive LES. Lower-esophageal-sphincter pressure is referenced to gastric pressure with the horizontal dotted line (0 mmHg) representing mean intragastric pressure. Note the abrupt increase in intra-abdominal pressure associated with coughing and the associated episode of intraesophageal acidification. Although it is difficult to be exact, it appears that the resting LES pressure at the time of reflux was 8 mmHg. (From Ref. 5, with permission.)

respectively (34). However, it should be noted that these studies were not controlled for the potential activity-limiting effect of the required instrumentation (recumbent subjects reading or watching television with a manometric assembly and a pH probe in their nose), or of a hiatal hernia.

A puzzling clinical observation and one that supports the importance of tLESRs is that only a minority of individuals with GERD have an LES pressure of less than 10 mmHg when determined by isolated fasting measurements (35,36). This observation can be somewhat reconciled when one considers the dynamic nature of LES pressure. The isolated fasting measurement is probably useful only in identifying patients with a grossly hypotensive LES, i.e., individuals constantly susceptible to strain-induced reflux and perhaps sometimes susceptible to free reflux. However, there is probably a larger group of patients with mild or moderate GERD susceptible to strain-induced reflux when their LES pressure has been temporarily diminished as a result of specific foods, drugs, or habits (5) (see below).

The Diaphragmatic Sphincter, Hiatal Hernia, and Other Anatomical Variables

The esophagus is normally anchored to the diaphragm such that the stomach cannot be displaced through the hiatus into the mediastinum. The main restraining structures are the phrenoesophageal ligament and an aggregation of posterior structures including the vagus nerve, tributaries of the left gastric vein, and branches of the left gastric artery (37,38). The phrenoesophageal ligament is formed from the fascia transversalis on the undersurface of the diaphragm and fused elements of the endothoracic fascia. This elastic membrane inserts circumferentially into the esophageal musculature, close to the squamocolumnar junction, and extends for about a centimeter above the EGJ at which point it thins and merges with the perivisceral fascia of the esophagus (39). The axial position of the squamocolumnar junction is normally within or slightly distal to the diaphragmatic hiatus (40). The diaphragmatic hiatus is most commonly formed by the right diaphragmatic crus, which originates from the anterior longitudinal ligament over the upper lumbar vertebrae and inclines forward to arch around the esophagus. Once muscle fibers emerge from this tendinous origin, they form two overlying bundles that diverge and then cross each other in a scissor-like fashion as they approach the hiatus. The lateral fibers of each hiatal limb insert into the central tendon of the diaphragm, but the medial fibers, which form the hiatal margins, incline toward the midline and merge anteriorly in front of the esophagus (41). Although variations of this pattern exist, the basic organization of two flattened muscle bundles first diverging like a scissor and then merging anterior to the esophagus is common to all arrangements with about a centimeter of muscle separating the anterior rim of the hiatus from the central tendon of the diaphragm (Fig. 3).

With sliding hiatal hernia, there is a widening of the muscular hiatal tunnel and circumferential laxity of the phrenoesophageal ligament, allowing the gastric cardia to herniate upward. In marginal instances, sliding hiatal hernia is an exaggeration of the normal phrenic ampulla. Owing to this subtle distinction, estimates of hernia prevalence in adults vary enormously, from 10% to 80% (42). With a large hernia, the esophageal hiatus abuts directly on the central tendon of the diaphragm and the anterior hiatal muscles are absent or very atrophic (41). Associated with this, the phrenoesophageal ligament becomes attenuated but, nonetheless, remains intact containing the herniated gastric cardia within the posterior mediastinum (42). When a sliding hiatal hernia enlarges, such that >3 cm of gastric pouch is herniated upward, its presence becomes obvious because gastric folds are evident traversing the diaphragm. Although there are instances in which trauma, congenital malformation, or surgical manipulation can be implicated, sliding hiatal hernias are usually acquired, typically in the fifth decade of life (43). Pregnancy is also an inciting factor (38,44). Conceptually, Marchand argues that the compounded stresses of age-related degeneration, pregnancy, and obesity

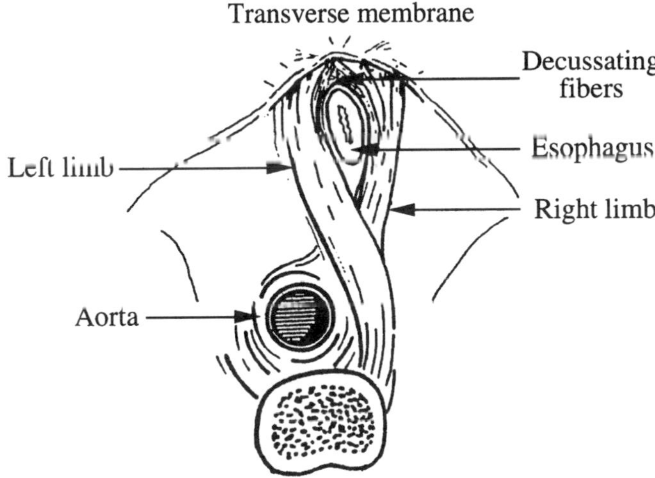

Figure 3 The most common anatomy of the diaphragmatic hiatus in which the muscular elements of the crural diaphragm derive from the right diaphragmatic crus. The right crus arises from the anterior longitudinal ligament overlying the lumbar vertebrae. Once muscular elements emerge from the tendon, two flat muscular bands form that cross each other in scissor-like fashion, form the walls of the hiatus, and decussate with each other anterior to the esophagus. (Modified from Ref. 41.)

take their toll on a relative weak point of the anatomy that is vulnerable to visceral herniation because it faces directly into the abdominal cavity. Furthermore, since the esophagus does not tightly fill the hiatus, the integrity of this opening depends upon its intrinsic structures, especially the phrenoesophageal ligament (41). Add to this vulnerability the repetitive stresses of coughing, respiration, Valsalva, vomiting, physiological herniation of swallowing, and postural change, and then compound the stress by packing the abdominal cavity with adipose tissue or a gravid uterus, and eventually the integrity of the hiatus is compromised. Another potential source of stress on the phrenoesophageal ligament is tonic contraction of the esophageal longitudinal muscle induced by reflux and mucosal acidification (45).

In contemplating the significance of hiatal hernia, it is instructive to read the work of Allison, who exhibited masterful understanding of the EGJ (43): ''and that the position of the stomach in relationship to the diaphragm is only important in so far as the diaphragm acts as a sphincter. . . . When the right crus of the diaphragm contracts, its action on the cardia is twofold: first, it compresses the walls of the esophagus from side to side, and second, it pulls down and increases the angulation of the esophagus.'' Allison also understood the analogy between the EGJ and the anal sphincters:

> The alimentary canal passes through two diaphragms, the thoracoabdominal and the pelvic. In each of these nature has adopted the same device to achieve continence. In each the canal is made to take a fairly abrupt bend, and at the bend is supported by an intrinsic and an extrinsic muscular mechanism. At the anorectal junction the internal sphincter is relatively well developed, but the main factor for continence is the puborectalis muscle which forms a lasso round the bend and hitches it forward to the back of the pubic bone. At the EGJ there is no thickening of the circular muscle fibers of the esophagus to form a sphincter, but the canal takes a bend forward and to the left, and this bend is lassoed and maintained by the right crus of the diaphragm which hitches it down to the lumbar spine.

As detailed below, recent investigations have now supported this ''two-sphincter hypothesis'' of EGJ competence (46,47).

Evidence of a specialized sphincteric role of the crural diaphragm begins with the observation that the costal and crural diaphragm can function independently. During esophageal distension, vomiting, and belching, electrical activity of the crural fibers is absent at the same time as the dome of the diaphragm is active, suggesting that the crural diaphragm is inhibited in some instances of LES relaxation (48,49). This reflex inhibition disappears with vagotomy (50). Conversely, crural contraction augments the EGJ with abrupt increases of intra-abdominal pressure as occur during inspiration, coughing, or abdominal straining (51). The importance of this mechanism was evident in studies of individuals with graded severity of hiatal hernia in whom the susceptibility to reflux with abrupt increases of intra-abdominal pressure depended upon both LES pressure and the presence of a hiatus hernia (52). When these data were modeled using a stepwise regression analysis that considered a host of anatomical and physiological factors as potential entry variables, the size of hiatal hernia was identified as having the highest correlation with the susceptibility to strain-induced reflux. The second significant factor was the instantaneous LES pressure, and the third was an interaction term between these two variables (Fig. 4) (52). The implication is that patients with hiatal hernia exhibit progressive impairment of EGJ compe-

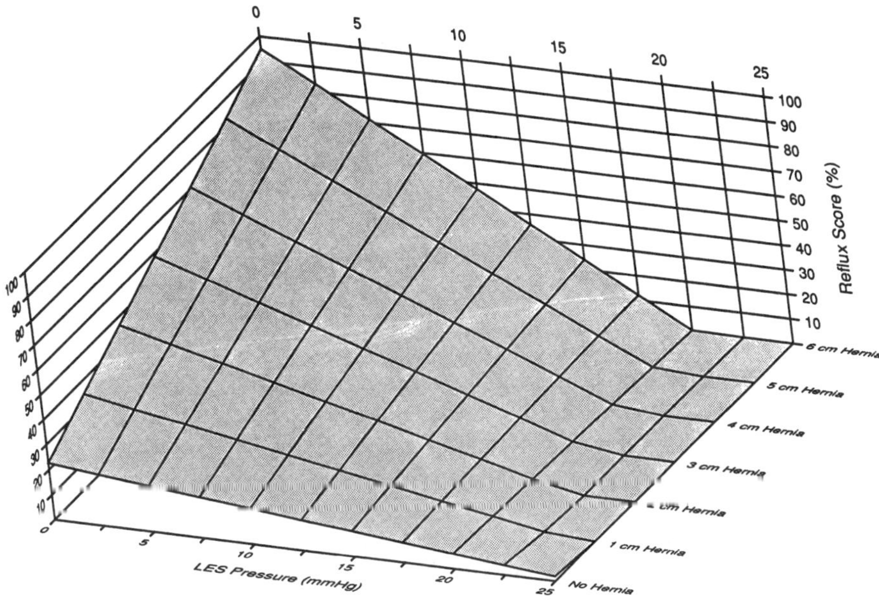

Figure 4 Model of the relationship between lower esophageal sphincter (LES) pressure, size of hernia and the susceptibility to gastroesophageal reflux induced by provocative maneuvers that increase intra-abdominal pressure as reflected by the reflux score on the Z-axis. The equation of the model is:

$$\text{Reflux score} = 22.64 + 12.05\,(\text{hernia size in cm}) - 0.83\,(\text{LESP}) - 0.65\,(\text{LESP} * \text{Hernia size})$$

The multiple correlation coefficient of this equation for the 50-subject data set was 0.86 ($r^2 = 0.75$). Thus, the susceptibility to stress reflux is dependent upon the interaction of the instantaneous LES pressure and the size of hiatal hernia. With progressive increase in the axial dimension of hiatal hernia, individuals are increasingly dependent upon the LES as an antireflux barrier and, hence, increasingly vulnerable to foods, habits, etc. that diminish the LES pressure. (From Ref. 52, with permission.)

tence proportional to the extent of axial herniation. Therefore, although neither hiatus hernia nor a hypotensive LES alone results in severe EGJ incompetence, the two conditions interact with each other according to the relationship graphed in Figure 4. This conclusion is consistent with the clinical experience that exercise, tight-fitting garments, and activities involving bending at the waist exacerbate heartburn in GERD in many patients (most of whom have a hiatal hernia), especially after having consumed meals that reduce LES pressure.

An interesting observation in the above investigation of hiatal hernia patients was that hiatal hernia size and LES pressure were inversely correlated suggesting that reduced LES pressure may be a consequence of hiatal hernia. Relevant animal data come from severing the phrenoesophageal ligament in dogs, analogous to the effect of axial hiatal hernia in which the ligament is stretched and its diaphragmatic attachments loosened (40,53). Severing the ligament substantially reduced peak EGJ pressure, which was then restored with reanastomosis (54). Analogous studies in humans include topographic analyis of the effect of hiatal hernia and hernia reduction on EGJ pressure (55). This was done with the aid of a mucosal clip, endoscopically placed at the squamocolumnar junction such that manometric, anatomical, and fluoroscopic data on the EGJ could be precisely correlated. As shown in Figure 5, topographic representation of the EGJ high-pressure zone of the hernia patients revealed separate intrinsic sphincter and hiatal canal pressure component, and repositioning the intrinsic sphincter back within this hiatal zone practically ''normalized'' the sphincter (55). These findings are consistent with an analysis by Klein et al. of the thoracoabdominal junction of 10 patients after resection of cancers at the EGJ; the ''sphincterless'' EGJ still exhibited an end-expiratory intraluminal pressure of 6 ± 1 mmHg (56). Perhaps, the only contradictory data are from diaphragmatic electromyographic (EMG) recordings, which support the notion of a phasic, but not tonic, diaphragmatic contribution to EGJ pressure (46,51,57). However, relying upon EMG recordings to completely represent the diaphragmatic contribution to EGJ pressure ignores the possible contribution of other forces such as diaphragmatic and ligamentous tension or elasticity to intraluminal pressure. Certainly, in the case of the upper-esophageal sphincter, such noncontractile forces contribute an intraluminal pressure of similar magnitude after experimental abolition of the myogenic tone (58).

The one aspect of the EGJ not normalized by the transposition illustrated in Figure 5 was the subdiaphragmatic segment, which was attenuated in the hiatal hernia subjects, even after transposition. This distal segment of the LES may be attributable to the sling fibers and clasp fibers of the gastric cardia, also referred to as the intra-abdominal segment of the esophagus (59,60). This is probably the most confusing segment of esophageal anatomy, referred to by Inglefinger as an anatomical and functional ''no-man's-land'' (61). Highlighting this confusion, Wolf remarked, ''It is indeed strange that, when normally located below the hiatus, the 'submerged segment' resembles the esophagus while, when displaced above the hiatus, it resembles stomach. In fact, when a large hiatal hernia is

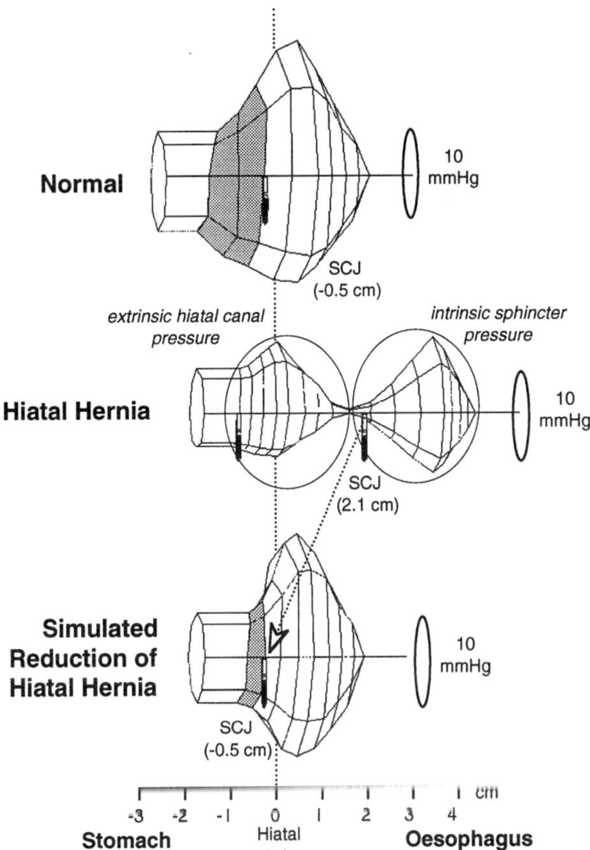

Figure 5 Pressure topography of the EGJ of normal subjects (top) and hiatal hernia patients (center). Position zero on the axial scale at the bottom is the midpoint of the diaphragmatic hiatus. The wire-frame representations are rotated such that the right anterior pressure is at the top and left posterior pressure is at the bottom, thereby accentuating the radial pressure asymmetry. The proximal clip indicates the median position of the squamocolumnar junction (SCJ) and the distal clip marks the median position of the intragastric aspect to the EGJ as imaged endoscopically. All values of length and pressure are the medians of the seven subjects in each subject group. Simulation of reducing the hiatus hernia (bottom) was done by algebraically repositioning the pressure values of the intrinsic LES (pressure peak proximal to the squamocolumnar junction) to within the extrinsically determined pressure of the hiatal canal. For each subject the positioning of the proximal high pressure zone was such that the squamocolumnar junction mucosal clip attained the median normal position, 0.5 cm distal to the hiatus. The shaded area indicates the portion of the sphincter segment distal to the squamocolumnar junction in the normals and in the transposed panels. All values of length and pressure are the medians of the subject groups. (From Ref. 55, with permission.)

present, the original submerged segment is incorporated into the hernia sac'' (62). Lieberman-Meffert et al. described a ''fold transition line,'' evident in postmortem specimens, which appears analogous to the intragastric margin of the EGJ as imaged endoscopically and related to the angle of His as identified externally (59). The squamocolumnar junction was 10.5 ± 4.4 mm proximal to the fold transition line when measured along the greater curvature. Although the relevance of this distal sphincter segment is controversial, Hill et al. found the integrity of this ''flap valve'' to correlate with EGJ competence against an antegrade pressure gradient in postmortem experiments (Fig. 6) (63). With progressive proximal

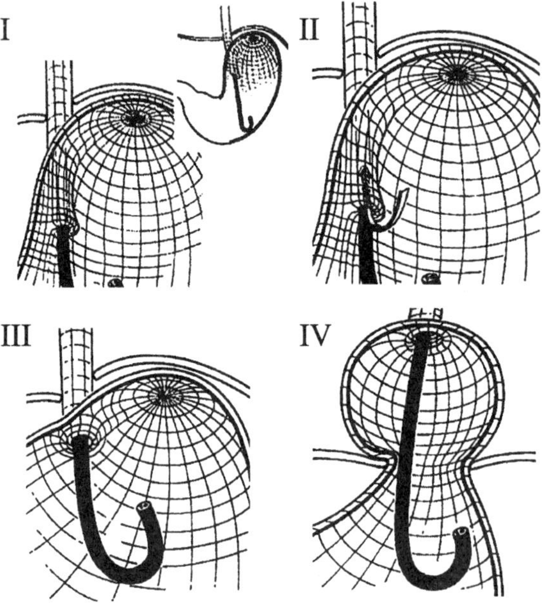

Figure 6 Three-dimensional representation of the progressive anatomical disruption of the gastroesophageal junction as occurs with development of an axial (sliding) hiatal hernia. In the grade I configuration (upper left), a ridge of muscular tissue is closely approximated to the shaft of the retroflexed endoscope. In the grade II configuration (upper right), the ridge of tissue is slightly less well defined and there has been slight orad displacement of the squamocolumnar junction along with widening of the angle of His. In the grade III appearance (lower left), the ridge of tissue at the gastric entryway is barely present and there is often incomplete luminal closure around the endoscope. Grade III deformity is nearly always accompanied by an obvious hiatal hernia. With grade IV deformity (lower right), no muscular ridge is present at the gastric entry. The gastroesophageal area stays open all the time, and squamous epithelium of the distal esophagus can be seen from the retroflexed endoscopic view. A hiatal hernia is always present. (Modified from Ref. 63.)

displacement of the squamocolumnar junction above the hiatus, this distal segment eventually becomes disrupted and splays open, creating a radiographically evident saccular structure identifiable as a nonreducing hiatal hernia (53). These observations suggest that shortening of the LES high-pressure zone commented on by surgeons as indicative of a mechanically defective sphincter (60,64,65) is probably related to anatomical changes in this region. In a recent investigation, Ismail et al. studied ''yield pressure'' of four subject groups graded by the visual integrity of the cardia when viewed endoscopically (64). They found a direct correlation between the ability of the cardia to withstand intragastric pressure and both the grade of cardia integrity and the size of hiatal hernia; no correlation was found with LES pressure.

Evident from the above discussion, retrograde competence of the EGJ is dependent upon several anatomical and physiological variables. Investigators have attempted to model EGJ competence in vitro using either excised cadaveric esophagi (66,67) or flaccid rubber tubes in pressure chambers (68). Although the precise findings vary with the details of the models, universal findings among investigators were that reflux frequency was inversely proportional to sphincter length and was exacerbated by an intrathoracic location of the sphincter. A model that included simulated respiration found that the associated cyclic pressure variations further increased the vulnerability to reflux (68). All models suggest that EGJ competence is a mechanical rather than a pharmacological or physiological process. However, this is not surprising because, by their very nature, in vitro models are limited in the physiological variables that can be introduced; none has attempted to simulate crural diaphragm contraction, dynamic changes in the angle of His, reflexive changes in LES tone, or the anatomical configuration of the cardia. Thus, although they provide useful data for understanding the contribution of some of the anatomical variables that contribute to EGJ competence, in vitro models cannot enhance our understanding of the complexities of the EGJ beyond that. Lacking are data on the interplay between anatomical variables and physiological responses. Obtaining these data will depend upon expanding our conceptualization of the EGJ beyond an ''either/or'' paradigm to a recognition that, just as GERD exists along a continuum of severity, so do the contributing pathophysiological factors. Only when these data are in hand will it be possible to truly model the integrity of the EGJ, and that will require mathematical simulation based on actual anatomical and physiological data.

ESOPHAGEAL ACID CLEARANCE

Following reflux, the period that the esophageal mucosa remains at a pH < 4 is defined as the acid clearance time. Acid clearance begins with emptying the refluxed fluid from the esophagus by peristalsis and is completed by titration of the residual acid by swallowed saliva (Fig. 7) (69). It takes about 7 mL of saliva to neutralize 1 mL of 0.1 N HCl with 50% of this neutralizing capacity attributable to salivary bicarbonate, and the typical rate of salivation is 0.5 mL/min (70). Thus, with normal esophageal emptying, increasing salivation with oral lozenges or gum chewing will hasten acid clearance. Of note, salivation virtually ceases during sleep, severely compromising the mechanism of acid clearance when re-

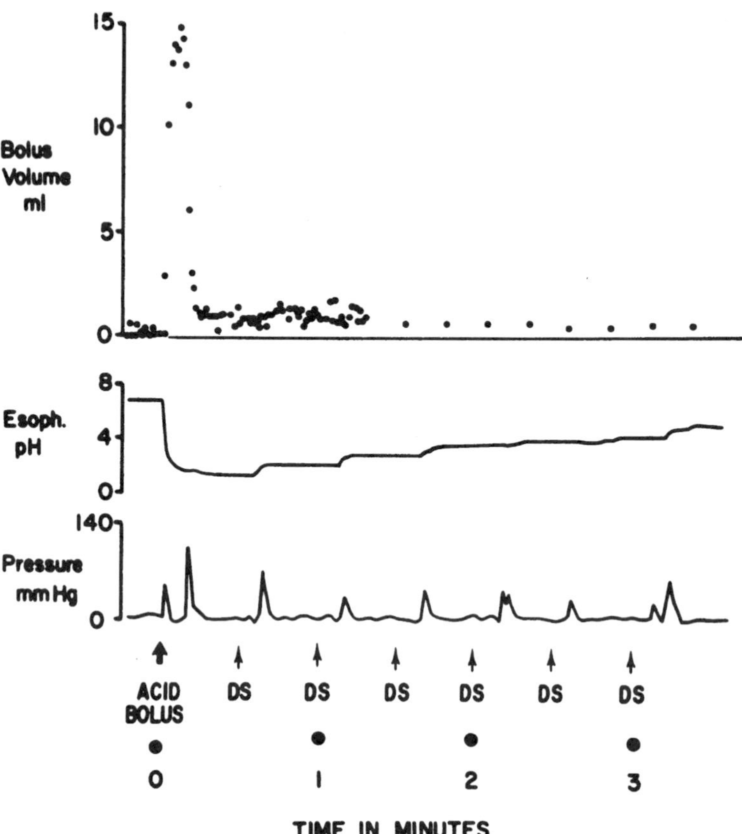

Figure 7 Relationship between esophageal peristalsis, distal esophageal pH, esophageal volume clearance, and esophageal acid clearance during an acid clearance test done with radiolabeled 0.1 N HCl. The calculation of bolus volume within the esophagus is derived from scintiscanning over the chest. DS denotes dry swallow. Note that, although all but about 1 mL of the infused fluid is cleared from the esophagus by the first peristaltic contraction, the distal esophageal pH remains unchanged. Stepwise increases in distal esophageal pH occur with subsequent swallows. (From Ref. 69, with permission.)

flux occurs during, or immediately prior to, sleep. However, some acid clearance is probably achieved during sleep by bicarbonate secretion from esophageal submucosal glands (71,72).

Prolongation of esophageal acid clearance among patients with esophagitis was demonstrated along with the initial description of an acid clearance test. Subsequent investigations have demonstrated heterogeneity within the patient population such that only about half of GERD patients have prolonged values. Of greatest relevance, a review of a large data set on 24-h esophageal pH recordings also suggested heterogeneity within the population of patients with symptomatic reflux disease such that individuals with known hiatal hernias tended to have the most prolonged recumbent acid clearance times (73). From what we know regarding the mechanisms of acid clearance, the two major potential causes of prolonged esophageal acid clearance are impaired esophageal emptying and impaired salivary function.

Esophageal Emptying in GERD

Patients with abnormal acid clearance show improvement with an upright posture suggesting that gravity can be used to augment impaired fluid emptying. Two mechanisms of impaired esophageal emptying have been identified: peristaltic dysfunction and "rereflux" associated with some hiatal hernias. Peristaltic dysfunction in esophagitis has been described by a number of investigators. Of particular significance are the occurrence of failed peristaltic contractions and hypotensive (<30 mmHg) peristaltic contractions that incompletely empty the esophagus (74). Peristaltic dysfunction is increasingly common with increasing severity of esophagitis (36). Recently, the term "ineffective esophageal motility" has been applied to this type of peristaltic dysfunction, defined by the occurrence of $\geq$30% ineffective contractions (amplitude < 30 mmHg or failed peristalsis) out of 10 test swallows. Patients with ineffective esophageal motility exhibit significantly greater recumbent esophageal acid exposure time and longer esophageal acid clearance time than individuals with normal esophageal motility, diffuse esophageal spasm, hypertensive LES, or "nutcracker esophagus" (75). Whether or not peristaltic dysfunction associated with peptic esophagitis is reversible is disputed. Most likely, acute dysfunction associated with active esophagitis is at least partially reversible but that associated with structuring or extensive fibrosis is not. Indeed, esophageal motor function was unchanged after healing of esophagitis by acid inhibition (76) or by antireflux surgery (77).

Hiatal hernias also impair esophageal emptying. Concurrent pH recording and scintiscanning show rereflux from the hernia sac during swallowing with most hiatal hernias (78). A more recent analysis categorized hernias as reducing or nonreducing depending upon whether they were evident only during peristalsis-induced esophageal shortening (79). Each subject performed 10 barium swallows and the outcome of each in terms of esophageal emptying was noted. Possible outcomes were of complete clearance, minimal clearance because of failed peristalsis, late retrograde flow of barium from the ampulla back up the tubular esophagus (Fig. 8), or early retrograde flow from the ampulla (rereflux) occurring coincident with LES relaxation (Fig. 9). The overall efficacy of esophageal emptying was significantly impaired in both hiatal hernia groups but it was especially

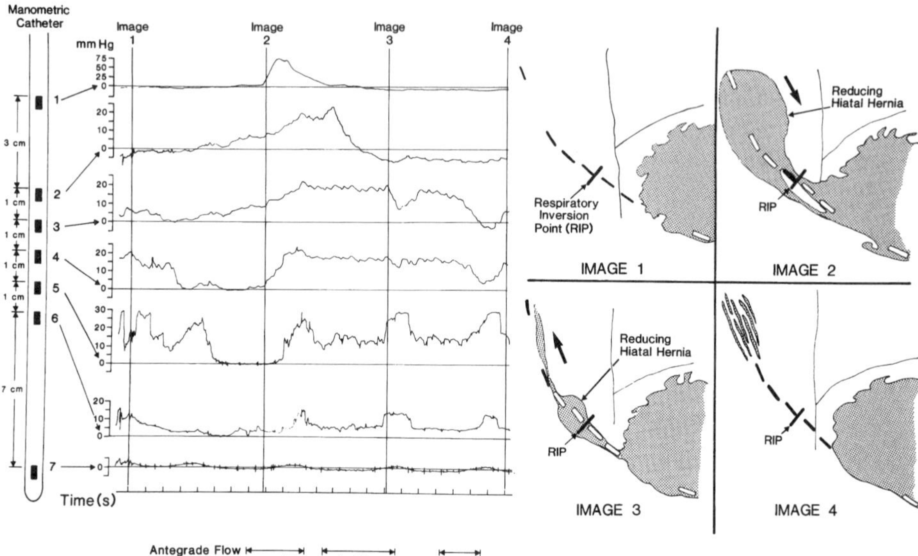

Figure 8 Concurrent manometric and videofluorographic recording of a 10-mL barium swallow in a subject with a reducing hiatal hernia characterized by late retrograde flow. The tracings from the video images on the right correspond to the four selected times from the swallowing sequence indicated by the numbers at the top of the vertical lines intersecting the manometric record. The schematic diagram to the left indicates the relative spacing of the pressure sensing ports (side holes located proximal to the markers in the fluoroscopic images). The lines at the bottom of the tracing indicate the timing and direction of barium flow. Image #1 depicts the instant of swallowing when barium was visible only in the stomach. Image #2 depicts the instant the stripping wave was at the level of the most proximal sensor; the hiatal hernia had formed and sensors #2, #3, and #4 were in a common cavity within the hernia. Image #3 depicts when retrograde flow began at which point sensors #2 and #3 were above the hernia, sensor #4 was measuring intrahernial pressure, sensors #5 and #6 were at the level of the diaphragm, and sensor #7 remained within the stomach. Image #4 shows residual barium in the distal esophagus and no hiatal hernia with sensors #3, #4, #5, and #6 now straddling the high-pressure zone comprised of the LES and diaphragm. (From Ref. 79, with permission.)

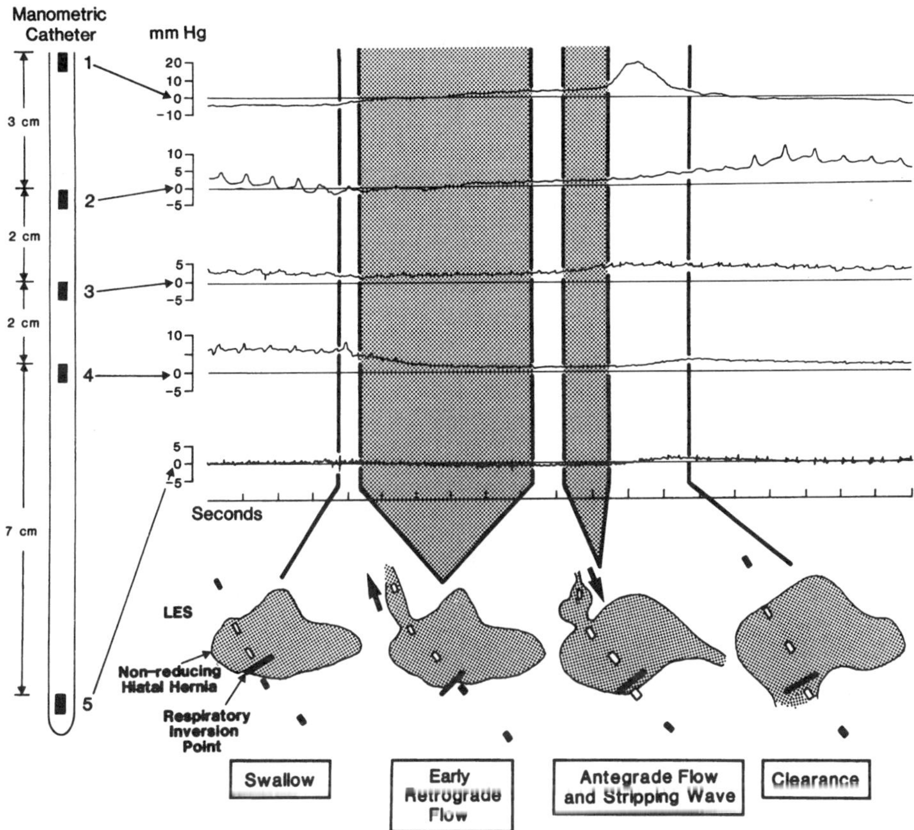

Figure 9 Concurrent manometric and fluoroscopic recording of a 10-mL barium swallow with early retrograde flow in a subject with a nonreducing hiatal hernia. Tracings below the manometric record correspond to the times on the manometric tracings intersected by the vertical lines. The schematic diagram to the left depicts the spacing of the pressure sensors. The arrows next to the images indicate the direction of barium flow. The first image to the far left shows a barium-filled hiatal hernia at the time of swallow with sensor #1 in the distal esophagus, sensor #2 in the LES, sensor #3 within the hernia, sensor #4 measuring crural contractile activity, and sensor #5 within the abdominal stomach. The second image, 1 s after the swallow, depicts the onset of retrograde flow; intrahernial pressure was 2 mmHg and LES pressure was 0 mmHg. Retrograde flow continued for 5 s until the peristaltic contraction reached the distal esophagus. The third image depicts antegrade flow with the stripping wave progressing down the esophagus and LES pressure increasing to equal intrahernia pressure (~4 mmHg). The final image to the far right shows barium cleared from the esophagus with the LES pressure now exceeding intrahernial pressure. (From Ref. 79, with permission.)

poor in the group with nonreducing hernias. The group with nonreducing hernias had complete emptying in only one-third of test swallows and exhibited early retrograde flow, a phenomenon unique to this group, in almost half.

Observations made on normal subjects offer some insight into the mechanism of early retrograde flow seen in nonreducing hernia patients (80). Under normal circumstances, LES relaxation is evident within 3 s of the swallow. However, sphincter (ampullary) opening is not evident until it is distended by the bolus being propelled by esophageal peristalsis, 5–10 s later. Thus, relaxation and opening of the LES do not occur simultaneously. Mechanistically, for opening to occur, pressure acting on the lumen of the sphincter must exceed the pressure surrounding the sphincter. However, because the normal position of the distal esophagus is intra-abdominal, intragastric pressure acting to open the sphincter is negated by the external pressure of equal magnitude. The effect of eliminating this intra-abdominal segment is evident with nonreducing hernias. Although hernia and nonhernia subjects demonstrated complete LES relaxation following each swallow, only the nonreducing hernia group demonstrated early retrograde flow. During early retrograde flow events, the LES opens from below immediately following swallow-induced LES relaxation. For this to occur, intragastric pressure within the sphincter must exceed the extrasphincteric pressure, indicating that the extrasphincteric pressure was less than intra-abdominal pressure (i.e., closer to intrathoracic pressure) in these individuals.

Another mechanism promoting EGJ competence during esophageal emptying is the crural diaphragm (79). In normal individuals the esophageal ampulla fills from above as the bolus is propelled ahead of the peristaltic contraction. As the peristaltic contraction arrives at the distal esophagus, intra-ampullary pressure increases to about 10 mmHg at which time ampullary emptying begins (80). During emptying, the diaphragmatic crura function as a one-way valve. During expiration, at which time the esophageal-gastric pressure gradient favors antegrade flow, the crus is relaxed and visibly open. However, during inspiration when intra-abdominal pressure increases, the crus contracts and closes, preventing gastroesophageal flow. The valvular effect of the crural diaphragm is impaired with nonreducing hernias because a gastric pouch persists above the diaphragm, thereby disabling this one-way valve function.

Salivary Function in GERD

Just as impaired esophageal emptying prolongs acid clearance, reduced salivary rate or diminished salivary neutralizing capacity has the same effect. Diminished salivation during sleep, for instance, explains why reflux events during sleep or immediately prior to going to sleep are associated with markedly prolonged acid clearance times. Similarly, chronic xerostomia is associated with prolonged esophageal acid exposure and esophagitis (81). However, there has been no convincing systematic difference found in the salivary function of GERD patients compared to controls (82). One group of subjects shown to have prolonged esophageal acid clearance times due to hyposalivation is cigarette smokers. Even those without symptoms of reflux disease were found to have acid clearance times 50% longer than those of nonsmokers and the salivary titratable base content of the smokers was only 60% of that of the age-matched nonsmokers (83). Reduced salivation of cigarette smokers is mediated by an anticholinergic effect similar to that observed in patients using anticholinergic medications.

In addition to bicarbonate, saliva contains a number of growth factors that have the potential to enhance mucosal repair. Epidermal growth factor (EGF), produced primarily in duodenal Brunner's glands and submaxillary ductal cells, has been the most extensively studied (84). In animal models, epidermal growth factor has been shown to provide cytoprotection against irritants, enhance the healing of gastroduodenal ulceration, and decrease the permeability of the esophageal mucosa to hydrogen ion (85–87). One group of investigators found reduced salivary EGF secretion in response to intraesophageal exposure to an acid/pepsin solution in patients with grade II esophagitis compared to controls (88). However, studies have not shown consistent differences in EGF concentration in esophagitis or Barrett's patients (89). Thus, at present it is not possible to implicate perturbations of EGF secretion (or other growth factors) in the pathogenesis of GERD or its complications.

SUMMARY

A fundamental abnormality in GERD is excessive reflux of gastric contents across the EGJ. Guarding against this, the EGJ is composed of a smooth muscle element (the LES), specialized anatomy, and the crural diaphragm. This high degree of anatomical and physiological specialization is designed to minimize reflux at rest, during dynamic stresses associated with increased intra-abdominal pressure, and during deglutitive LES relaxation, while at the same time selectively permitting belching. When reflux does occur, it is attributable to tLESRs, abdominal straining, or extreme LES hypotension. Virtually all reflux events occurring during periods of normal LES pressure occur by tLESR. Susceptibility to strain-induced reflux (abrupt increase in intra-abdominal pressure) is inversely proportional to LES pressure. Furthermore, this susceptibility is increased by anatomical compromise of the EGJ, exemplified by hiatal hernia. In addition to the occurrence of reflux events, esophageal acid exposure is also related to the process of acid clearance, which depends upon effective esophageal emptying and neutralization of residual acid by swallowed saliva. Esophageal emptying can be impaired in GERD patients either because of impaired peristalsis or because of hiatal hernia. Failed peristalsis and hypotensive peristalsis are common in chronic

GERD. Hiatal hernias also impair the process of esophageal emptying (and consequently acid clearance) by permitting retrograde flow of gastric juice during deglutitive LES relaxation. These functional impairments of the EGJ associated with hiatal hernia lead to increased esophageal acid exposure and offer one explanation for the observed chronicity of reflux disease.

REFERENCES

1. Barham CP, Gotley DC, Alderson D. Precipitating causes of acid reflux episodes in ambulant patients with gastro-oesophageal reflux disease. Gut 1995; 36:505–510.
2. Dent J, Dodds WJ, Friedman RH, Sekiguchi T, Hogan WJ, Arndorfer RC, Petrie DJ. Mechanism of gastroesophageal reflux in recumbent asymptomatic human subjects. J Clin Invest 1980; 65:256–267.
3. Dodds WJ, Dent J, Hogan WJ, Helm JF, Hauser RG, Patel GW, Egide M. Mechanisms of gastroesophageal reflux in patients with reflux esophagitis. N Engl J Med 1982; 307:1547–1552.
4. Mittal RK, Holloway RH, Penagini R, Blackshaw LA, Dent J. Transient lower esophageal sphincter relaxation. Gastroenterology 1995; 109:601–610.
5. Kahrilas PJ, Gupta RR. Mechanisms of acid reflux associated with cigarette smoking. Gut 1990; 31:4–10.
6. Holloway RH, Penagini R, Ireland AC. Criteria for objective definition of transient lower esophageal sphincter relaxation. Am J Physiol 1995; 268:G128–G133.
7. Kahrilas PJ, Dodds WJ, Dent J, Wyman JB, Hogan WJ, Arndorfer RC. Upper esophageal sphincter function during belching. Gastroenterology 1986; 91:133–140.
8. Wyman JB, Dent J, Heddle R, Dodds WJ, Toouli J, Downton J. Control of belching by the lower esophageal sphincter. Gut 1990; 31:639–646.
9. Martin C, Dodds WJ, Liem H, Dantas R, Layman R, Dent J. Diaphragmatic contribution to gastroesophageal competence and reflux in dogs. Am J Physiol 1992; 263: G551–G557.
10. Trifan A, Shaker R, Ren JL, Mittal RK, Saeian K, Dua K, Kusano M. Inhibition of resting lower esophageal sphincter pressure by oropharyngeal water stimulation in humans. Gastroenterology 1995; 108:441–446.
11. Mittal RK, Chiareli C, Liu J, Shaker R. Characteristics of lower esophageal sphincter relaxation induced by pharyngeal stimulation with minute amounts of water. Gastroenterology 1996; 111:378–384.
12. Mittal RK, Stewart WR, Schirmer BD. Effect of a catheter in the pharynx on the frequency of transient lower esophageal sphincter relaxations. Gastroenterology 1992; 103:1236–1240.
13. Boulant J, Fioramonti J, Dapoigny M, Bommelear G, Bueno L. Cholecystokinin and nitric oxide in transient esophageal sphincter relaxation to gastric distention in dogs. Gastroenterology 1994; 107:1059–1066.
14. Boulant J, Mathieu S, D'Amato M, Abergel A, Dapoigny M, Bommelear G. Cholecystokinin in transient lower oesophageal sphincter relaxation duo to gastric distension in humans. Gut 1997; 40:575–581.

15. Boeckxstaens GE, Hirsh DP, Fakhry N, Holloway RH, D'Amato M, Tytgat GNJ. Involvement of cholecystokinin A receptors in transient lower esophageal sphincter relaxations triggered by gastric distension. Am J Gastroenterol 1998; 93:1823–1828.
16. Clave P, Gonzalez Moreno A, Lopez R, Farre A, Cusso X, D'Amato M, Azipiroz F, Lluis F. Endogenous cholecystokinin enhances postprandial gastroesophageal reflux in humans through extrasphincteric receptors. Gastroenterology 1998; 115:597–604.
17. Zerbib F, Bruley des Varannes S, D'Amto M, Scarpignato C, Galmiche JP. Effect of the CCK-A receptor anatagonist Loxiglumide on gastric tone and transient lower esophageal sphincter relaxations in humans. Gastroenterology 1997; 112:A857.
18. Zerbib F, Bruley des Varannes S, D'Amto M, Scarpignato C, Galmiche JP. Effect of Loxiglumide on lower esophageal sphincter motor events and gastric relaxation induced by duodenal infusion of a liquid meal in healthy subjects. Gastroenterology 1998; 114:A863.
19. Ledeboer M, Masclee AAM, Batatra MR, Jansen JBMJ, Lamers CBHW. Effect of cholecystokinin on lower oesophageal sphincter pressure and transient lower oesophageal sphincter relaxations in humans. Gut 1995; 36:39–44.
20. Fioramonti J, Bueno J, Boulant J, Dapoigny M, Bommelaer G. Cholecystokinin and transient lower oesophageal sphincter relaxation (letter; comment). Gut 1995; 37: 298.
21. Penagini R, Bianchi PA. Effect of morphine on gastroesophageal reflux and transient lower esophageal sphincter relaxation. Gastroenterology 1997; 113:409–414.
22. Mittal RK, Holloway R, Dent J. Effect of atropine on the frequency of reflux and transient lower esophageal sphincter relaxation in normal subjects. Gastroenterology 1995; 109:1547–1554.
23. Mittal RK, Chiareli C, Liu J, Holloway RH, Dixon Jr W. Atropine inhibits gastric distension and pharyngeal receptor mediated lower oesophageal sphincter relaxation. Gut 1997; 41:285–290.
24. Lidums I, Checklin H, Mittal RK, Holloway RH. Effect of atropine on gastro-oesophageal reflux and transient lower oesophageal sphincter relaxations in patients with gastro-oesophageal reflux disease. Gut 1998; 43:12–16.
25. Dodds WJ, Dent J, Hogan WJ, Arndorfer RC. Effect of atropine on esophageal motor function in humans. Am J Physiol 1981; 240:G290–G296.
26. Diamant NE. Physiology of the esophagus. In: Sleisenger MH, Fordtran JS, eds. Gastrointestinal Disease-Pathophysiology, Diagnosis, Management, 4th ed. Philadelphia: WB Saunders, 1989: 548–559.
27. Goyal RK, Rattan S. Genesis of basal sphincter pressure: effect of tetrodotoxin on lower esophageal sphincter pressure in opossum in vivo. Gastroenterology 1976; 71:62–67.
28. Asoh R, Goyal RK. Electrical activity of the opossum lower esophageal sphincter in vivo. Gastroenterology 1978; 74:835–840.
29. Zelcer E, Weisbrodt NW. Electrical and mechanical activity of the lower esophageal sphincter in the cat. Am J Physiol 1984; 246:G243–G247.
30. Dektor DL, Ryan JP. Transmembrane voltage of opossum esophageal smooth muscle and its response to electrical stimulation of intrinsic nerves. Gastroenterology 1982; 82:301–308.

31. Kannan MS, Jagler LP, Daniel EE. Electrical properties of smooth muscle cell membrane of opossum esophagus. Am J Physiol 1985; 248:G342–G346.
32. Schulze K, Hajjar JJ, Christensen J. Regional differences in potassium content of smooth muscle from opossum esophagus. Am J Physiol 1978; 235:E709–E713.
33. Schlippert W, Schulze K, Forker EL. Calcium in smooth muscle from the opossum esophagus. Proc Soc Exp Biol Med 1979; 162:354.
34. Dent J, Dodds WJ, Hogan WJ, Toouli J. Factors that influence induction of gastroesophageal reflux in normal human subjects. Dig Dis Sci 1988; 33:270–275.
35. Behar J, Biancani P, Sheahan DG. Evaluation of esophageal tests in the diagnosis of reflux esophagitis. Gastroenterology 1976; 71:9–15.
36. Kahrilas PJ, Dodds WJ, Hogan WJ, Kern M, Arndorfer RC, Reece A. Peristaltic dysfunction in peptic esophagitis. Gastroenterology 1986; 91:897–904.
37. Barrett NR. Discussion on hiatus hernia. Proc R Soc Med 1932; 122:736–796.
38. Rigler LG, Eneboe JB. Incidence of hiatus hernia in pregnant women and its significance. J Thorac Surg 1935; 4:262–268.
39. Low A. A note on the crura of the diaphragm and the muscle of Treitsz. J Anat Lond 1907; 42:93–96.
40. Kahrilas PJ, Wu S, Lin S, Pouderoux P. Attenuation of esophageal shortening during peristalsis with hiatus hernia. Gastroenterology 1995; 109:1818–1825.
41. Marchand P. The anatomy of esophageal hiatus of the diaphragm and the pathogenesis of hiatus herniation. Thorac Surg 1959; 37:81–92.
42. Skinner DB, Roth JLA, Sullivan BH, Stein GN, Levine M. Reflux Esophagitis. In: Berk, JE editor in chief. Gastroenterology, 4th ed. Philadelphia: WB Saunders, 1985: 717–768.
43. Allison PR. Reflux esophagitis, sliding hiatal hernia, and the anatomy of repair. Surg Gynecol Obstet 1951; 92:419–431.
44. Evans JR, Bouslog JS. Hiatus hernia. Radiology 1940; 34:530–535.
45. Paterson WG, Kolyn DM. Esophageal shortening induced by short-term intraluminal acid perfusion in opossum: a cause of hiatus hernia? Gastroenterology 1994; 107: 1736–1740.
46. Boyle JT, Altschuler SM, Nixon TE, Tuchman DN, Pack AI, Cohen S. Role of the diaphragm in the genesis of lower esophageal sphincter pressure in the cat. Gastroenterology 1985; 88:723–730.
47. Mittal RK, Balaban DH. The esophagogastric junction. N Engl J Med 1997; 336: 924–932.
48. Altschuler SM, Boyle JT, Nixon TE, Pack AI, Cohen S. Simultaneous reflex inhibition of lower esophageal sphincter and crural diaphragm in cats. Am J Physiol 1985; 249:G586–G591.
49. Monges H, Salducci J, Naudy B. Dissociation between the electrical activity of the diaphragmatic dome and crura muscular fibers during esophageal distension, vomiting and eructation, an electromyographic study in the dog. J Physiol Paris 1978; 74:541–554.
50. De Troyer A, Rosso J. Reflex inhibition of the diaphragm by esophageal afferents. Neurosci Lett 1982; 30:43–46.
51. Mittal RK, Fisher M, McCallum RW, Rochester DF, Dent J, Sluss J. Human lower

esophageal sphincter pressure response to increased intra-abdominal pressure. Am J Physiol 1990; 258:G624–G630.
52. Sloan S, Rademaker AW, Kahrilas PJ. Determinants of gastroesophageal junction incompetence: hiatus hernia, lower esophageal sphincter, or both? Ann Intern Med 1992; 117:977–982.
53. Friedland GW. Historical review of the changing concepts of lower esophageal sphincter anatomy. Am J Roentgenol 1978; 131:373–388.
54. Michelson E, Siegel CI. The role of the phrenico-esophageal ligament in the lower esophageal sphincter. Surg Gynecol Obstet 1964; 118:1291–1294.
55. Kahrilas PJ, Lin S, Chen J, Manka M. The effect of hiatus hernia on gastro-oesophageal junction pressure. Gut 1999; 44:483–489.
56. Klein WA, Parkman HP, Dempsey DT, Fisher RS. Sphincterlike thoracoabdominal high pressure zone after esophagogastrectomy. Gastroenterology 1993; 105:1362–1369.
57. Mittal RK, Rochester DF, McCallum RW. Electrical and mechanical activity in the human lower esophageal sphincter during diaphragmatic contraction. J Clin Invest 1988; 81:1182–1189.
58. Asoh R, Goyal RK. Manometry and electromyography of the upper esophageal sphincter in the opossum. Gastroenterology 1978; 74:514–520.
59. Lieberman-Meffert D, Allgöwer M, Schmid P, Blum AL. Muscular equivalent of the lower esophageal sphincter. Gastroenterology 1979; 76:32–38.
60. Zaninotto G, DeMeester TR, Schwizer W, Johansson KE, Cheng JC. The lower esophageal sphincter in health and disease. Am J Surg 1988; 155:104–111.
61. Ingelfinger FJ. Esophageal motility. Physiol Rev 1958; 38:533–584.
62. Wolf BS. Sliding hiatal hernia: the need for redefinition. Am J Roentgenol 1973; 117:231–247.
63. Hill LD, Kozarek RA, Kraemer SJM, Aye RW, Mercer CD, Low DE, Pope II CE. The gastroesophageal flap valve: in vitro and in vivo observations. Gastrointest Endosc 1996; 44:541–547.
64. Ismail T, Bancewicz J, Barlow J. Yield pressure, anatomy of the cardia and gastrooesophageal reflux. Br J Surg 1995; 82:943–947.
65. Stein HJ, DeMeester TR, Naspetti R, Jamieson J, Perry RE. Three-dimensional imaging of the lower esophageal sphincter in gastroesophageal reflux disease. Ann Surg 1991; 214:374–384.
66. Bonavina L, Evander A, DeMeester TR, Walther B, Cheng SC, Palazzo L, Concannon JL. Length of the distal esophageal sphincter and competency of the cardia. Am J Surg 1986; 151:25–34.
67. DeMeester TR, Wernly JA, Bryant GH, Little AG, Skinner DB. Clinical and in vitro determinants of gastroesophageal junction competence: a study of the principles of antireflux surgery. Am J Surg 1979; 137:39–46.
68. Kadirkamanathan SS, Evans DF, Swain CP. The mechanical model of gastroesophageal reflux: what are the most important factors causing gastroesophageal reflux? In: Giuli R, Galmiche JP, Jamieson GG, Scarpignato C, eds. The Esophagogastric Junction 420 Questions—420 Answers. Montrouge, France: John Libbey Eurotext, 1998:340–345.
69. Helm JF, Dodds WJ, Pelc LR, Palmer DW, Hogan WJ, Teeter BC. Effect of esopha-

geal emptying and saliva on clearance of acid from the esophagus. N Engl J Med 1984; 310:284–288.
70. Helm JF, Dodds WJ, Hogan WJ, Soergel KH, Egide MS, Wood CM. Acid neutralizing capacity of human saliva. Gastroenterology 1982; 83:69–74.
71. Myers RL, Orlando RC. In vivo bicarbonate secretion by human esophagus. Gastroenterology 1992; 103:1174–1178.
72. Singh S, Bradley LA, Richter JE. Determinants of oesophageal ''alkaline'' pH environment in controls and patients with gastro-oesophageal reflux disease. Gut 1993; 34:309–316.
73. Johnson LF. 24-hour pH monitoring in the study of gastroesophageal reflux. J Clin Gastroenterol 1980; 2:387–399.
74. Kahrilas PJ, Dodds WJ, Hogan WJ. Effect of peristaltic dysfunction on esophageal volume clearance. Gastroenterology 1988; 4:73–80.
75. Leite LP, Johnston BT, Barrett J, Castell JA, Castell DO. Ineffective esophageal motility (IEM): the primary finding in patients with nonspecific esophageal motility disorder. Dig Dis Sci 1997; 42:1859–1865.
76. Timmer R, Breumelhof R, Nadorp JH, Smout AJ. Oesophageal motility and gastrooesophageal reflux before and after healing oesophagitis. A study using 24 hour ambulatory pH and pressure monitoring. Gut 1994; 35:1519–1522.
77. Rydberg L, Ruth M, Lundell L. Does oesophageal motor function improve with time after successful antiflux surgery? Results of a prospective, randomised clinical study. Gut 1997; 41:82–86.
78. Mittal RK, Lange RC, McCallum RW. Identification and mechanism of delayed esophageal acid clearance in subjects with hiatus hernia. Gastroenterology 1987; 92: 130–135.
79. Sloan S, Kahrilas PJ. Impairment of esophageal emptying with hiatal hernia. Gastroenterology 1991; 100:596–605.
80. Lin S, Brasseur JG, Pouderoux P, Kahrilas PJ. The phrenic ampulla: distal esophagus or potential hiatal hernia? Am J Physiol 1995; 268:G320–G327.
81. Korsten MA, Rosman AS, Fishbein S, Shlein RD, Goldberg HE, Beiner A. Chronic xerostomai increases esophageal acid exposure and is associated with esophageal injury. Am J Med 1991; 90:701–706.
82. Sonnenberg A, Steinkamp U, Weise A, Berges W, Weinbeck M, Rohner HG, Peter P. Salivary secretion in reflux esophagitis. Gastroenterology 1982; 83:889–895.
83. Kahrilas PJ, Gupta RR. The effect of cigarette smoking on salivation and esophageal acid clearance. J Lab Clin Med 1989; 114:431–438.
84. Konturek JW, Bielanski W, Konturek J, Bogdal J, Oleksy J. Distribution and release of epidermal growth factor in man. Gut 1989; 30:1194–1197.
85. Konturek SJ, Radecki T, Brzozowski T, Piastucki I, Dembinski A, Dembinska-Kiec A, Zmuga A, Gryglewski R, Gregory H. Gastric cytoprotection by epidermal growth factor, role of endogenous prostaglandins and DNA synthesis. Gastroenterology 1981; 81:438–443.
86. Olsen SP, Poulsen S, Therkelsen K, Nexo E. Oral administration of synthetic human urogastrone promotes healing of chronic duodenal ulcers in rats. Gastroenterology 1986; 90:911–917.
87. Sarosiek J, Feng T, McCallum R. The interrelationship between salivary epidermal

growth factor and the functional integrity of the esophageal mucosa. Am J Med Sci 1991; 302:359–362.
88. Rourk RM, Namiot Z, Sarosiek J, Yu Z, McCallum RM. Impairment of salivary epidermal growth factor secretory response to esophageal mechanical and chemical stimulation in patients with reflux esophagitis. Am J Gastroenterol 1994; 89:237–244.
89. Maccini D, Veit B. Salivary epidermal growth factor in patients with and without acid peptic disease. Am J Gastroenterol 1990; 85:1102–1104.

6

Pathophysiology of Gastroesophageal Reflux Disease

Offensive Factors and Tissue Resistance

Roy C. Orlando
Tulane University Medical School, New Orleans, Louisiana

Gastroesophageal (acid) reflux is an almost universal and daily occurrence, even in asymptomatic healthy subjects. Nevertheless, only a small percentage of the population at risk—which is everyone—develops gastroesophageal reflux disease (GERD), the latter heralded by symptoms, such as heartburn, or (microscopic and/or macroscopic) signs of damage to the esophageal mucosa (1). This attests to the effectiveness of the three-tiered esophageal defense against injury to the esophageal mucosa from the noxious factors within gastric juice (Fig. 1). The first, and most well-studied, tier of the defense is the antireflux barrier. Comprised primarily of the lower esophageal sphincter and diaphragmatic support, the antireflux barriers are designed to *limit the frequency and volume* of contact between refluxate and esophageal epithelium. When these barriers fail, the second tier of defense, known as the esophageal luminal clearance mechanisms come into play to *limit the duration* of contact between refluxate and esophageal epithelium. These consist of esophageal peristalsis and gravity, for volume clearance, and swallowed salivary secretions and secretions from esophageal submucosal glands, for acid clearance and restoration of a neutral pH. However, esophageal clearance, even under optimum circumstances, is not instantaneous, usually requiring 3–5 min to restore pH to neutrality after a single episode of reflux (2). Moreover clearance of the refluxate is often considerably slower at night since all

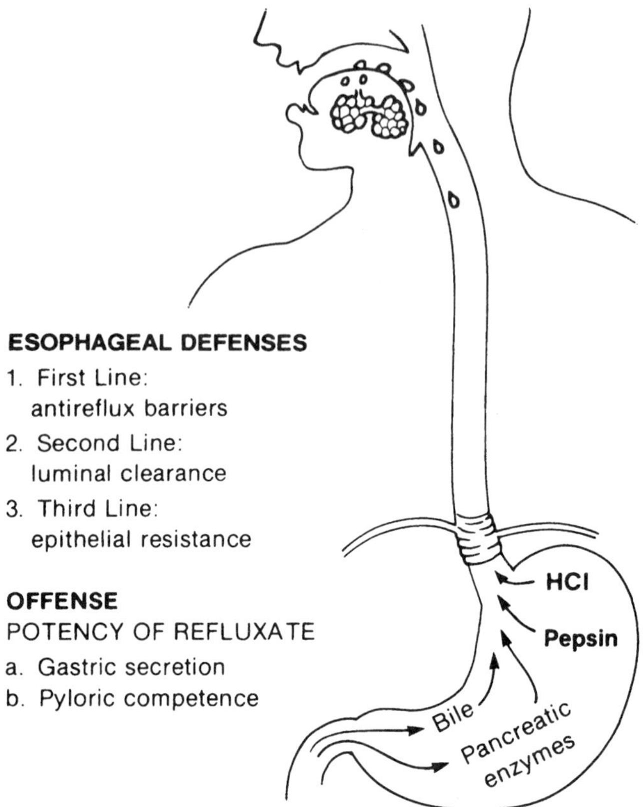

Figure 1 The esophagus protects itself from reflux-induced mucosal injury through a three-tiered system: antireflux barriers, luminal clearance mechanisms, and epithelial resistance. (Reprinted with permission from Orlando RC. Reflux esophagitis. In: Yamada T, Alpers DH, Laine L, Owyang G, Powell DW, eds. Textbook of Gastroenterology. Philadelphia: Lippincott Williams & Wilkins, 1999:1235–1263.)

investigated components (submucosal glands are yet to be studied) are inoperable during rapid-eye-movement sleep (3–5). On average, the daily dwell time for acid within the lumen of the esophagus is on the order of 2 h or more. For this reason, a third tier of defense is needed to maintain the health and integrity of the esophageal epithelium; this is known as "*tissue resistance*." Tissue resistance includes those factors associated with the mucosa that are designed to *limit damage during contact of refluxate with esophageal epithelium* (6). Ultimately, the interplay between the noxious luminal factors and epithelium are the final arbiters of disease—disease heralded clinically by heartburn and morphological changes within the epithelium. This chapter reviews the mechanisms comprising tissue resistance and their respective roles in preventing injury during contact with noxious elements in the refluxate. It also describes the pathophysiological sequence by which acid and acid-pepsin overcomes tissue resistance to lead to esophagitis and, based on this knowledge, provides an alternative hypothesis to lower esophageal sphincter (LES) dysfunction to account for the development of GERD in patients with normal acid contact time on 24-h pH monitoring.

NOXIOUS FACTORS IN THE REFLUXATE

The evidence that GERD is an appropriately named disorder is derived from the success of surgical fundoplication. Fundoplication controls GERD by mechanically altering access of gastric contents to the esophagus. Since it does not alter what is ingested or present within the stomach, the implication is that contact of the esophageal epithelium with gastric contents is essential for the development of GERD. Among the substances in gastric juice that may be noxious to the esophagus are: hydrochloric acid, pepsin, conjugated and unconjugated bile salts, and a host of pancreatic enzymes, especially trypsin. Nonetheless, the most noxious component in the refluxate is gastric (hydrochloric) acid. This is evident by the observation that heartburn can be relieved by ingestion of antacids and controlled by medication that inhibits acid secretion, i.e., H_2-receptor antagonists and proton pump inhibitors (1). While this establishes gastric acid as a key component in the development of GERD, it does not exclude acid acting in concert with other elements in the refluxate.

Other elements within the refluxate that may assist in mucosal damage are pepsin, a gastric protease secreted by chief cells, bile salts (conjugated and unconjugated), detergents secreted by liver and entering stomach via duodenogastric reflux, and pancreatic enzymes, e.g., proteases such as trypsin, that also enter the stomach by duodenogastric reflux. Under conditions in which gastric pH (and so the refluxate) is acidic, pancreatic enzymes are inactive and unconjugated bile salts insoluble, making these agents unlikely candidates to contribute to (esophageal) mucosal damage (7,8).

In contrast to pancreatic enzymes and unconjugated bile salts, the addition of pepsin to acidic solutions of pH < 3.0 increases the rate and degree of esophageal damage (9,10). This makes it a likely contributor to acid damage in GERD, though the magnitude of the contribution is unclear because agents that control acidity also inactivate pepsin. Ideally, the contribution of pepsin to damage in GERD is best determined by a drug that is purely antipepsin but not antiacid. However, no such therapy is currently available. Despite this uncertainty, the primacy of acid remains unchallenged since acid alone at physiological concentrations ($pH < 2.0$) can damage the esophagus while pepsin without acid (i.e., $pH \geq 3$) is innocuous in the esophagus (76).

Conjugated bile salts can also contribute to acid damage in GERD. This is because they are usually present in gastric juice and their addition, experimentally, to acid solutions increases the rate and degree of damage to the esophagus over that of acid alone (8,11). Yet, the clinical relevance of these observations remains uncertain because the bile salt concentrations in gastric juice of GERD patients are at levels that are noncytotoxic, ranging from 0.05 to 0.5 mM (vs. cytotoxic levels of 5 mM shown for sodium taurocholate experimentally) (12). However, noncytotoxic concentrations of conjugated bile salts at acidic pH may still accumulate in esophageal epithelium to reach cytotoxic concentrations. This occurs because at acid pH these molecules are lipid soluble and can cross the cell membrane. Once in the cell, they ionize at neutral pH and so are effectively trapped within the cytoplasm. Nonetheless, though plausible, this sequence remains unsupported by quantitative studies documenting increased bile salts in the esophageal epithelium of GERD patients or by morphological studies showing unique morphological changes within esophageal epithelium injured by bile salts. These changes, or pathological footprints, include both bile salt deposition within esophageal epithelial cells, apparent on light microscopy, and microvesiculation of cell membranes, a finding demonstrable by electron microscopy (13,14). In effect, the pathological features of GERD do not reflect those predicted were bile salts a major injurious factor, and remain entirely consistent with that due to contact of the epithelium with acid and pepsin (detailed later).

TISSUE RESISTANCE

Tissue resistance refers to the structural and functional elements within the esophageal mucosa that protect the epithelium against damage. In the context of GERD, the focus is on those elements of defense that protect against the luminal attack by acid and acid-pepsin. Tissue resistance against luminal acid is considerable. This is evident by the absence of damage to esophageal epithelium despite continuous exposure to HCl, pH 2.0, for 3.5 h in rabbits and by absence of symptoms or signs of damage despite continuous exposure to HCl, pH 1.1, for 30 min in humans (Bernstein test) (10,15). The ability of the epithelium to tolerate such acidity is multifactorial and the factors are best understood by viewing mucosal defense as a three-compartment model. The first compartment, *preepithelial defense*, includes those factors that reside on the lumen side of the epithelium; the second compartment, *epithelial defense*, includes those factors within the epithelium proper; and the third compartment, *postepithelial defense*, includes those factors that reside on the serosal or blood side of the epithelium (Table 1).

Table 1 Potential Components of Tissue Resistance Against Acid Injury in the Esophagus

Preepithelial defense
1. Mucous layer
2. Unstirred water layer
3. Surface bicarbonate ion concentration

Epithelial defense
4. Structures
    a. Cell membranes
    b. Intercellular junctional complexes (tight junctions, glycoconjugates)
5. Functions
    a. Epithelial transport (e.g., Na^+/H^+ exchanger, Na^+-dependent Cl^-/HCO_3^- exchanger)
    b. Intracellular and extracellular buffers
    c. Cell replication

Postepithelial defense
6. Blood flow
7. Tissue acid-base status

Source: Adapted with permission from Orlando RC. Esophageal epithelial resistance. In: Castell DO, Wu WC, Ott DJ, eds. Gastroesophageal Reflux Disease: Pathogenesis, Diagnosis, Therapy. Mount Kisco, NY: Futura Publishing Co., 1985:55.

Preepithelial Defense

The preepithelial defense against acid damage to stomach and duodenum has been most thoroughly studied, and consists of a surface mucous and unstirred water layer rich in bicarbonate ions (Fig. 2). This defense is largely created by secretion of both mucus and bicarbonate from epithelial surface cells and (in duodenum) Brunner's glands, and by paracellular diffusion of bicarbonate from blood to lumen. The result is an alkaline microenvironment interposed between highly acidic gastric juice and the epithelial surface (16,17). Mucus, comprised of high-molecular-weight glycoproteins, is a viscoelastic substance with gel-like properties that can physically trap and hinder pepsin diffusion from lumen to epithelial surface. Though an ineffective barrier to H^+, mucus protects against H^+ by expanding the unstirred water layer and its capacity for entrapping bicarbonate ions. Consequently, the preepithelial defense in stomach and duodenum has considerable capacity, being able to maintain a neutral or near-neutral cell-surface pH even when luminal acidity is as low as pH 2.0 (18).

The preepithelial defense in esophagus has been less well characterized, but the data that exist indicate that it has limited capacity for protection of the epithelial surface against exposure to acid in both humans and animals (rabbit, opossum). For example, Quigley and Turnberg showed that in vivo perfusion of

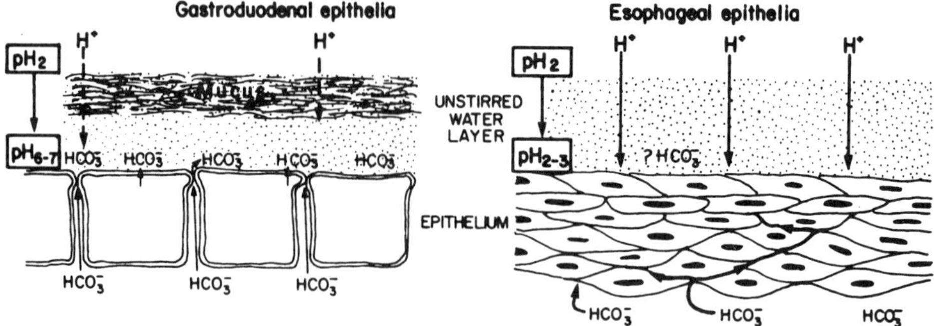

Figure 2 Preepithelial defense. In gastric and duodenal epithelia, H^+ must cross the mucus–unstirred water layer–bicarbonate barrier before contact can be made with the surface of the epithelium. Diffusion of pepsin but not H^+ is blocked by mucus; however, H^+ can be neutralized by HCO_3^- residing in the unstirred water layer. In contrast to gastric and duodenal epithelia, the preepithelial defense in the esophagus is poorly developed, having an ineffective mucus-HCO_3^- barrier to buffer backdiffusing H^+. [Reprinted with permission from Orlando RC. Esophageal epithelial defense against acid injury. J Clin Gastroenterol 1991; 13(suppl 2):1–5.]

the human esophagus with acid (HCl) resulted in a lumen:surface pH gradient of only 10:1; i.e., at luminal pH 2.0 the surface pH dropped to 3.0 (18). Moreover, in an in vitro comparative study in the submucosal gland-free rabbit esophagus and submucosal gland-bearing opossum esophagus, neither the rabbit nor the opossum was able to sustain a lumen:surface pH gradient when luminally perfused with HCl, pH 2.0 (19). Yet, the opossum, but not the rabbit, could sustain a luminal:surface pH gradient at a luminal pH of 3.5, and this could be enhanced by exposure to carbachol. These observations suggest that submucosal gland secretions contribute to the preepithelial defense, but its protective capacity is limited to acidity $\geq$ pH 2.0. Why this defense is so poorly developed in esophagus is unclear, but possible reasons include: (1) lack of a surface mucous layer to trap bicarbonate, (2) lack of bicarbonate secretion by stratified squamous epithelium, and (3) low rates of bicarbonate diffusion across the junctions in this ''electrically tight'' tissue (20–22). The apparent lack of a surface mucous layer is notable given esophageal exposure to mucins secreted by salivary and submucosal glands. Yet, either these soluble proteins lack the capacity to cross-link to form a viscoelastic layer or the underlying epithelium lacks the requisite chemistry for fixation of mucus to its surface. Irrespective of cause, however, the inadequacy of the preepithelial defense in esophagus shifts the burden of defense against luminal acidity directly onto the epithelium proper. This shift, moreover, has clinical consequences and likely explains the need for greater levels of control over gastric acid secretion in patients with GERD than required for patients with peptic ulcer disease of the duodenum or stomach (23). Specifically, epithelial repair requires an environment in the tissue of neutral or near-neutral pH. Therefore, in the presence of an effective preepithelial defense as for stomach and duodenum, gastric acid secretion needs only moderate inhibition—as afforded by H_2-receptor antagonists—to achieve this pH, while in the absence of an effective defense, gastric acid secretion needs to be more tightly controlled—as afforded by proton pump inhibitors—to achieve such a pH.

Epithelial Defense

Structural Components

Epithelial defense comes into play when acid or acid-pepsin penetrates the preepithelial defense and consists of structural and functional elements within the epithelium proper. In human esophagus the epithelium proper is a *nonkeratinized*, stratified squamous epithelium, whose 30–40 cell layers are subdivided into three regions: stratum corneum, stratum spinosum, and stratum (basalis) germinativum (24). The stratum corneum consists of 5–10 layers of flat, pancake-shaped cells lining the luminal surface. These cells are in varying stages of degeneration and serve as a barrier layer for protection against both physical and chemical injury (25,26). Below the stratum corneum is the stratum spinosum. It consists of 10–20 layers of mature, somewhat less flattened cells. These cells are metabolically active and principally responsible for the active epithelial transport of sodium ions (Na) from lumen to blood. In addition, these cells are transitional, migrating upward as they mature to replace the degenerating surface cells of the barrier layer as they slough into the lumen. The stratum germinativum consists of the lowest one to two cell layers. These cells, which are cuboidal to columnar in shape, are attached to the basement membrane by hemidesmosomes and represent the only cells within the epithelium capable of mitosis and replication.

The structural defense within esophageal epithelium viewed at the cellular level consists of a ''fence-like'' formation of cell membranes and intercellular junctions. The intercellular junctions are comprised of a series of tight junctions between which are sandwiched an intercellular glycoprotein matrix (Fig. 3) (25,26). Together these structures are responsible for the epithelium's high electrical resistance (1000–3000 ohms/cm^2) and protect by creating throughout the stratum corneum a barrier to diffusion of acid-pepsin into the epithelium. The lumen-facing, apical cell membrane, in particular, is highly impermeant to H^+, despite possession of Na channels, discussed below (27,28). The junctions are also effective at limiting the rate of acid entry into the tissue through the paracellular route. This is achieved by tight junctions via the formation of protein bridges between neighboring cell membranes, such bridges encircling all cells within the

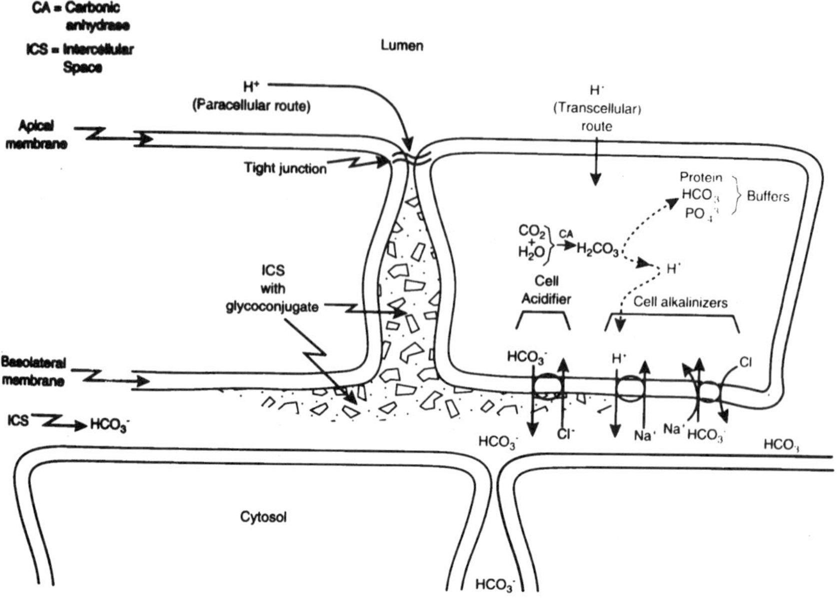

Figure 3 Epithelial defense. Some of the recognized epithelial defenses against acid injury are illustrated. Structural barriers to H^+ diffusion include the cell membrane and intercellular junctional complex. Functional components include intracellular buffering by negatively charged proteins and HCO_3^- and H^+ extrusion processes (Na^+/H^+ exchange and Na^+-dependent Cl^-/HCO_3^- exchange) for regulation of intracellular pH. (Adapted from Orlando RC. Esophageal epithelial resistance. In: Castell DO, Wu WC, Ott DJ, eds. Gastroesophageal Reflux Disease: Pathogenesis, Diagnosis, Therapy. Mount Kisco, NY: Futura Publishing Co., 1985:55.)

layer. The junctions, however, are not completely impermeant as they permit diffusion of small ions and water-soluble molecules across them (22,29). Also, the junctions are lined by negative charges (e.g., carboxyl, phosphate, and sulfate groups) and so tend to be cation selective. While this would initially appear to favor the passage of H^+, there is evidence that suggests that at low luminal pH, this pathway changes its permselectivity from cation to anion selective and thus prevents further H^+ diffusion through this route (22,29,30).

Noteworthy is that the rabbit and human esophageal tight junctions have in freeze-fracture replicas only a few bridging strands per cell layer. As strand number generally correlates with electrical tightness, this seemed inconsistent with the esophageal epithelium having a high electrical resistance. Yet complementing the barrier function of the tight junctions of the stratum corneum in esophagus is the intercellular glycoprotein matrix. Its contribution was demonstrable in rabbit esophagus using the electron-dense tracer lanthanum, and a similar substance observed in the stratum corneum of human esophagus (26,31). The precise nature of the glycoproteins remains unknown, but it is apparent that they are synthesized and secreted as membrane-coating granules from the cells of the stratum spinosum into the intercellular space (25). In the intercellular space, this matrix synergizes with the tight junctions to form the barrier to H^+ diffusion for the paracellular pathway. In effect, the structural defense in esophageal epithelium provides the physical barrier to H^+ and pepsin diffusion into the epithelium, with apical cell membranes controlling transcellular diffusion and junctional proteins controlling paracellular diffusion. By slowing the rate of H^+ diffusion, this defense works in concert with functional elements, discussed below, which buffer and transport H^+ from the tissue for removal by the blood stream.

Functional Components

The functional components of the epithelial defense consist primarily of cellular and intercellular buffers and basolateral membrane transport proteins. These protect by neutralizing H^+ within cytoplasm and intercellular space and by transporting H^+ from cytoplasm to intercellular space (Fig. 3). Buffering substances within the epithelium include proteins, phosphates, and bicarbonate ions. Within the cytoplasm, bicarbonate generation from water and carbon dioxide is catalyzed by carbonic anhydrase while extracellular bicarbonate is derived in large measure by diffusion from the blood supply (1,32). Bicarbonate and other buffers act within the cytoplasm to prevent a drop in pHi as H^+ enters across the membrane. When the cytosolic buffer capacity is exceeded and pHi becomes acidic, two acid extruding basolateral membrane proteins, the Na/H exchanger (NHE-1 isotype) and *Na-dependent* Cl/HCO_3 exchanger, operate at increased rate to transport excess H^+ from cytoplasm to intercellular space (33–35). Both transporters are driven by the Na gradient across the cell membrane, with the Na/H exchanger transporting H^+ for extracellular Na and the Na-dependent Cl/HCO_3 exchanger transporting Cl in exchange for extracellular HCO_3. (HCO_3 entry into the cytoplasm is, through H^+ buffering, the equivalent to H^+ removal from the cytoplasm.) The end-result of transporter activity is to raise low pHi back to neutrality by dumping H^+ into the intercellular space. Notably, this process works well as long as there remains adequate buffer within the intercellular space (see below).

Squamous epithelial cells come equipped with a third basolateral membrane transporter that is important for regulation of pHi, and that is the *Na-independent* Cl/HCO_3 exchanger (34). Under physiological conditions, this transporter operates to restore pHi to neutrality when pHi becomes too alkaline. This is done by exchanging HCO_3 for extracellular Cl, and since HCO_3 removal equates to H^+ gain, the transporter effectively lowers pHi by absorption of HCl. In the context of GERD, one situation in which this mechanism may come into play is during recovery following cell acidification—the exuberance of the mechanisms for acid extrusion overshooting as it were by extruding more H^+ than necessary to restore neutral pHi. Restoration of pHi then is achieved by activation of the Na-independent Cl/HCO_3 exchanger to compensate for the overshoot. In effect, pHi of squamous cells is a highly regulated process, being restored to and maintained at a neutral set point by changes in rates of acid extruders and acid absorber.

Postepithelial Defense

The postepithelial defense is created by the blood supply, and is the foundation upon which all other components depend for their existence. For example, an adequate blood supply is essential for regulation of tissue acid-base balance as well as for providing oxygen and nutrients for cell metabolism, growth, and repair. With respect to acid-base balance, the blood supply provides a high concentration of bicarbonate to the tissue for neutralization of excess H^+ resulting from both cell metabolism and back-diffusion from the lumen during acid reflux. Further, the blood supply is adaptable, with flow rates being shown to increase during periods of low luminal pH, presumably to enhance its capacity for removal of excess H^+ (36). The mediator of this increase in flow, at least in the opossum, appears to involve the release of nitric oxide and histamine, the latter derived from mast cells within the tissue (37). The essential value of blood-derived bicarbonate is best illustrated by experiments in which esophageal epithelium is mounted in Ussing chambers and exposed to an innocuous concentration of luminal acidity, HCl pH 2.0. Tissues in which bicarbonate is present on the serosal (blood) side tolerate such luminal acidity for hours without injury while similarly handled tissues deprived of serosal bicarbonate (or other buffer) develop extensive necrosis (38).

PATHOPHYSIOLOGY OF ACID INJURY

The pathophysiology of acid injury has been most thoroughly explored using the rabbit esophageal epithelium as a model for human esophageal epithelium. This is because, like human esophageal epithelium, that of the rabbit is a Na-absorbing, ''electrically tight,'' stratified squamous epithelium whose junctional complexes consist of tight junctions with few strands and intercellular glycoprotein matrix. Moreover, rabbit, like human, esophageal epithelium responds to high luminal acidity with a time-dependent biphasic change in transepithelial potential difference (PD) (see below), whose individual squamous cells utilize a basolateral membrane, acid-extruding, Na/H exchanger (NHE-1 isotype) as a principal mechanism for regulation of pHi. Two dissimilarities between rabbit and human esophagus are notable, but neither impacts negatively on using rabbit esophageal epithelium as a model for studies on the mechanism of acid injury. One is in the degree of epithelial keratinization, rabbit being partially keratinized and human being nonkeratinized, and the other is that the human, but not the rabbit, esophagus contains submucosal glands. Submucosal glands secrete mucin and bicarbonate, so quantitative differences should exist between human and rabbit esophagus with respect to rate of luminal acid clearance and magnitude of the lumen-to-surface pH gradient—such differences already shown between the gland-free rabbit and gland-bearing opossum esophagus (19). Nonetheless, since the capacity of the contribution of submucosal gland secretion to the preepithelial defense is limited, studies using high luminal acidity, pH < 2.0, result in patterns of damage that are remarkably similar for human and rabbit esophageal epithelia (as described below).

With rabbit as model, the mechanisms by which luminal acid damages the esophageal epithelium were initially elucidated by a combination of morphological and electrophysiological studies (39–41). Perfusion of rabbit esophagus in vivo with HCl, pH 1.4, resulted in a biphasic pattern in esophageal PD—PD increasing initially, then, declining progressively to zero (Fig. 4). Ussing chamber experiments subsequently established that the *first stage* of increasing PD was due to H^+ diffusion from lumen to serosa, the *second stage* of declining PD was due to increased epithelial permeability, and the *third stage* was due to increased epithelial permeability coupled with inhibited ion transport. By filling in the details at these various stages one obtains a fairly clear picture of how high luminal acidity ultimately gets translated into symptoms and signs of epithelial damage. For example, when H^+ diffuses from lumen to serosa, it must traverse the epithelium via the transcellular pathway, paracellular pathway, or both. Using intracellular pH microelectrodes it is evident that little or no H^+ enters the cytoplasm of esophageal epithelial surface cells across the apical cell membrane. This is obvious in that exposure to luminal acid, pH ≥ 2.0 results in no significant change in pHi (27). This observation, as noted previously, is also somewhat surprising since the apical cell membrane contains cation channels that permit Na^+ to diffuse across the apical membrane to enter the cytosol and at far lower concentration gradients. Yet, studies have shown that luminal pH ≥ 2.0 inhibit the cation channel in such a manner as to block the movement through it of *all cations, including H^+ itself* (28). Moreover, since at pH ≥ 2.0 there is no evidence for a H^+ diffusion potential across the epithelium, the implication is that at these luminal concentrations H^+ can traverse neither the transcellular nor the paracellular pathway. This in effect is a testament to the potency of the barrier characteristics of the healthy esophageal epithelium. So why does PD rise when the tissue is exposed to pH ≤ 2.0? The answer is that at these concentrations H^+ breaks the barrier, creating

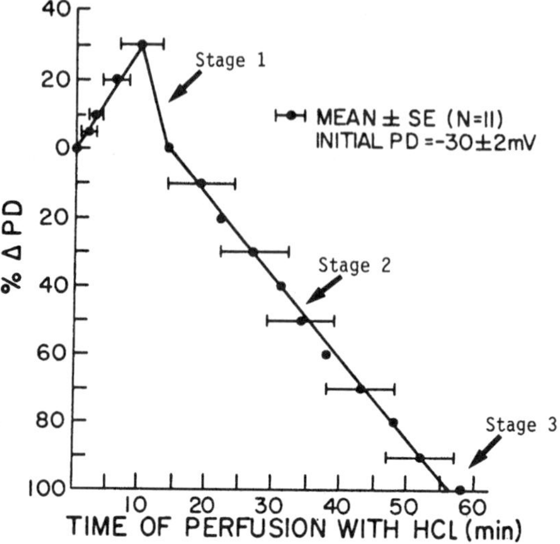

Figure 4 The percent change in rabbit esophageal transmural potential difference (ΔPD) is shown plotted against the time of exposure to 80 mmol HCl–80 mmol NaCl. A transient increase in PD occurs during the first 10 min. This is followed by a progressive decline in PD until it reaches zero at 1 h. Values are means ± standard error, $n = 11$. PD $= -30$ mV ± 2 mV. (Reprinted with permission from Orlando RC, Powell DW, Carney CN. Pathophysiology of acute acid injury in rabbit esophageal epithelium. J Clin Invest 1981; 68:286–293.)

a H^+ diffusion potential across the epithelium. The pathway that H^+ takes across the epithelium will become clear from studies focusing on the second stage of the model.

The *second stage* of declining PD during luminal acid exposure at pH ≤ 2.0, as defined in Ussing chamber experiments, is due to an increase in epithelial permeability, a reflection of a broken barrier. Moreover, this increase in permeability was due to an increase in ion permeation via the paracellular, and not the transcellular, route. Support for these conclusions was obtained by mounting tissues in Ussing chambers—after perfusion with acid in vivo until the PD was 50% below initial values—and showing that the decline in electrical resistance correlated with an increase in transepithelial mannitol flux (39–41). Moreover, these same tissues appeared normal macroscopically and histologically on light microscopy, and had normal short-circuit currents in the Ussing chamber indicating that transcellular Na transport remained intact. These data, en toto, suggest that the acid-induced decline in PD—indicating a break in the barrier—is the result of acid damage to the junctional complex rather than to the cell and its membranes. A similar conclusion, i.e., that acid or acid-pepsin damage to the esophageal epithelium begins with a *direct (extracellular) attack on the junctions*, was also reached when acid- or acid-pepsin-damaged tissues were subjected to circuit analysis (42). Before completely accepting this hypothesis, however, it is important to note that when PD declined, pHi, as monitored by intracellular microelectrodes, simultaneously declined by 1 pH unit, i.e., from neutral levels, pH 7.4, to pH 6.4. This at least raised the possibility that the change in junctional permeability was not primary but secondary to cell acidification—presumably luminal acidity of pH < 2.0 enabling sufficient H^+ to diffuse directly across the apical membrane. Nonetheless, one way that this possibility was excluded was by demonstrating that acidification of surface cells with HCl to pH 6.4 by means other than using such high luminal acidity did not increase junctional permeability (27). (The means chosen was by acidification of the serosal solution with HCl, pH 3.0—see details below.)

The data above establish that the *second stage* of acid damage to esophageal epithelium—when PD declines—is the result of an increase in paracellular permeability. Notably, at this stage the esophagus appeared normal grossly and by light microscopy. However, transmission electron microscopy (TEM) showed the epithelium to be abnormal, with prominently *dilated intercellular spaces*, such dilatations presumably a reflection of increased salt and water flow across more leaky junctions (Fig. 5). As TEM revealed no apparent morphological change to cells or the membrane region of the junctions, dilated intercellular spaces can be viewed as the earliest morphological evidence of acid damage in esophageal epithelium.

When there is continued perfusion of rabbit esophagus with HCl, pH $<$ 2.0, the second stage of acid damage proceeds inexorably to the *third stage* of acid damage. The third stage is recognized by the continued decline in the in vivo PD effectively to zero (39–41). The third stage is also readily recognizable morphologically by the appearance of macroscopic erosions and ulceration and light microscopically by the presence of extensive cell edema and necrosis. How this evolution takes place is both fascinating and clinically important since without necrosis the development of such complications of esophagitis as peptic stricture and Barrett's esophagus is unlikely. Fundamentally the transition from second to third stage occurs when the rate of acid diffusion across the damaged junctions is sufficient to overcome intercellular buffer capacity, resulting in *acidification of the intercellular space*. The consequences of intercellular acidification become most apparent in experiments in which healthy esophageal epithelium mounted in Ussing chambers is exposed to high luminal acidity in the presence or absence of buffer (bicarbonate) in the serosal solution. Notably, though both exposures result in similar increases in paracellular permeability as reflected by a decline in R, only the tissues exposed to bicarbonate-free solution exhibit cell necrosis. Moreover, similar and equal protection against acid-induced necrosis

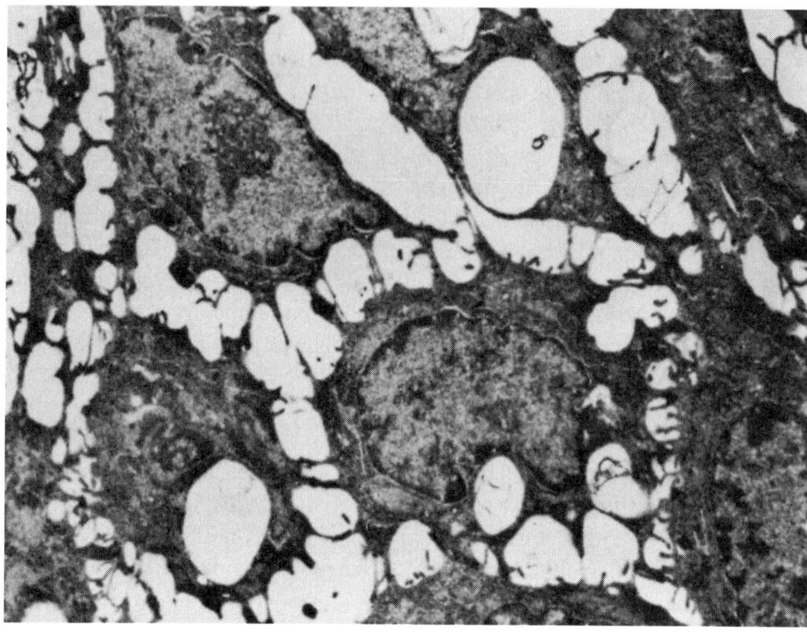

Figure 5 Electron micrograph of lower stratum spinosum in rabbit esophagus after in vivo HCl exposure lowered potential difference by 50% (perfusion time approximately 30 min). There is prominent dilatation of the intercellular spaces, but the cells themselves show no evidence of damage. Original magnification ×6375. (Reprinted with permission from Carney CN, Orlando RC, Powell DW, Dotson MM. Morphologic alterations in early acid-induced epithelial injury of the rabbit esophagus. Lab Invest 1981; 45:198–208.)

is afforded by serosal HEPES, a buffer that is cell-impermeant and confined to the intercellular space (38). These effects support the following two conclusions. One is that acid protection by buffer in this model was afforded below the level of the junctions (since acid reduced R similarly in buffered and unbuffered solutions), and two, a prerequisite for the development of cell necrosis is for H^+ to enter and acidify the intercellular space. A third supposition that can be made from this study is that acid-induced cell necrosis occurs after acidification of the intercellular space because H^+ comes in contact with and crosses the basolateral membrane (producing intracellular acidification) more efficiently than across the apical membrane (Fig. 6). Direct support for this latter concept was subsequently obtained by showing with intracellular pH microelectrodes that serosal acidification—with direct access of H^+ to the basolateral membrane—leads to cell acidification at levels of acidity (pH $\leq$ 6 to 2) that have essentially no effect on pHi when in contact with the epithelium from the luminal side where H^+ have direct

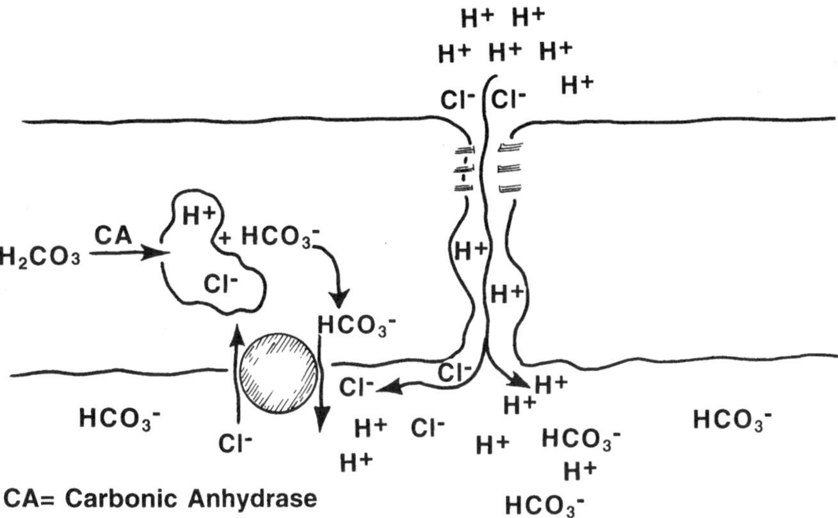

Figure 6 The pathway is depicted by which luminal HCl attacks and damages the cells within esophageal epithelium. Initially, high luminal acidity directly attacks and damages the intercellular junctional barrier, resulting in increased rates of acid diffusion into the intercellular space. Subsequent acidification of the intercellular space results in acidification of the cell cytosol by the access of HCl to the acid-permeant basolateral cell membrane. One important mechanism for acid absorption across the basolateral cell membrane is through operation of the (Na-independent) Cl^-/HCO_3^- exchanger.

access to the apical membrane (27). Another point of interest here is to recall that luminal pH 1.6, after increasing junctional permeability, lowers pHi by 1 pH unit. Since serosal acidity of pH 3.0 similarly results in a 1-pH-unit decline in pHi of surface cells, one can infer that luminal pH 1.6 lowered pHi by first acidifying the intercellular space to approximately pH 3.0.

To summarize: High luminal acidity directly attacks and damages the junctions, increasing paracellular permeability. This increase in permeability leads to greater H^+ diffusion and acidification of the intercellular space, and acidification of the intercellular space readily acidifies the cell cytosol because of H^+ contact with the more acid-permeant basolateral membrane. Acidification of the cytosol is then the crucial event that promotes cell edema and necrosis.

Additional details of this model have also been forthcoming in that the greater permeability of the basolateral membrane to H^+ has been attributed to its possession of a Na-independent, Cl/HCO_3 exchanger (43). This transmembrane transporter, as previously discussed, normally serves to extrude *excess* bicarbonate from the cytosol, restoring an alkaline pHi to neutrality. Noteworthy, however, is that it is extracellular serosal pH—normally a direct reflection of that of blood—that governs what the cell cytosol considers neutrality. Consequently, when serosal pH falls to acidic levels—as occurs when acid acidifies the intercellular space—pHi falls to a new lower set point, achieving what it perceives as the new level of "neutrality." The level of reduction in pHi in this situation directly reflects the degree of intercellular acidity because for each HCO_3 exchanging out of the cell along its gradient, the cell accumulates a H^+ (this is due to carbonic acid being the source of the lost HCO_3 so that its loss equates directly to H^+ gain). Moreover, since Cl is the counterion to bicarbonate, each lost HCO_3 or gained H^+ is associated with gain of a Cl ion, resulting effectively in cell absorption of extracellular HCl (Fig. 6). The major reason that intercellular acidity does not ultimately translate into similarly low levels of pHi is the direct opposition and continued activity of the basolateral membrane Na/H exchanger, the latter extruding excess intracellular H^+ for extracellular Na (see above). This is supported by the ability of amiloride, an inhibitor of Na/H exchange, to result in greater lowering of pHi at a fixed level of extracellular acidity (43,44). Additional experimental data in support of this overall schema for cell acidification and necrosis are the ability to prevent acidification of esophageal cells in primary culture and cell necrosis in intact sections of esophageal epithelium exposed to serosal acidity by inhibitors of Cl/HCO_3 exchange, e.g., the disulfonic stilbene derivative DIDS or SITS, and by use of a Cl-free solution (43).

Another facet of the model that has been explored is the mechanism by which the acid-induced reduction in pHi that occurs with the lowering of intercellular pH produces cell swelling and edema. Using both primary cultures of esophageal cells and whole sections of esophageal epithelium from the rabbit, cell swelling was identifiable when extracellular pH was lowered to pH < 2.0 (45,46). The mechanism for this occurrence appears to involve the ability of low pHi to elevate intracellular calcium, the latter then activating a transmembrane, bumetanide-sensitive, basolateral membrane NaK2Cl cotransporter. Activation of this cotransporter results in increased cytosolic uptake of Na, K, and Cl ions, and at a time that low pHi inhibits mechanisms for ion extrusion that are critical for volume regulation, e.g., basolateral membrane Na,K,ATPase and K channels (40,41,47). Consequently, ions enter in excess of loss resulting in an osmotic force favoring net water uptake and cell swelling. In one respect cell swelling can be viewed as an extraordinary means, through dilution, at protection against a highly acidic intracellular environment—the cell effectively sacrificing volume regulation to defend its internal pH. Moreover, cell swelling, taken to the extreme of membrane rupture, may be one means that acid-exposed esophageal cells eventually undergo necrosis. Alternatively, cell necrosis due to low pHi may produce cell edema and cell death through parallel but independent pathways. For instance, cell death at low pHi, as described in hepatocytes, may induce necrosis or apoptosis via activation of the mitochondrial permeability transition. The mitochondrial permeability transition occurs by the generation of high-conductance, cyclosporin A–inhibitable pores within the inner mitochondrial membrane. These pores nonselectively permit large numbers of small solutes to penetrate the mitochondria, resulting in mitochondrial depolarization, uncoupling of oxidative phosphorylation, and mitochondrial swelling. Depending, then, upon the presence or absence of ATP, the induction of the mitochondrial permeability transition is followed by necrotic or apoptotic cell death, respectively (48). While such a sequence has not been established in esophageal epithelial cells, apoptosis as a means of cell death is known to occur in healthy (human) esophageal epithelium. Moreover, there is evidence that this is in part mediated by the interaction of Fas ligand with Fas receptors on squamous cells (49). Nonetheless, whether luminal acid exposure increases esophageal cell death through the apoptotic process remains to be established.

Although acid-induced cell death (necrosis and/or apoptosis) represents the end of life for the cell, this alone should not pose a problem to the otherwise intact epithelium, particularly if it has the capacity for rapid repair. Unfortunately, the multilayered esophageal epithelium, unlike gastric or duodenal epithelium, lacks the means for "epithelial restitution." Epithelial restitution is the process whereby viable cells adjacent to an injury rapidly migrate over and seal a defect, and usually can do so in 30–60 min (50,51). The speed of healing in this case reflects the fact that "restitution" does not require protein synthesis. Restitution, however, requires the presence of an intact basement membrane to serve as scaffold for cell attachment and migration, access to such a structure lacking for all but the lowest of this multilayered epithelium. In addition, restitution requires the support of an effective preepithelial defense to maintain regional pH in a near-neutral range. This is evident in that restitution is markedly inhibited if the mucus layer overlying the damaged epithelium is removed either mechanically or chemically. Since the esophageal epithelium, as noted previously, lacks a mucus layer, were restitution possible, it would likely be limited by the inability to maintain a neutral or near-neutral pH in the injured region (20). Instead of restitution, then, the esophageal epithelium must rely on cell replication and migration lumenward from the basal layers to seal its defects. This unfortunately takes considerably longer than the normal cell turnover of 5–8 days (52,53), and even though shortened somewhat in acid-exposed tissues due to increased cell turnover (54,55), there remains ample time (clinically) for repeat exposure to acidic refluxates for H^+ to penetrate the broken barrier and damage cells of ever-deeper layers. The end result of this cumulative process is conversion of focal areas of microscopic necrosis into macroscopic defects known as erosions.

A characteristic of the transition from microscopic (nonerosive) to macroscopic (erosive) disease is the presence of acute and chronic inflammatory cells within the acid-damaged epithelium and subepithelial layers of esophagus. This, on the one hand, is an expected response to injury, migration of cells triggered by the release of, yet to be defined, cytokines and chemokines from both injured and uninjured squamous cells and resident immune cells within the tissue. These cells, as part of the containment and repair process, are presumably programmed for digestion and removal of necrotic debris. Yet, these same inflammatory cells may act indiscriminantly, at times serving to amplify, instead of reducing, the epithelial injury. For example, it was shown in acid-perfused rabbit esophagus in vivo that pretreatment with ketotifen to inhibit white-cell migration reduced the degree of macroscopic and microscopic injury to the epithelium (56). Further, since pretreatment in this same model with superoxide dismutase, and to a lesser extent catalase, could also reduce the degree of injury, white-cell production of oxygen-derived free radicals, especially superoxide anion and hydrogen peroxide,

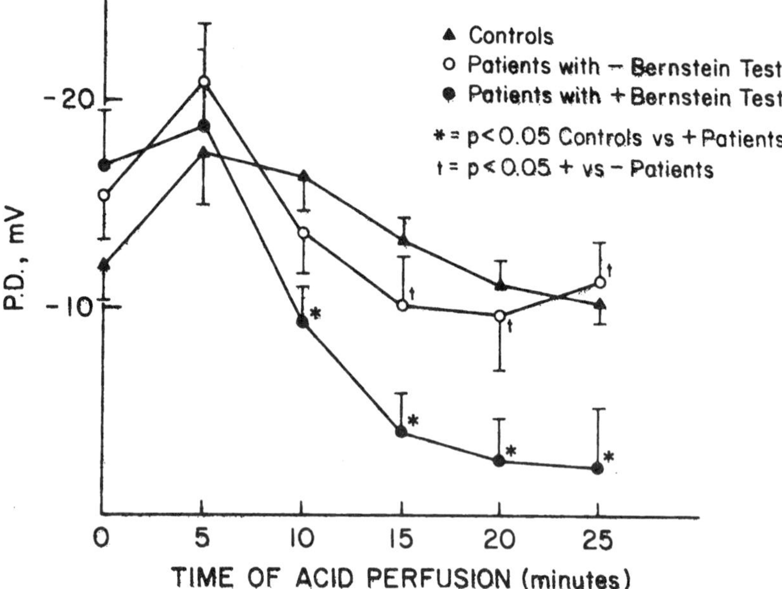

Figure 7 The effects of continuous esophageal acid perfusion (0.1N HCl) on esophageal transmural electrical potential difference (PD) in patients with positive (+), $n = 11$, and negative (−), $n = 8$, Bernstein tests and healthy control subjects, $n = 10$. Esophageal PD increases early during acid perfusion, and then falls progressively toward zero. The fall toward zero PD is noted to be most dramatic for the endoscopy negative patients with a positive Bernstein test suggesting the presence of impaired epithelial barrier function. (Reprinted with permission from Orlando RC, Powell DW. Studies of esophageal epithelial electrolyte transport and potential difference in man. In: Allen A, Flemstrom G, Garner A, Silen W, Turnberg LA, eds. Mechanisms of Mucosal Protection in the Upper Gastrointestinal Tract. New York: Raven Press, 1984: 75–79.)

was believed to be an important contributor to their toxic action. From this perspective, it is apparent that there are both intrinsic (inflammatory cells) and extrinsic (acid reflux) means for perpetuation and amplification of the epithelial injury, and when chronic and uncontrolled, this injury may progress to complications. The complications include ulceration with either hemorrhage and/or perforation (rare) or formation of a peptic stricture and/or a specialized columnar-lined lower (Barrett's) esophagus (common). Although the precise mechanisms responsible for stricture formation and Barrett's esophagus remain unknown, both can be viewed as aberrant attempts at repair (1).

Parallels Between the Rabbit Model and GERD

Two key observations in humans support a similar pathogenesis for acid injury to esophageal epithelium as defined in the rabbit model. First, luminal perfusion in vivo with high concentrations of HCl (Bernstein test) produces in humans a similar biphasic pattern in esophageal potential difference (PD). This is evident in healthy and mildly acid-damaged (nonerosive GERD) esophageal epithelium (Fig. 7) while PD is abolished in severely damaged human esophageal epithelium as in those with erosive GERD (57,58). Second, patients with both erosive and nonerosive GERD have the same morphological hallmark of early acid damage to esophageal epithelium, i.e., dilated intercellular spaces (Fig. 8) (59). The clinical

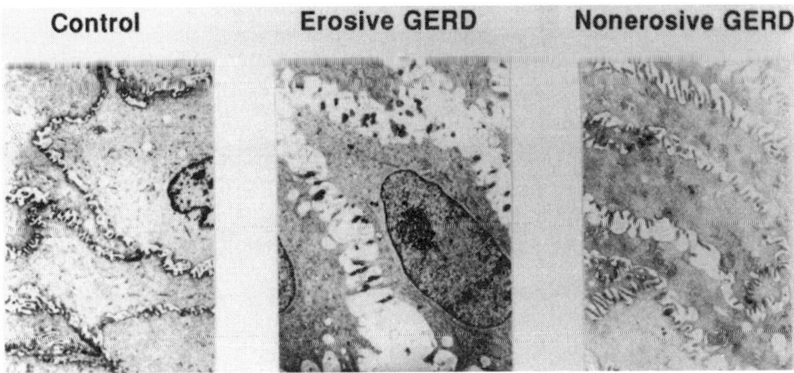

Figure 8 Transmission electron photomicrographs of an esophageal mucosal biopsy from a (control) subject without esophageal disease, a subject with heartburn and erosive esophagitis, and a subject with heartburn and nonerosive esophagitis on endoscopy. Note the widened intercellular spaces in the two subjects with heartburn. Original magnification ×3000. (Modified and reprinted with permission from Tobey NA, Carson JL, Alkiek RA, Orlando RC. Dilated intercellular spaces: a morphological feature of acid reflux-damaged human esophageal epithelium. Gastroenterology 1996; 111:1200–1205.)

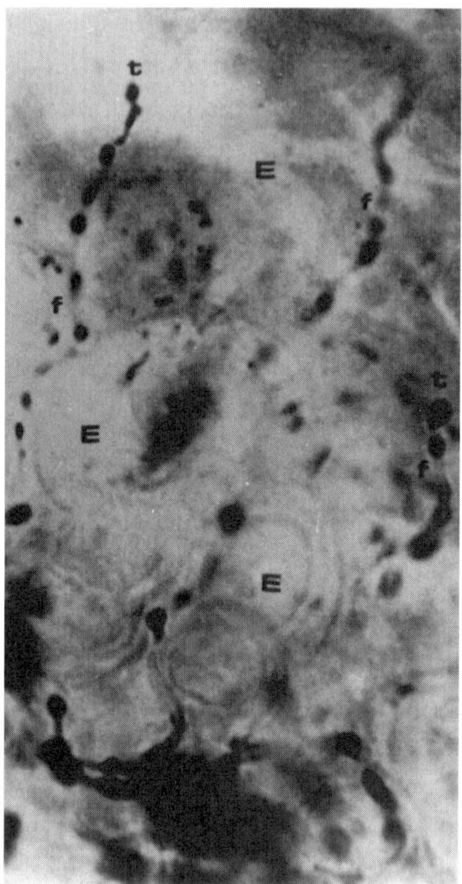

Figure 9 Photomicrograph showing the nerve fibers (f) traversing the intercellular spaces of esophageal epithelium in macaque. OsO_4-ZnI_2 solution. ×320. (Reprinted with permission from Rodrigo J, Hernandez CJ, Vidal MA, Pedrosa JA. Vegetative innervation of the esophagus. III. Intraepithelial endings. Acta Anat 1975; 92:242–258.)

implications of finding both a similar PD pattern during acid perfusion and similar morphological changes is considerable because *it suggests that, as in the rabbit model, the pathogenesis of GERD involves the direct attack and damage of the intercellular junctions by refluxed gastric acid-pepsin*. If acid initially damages the junctions and increases their permeability, it follows that *the occurrence of heartburn in nonerosive GERD reflects the greater accessibility of luminal H^+ to the afferent (sensory) nerves in esophageal epithelium*. These afferent sensory

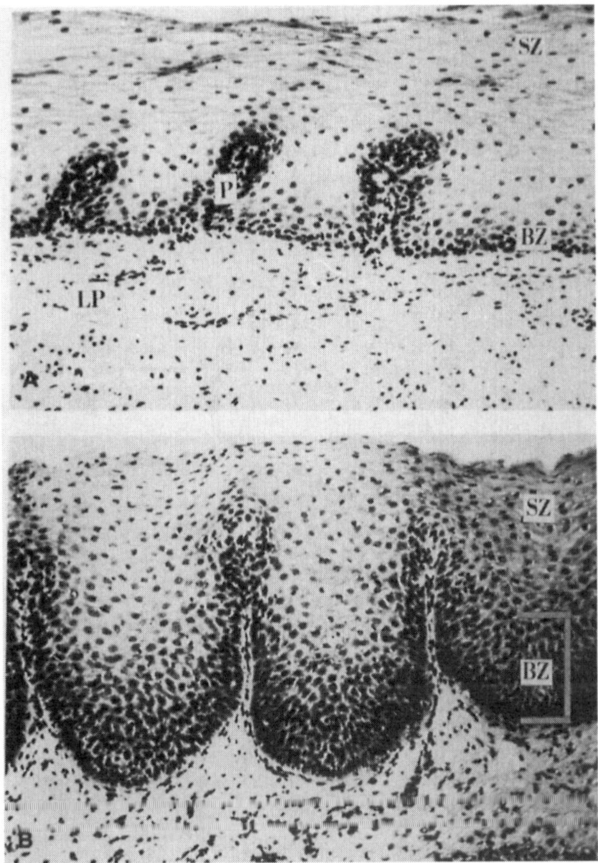

Figure 10 (A) Normal esophageal suction biopsy from a healthy subject without esophagitis. Basal zone thickness is approximately 10% of total epithelial thickness; papillae extend approximately one-half the distance to the epithelial surface. (B) Abnormal suction biopsy from a subject with symptomatic reflux. Basal zone thickness is approximately 35% of total epithelial thickness; papillae extend over two-thirds of the distance to the epithelial surface. BZ: basal zone; SZ: stratified zone; P: papillae; LP: lamina propria. Hematoxylin and eosin ×170. (Reprinted with permission from Ismail-Beigi F, Horton PF, Pope CE II. Histological consequences of gastroesophageal reflux in man. Gastroenterology 1970; 58:163–174.)

terminals are calcitonin-gene-related peptide positive and known to be accessible since they reside within the intercellular space just below the surface cell layers (Fig. 9) (60,61). Further, vagal sensory afferents—as shown in airway epithelia—will signal in response to acidic pH < 6.2 and signal maximally at acidic pH of 5.0 (62). Also, given their accessibility to luminal contents, vagal afferents may also signal in response to, for example, hypertonicity, and this may account for the development of heartburn during esophageal perfusion with tomato juice at neutral pH (63). Moreover, these observations provide a compelling argument against the phenomenon of esophageal visceral hypersensitivity as the cause for the ''acid-sensitive'' esophagus in patients with nonerosive GERD (64). In this instance visceral hypersensitivity is inappropriate since the sensory nerve endings in patients with nonerosive GERD respond appropriately to an excess level of intercellular acidity. *Further, if acid initially damages the junctions, a means is provided as to how repeated H^+ exposure can progress from nonerosive to erosive GERD* (Fig. 6). This occurs when excess H^+ entry across the ''leaky'' junctions acidifies the intercellular space to access the more acid-permeable basolateral membrane. Interestingly, as acid injures the surface cells and they are shed into the lumen, two additional morphological changes may occur in human esophageal epithelium that have previously been recognized as ''early'' hallmarks of GERD (65). One is elongation of the rete pegs, the rete pegs appearing closer to the esophageal lumen—due to the greater rate of surface cell layer damage and desquamation—and the other is basal cell hyperplasia—due to increased rates of cell replication, a reparative attempt in response to increased loss of surface cells (Fig. 10). *Finally, if acid initially damages the junctions, it also explains in part the stimulus for basal cell hyperplasia, and that is by the ability of swallowed salivary EGF to now access the EGF receptors located on the basolateral membranes of basal cells* (66).

GERD—AN EPITHELIAL DISEASE?

Traditionally, reflux esophagitis has been considered exclusively a motor disease, the major motor disturbance being increased frequency of transient lower esophageal sphincter relaxations (1). However, a case can be made that GERD is, at least in part, due to an impairment in epithelial resistance. The most compelling evidence for this is the observation that up to 50% of patients with nonerosive disease and 30% with erosive disease have normal acid contact times on 24-h pH monitoring (Fig. 11) (67–69). Since normal acid contact time implies that the antireflux and luminal clearance mechanisms are functioning normally, esophagitis in these patients must result from either an excessively noxious refluxate or a defect in epithelial resistance. As the data suggest that the potency of the refluxate in GERD patients is no different than that of healthy subjects—and specifically patients with GERD and healthy subjects have similar rates of

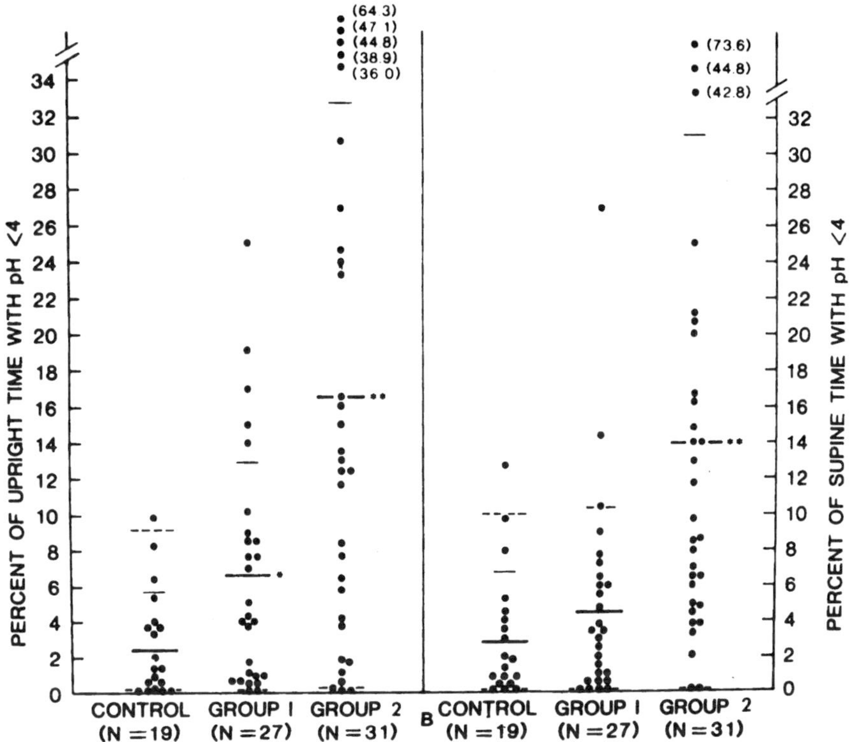

Figure 11 Upright and supine esophageal acid exposure times are shown in A and B, respectively. Although supine acid exposure time did not differ between control patients and patients with reflux symptoms and a normal endoscopy (group 1), there was a significant difference in their upright acid exposure times. Patients with reflux symptoms and erosive esophagitis (group 2) had significantly more acid exposure time in both positions than the first two groups. Despite this, marked overlap was seen between all groups. Mean + 1 SD is shown for each group. Two standard deviations above the mean is shown for controls (---). $*p < 0.05$ versus control. $**p < 0.01$ versus control group 1. (Reprinted with permission from Schlesinger PK, Donahue PE, Schmid B, Layden TJ. Limitations of 24-hour intraesophageal pH monitoring in the hospital setting. Gastroenterology 1985; 89:797.)

acid and pepsin secretion (70)—the likely explanation is the presence of impaired epithelial resistance. Moreover, there are many ways that the epithelium can develop defects that would subsequently predispose it to damage upon contact with gastric acid during physiological reflux. Among these are esophageal exposure to alcohol, heat, hypertonic solutions, cigarette smoke, or medications such as nonsteroidal anti-inflammatory drugs (71–75). All of these factors have been shown to impair one or more important tissue defenses described above. For example, alcohol, hypertonicity, and heat can all increase the permeability of the junctions, making them effectively more leaky to H^+. Cigarette smoking, however, has no effect on epithelial permeability but can inhibit active sodium transport. The consequence of inhibition of Na transport is to impair the activity of enzymes dependent on the transmembrane Na gradient, e.g., the acid-extruding mechanisms such as Na/H exchange. Consequently, epithelium exposed to cigarette smoke would have difficulty restoring pHi to neutrality following acidification. In the case of those that increase junctional permeability to H^+, e.g., hypertonicity, such exposures have the capacity to lower epithelial resistance so that previously innocuous concentrations of H^+ can become noxious. For example, prior exposure to hypertonic urea (1200 mosm/Kg.H_2O) can take a nondamaging luminal acidity, HCl, pH 2.0, and convert it into one that produces tissue necrosis (74). Based on these observations, it is clear that even common exposures at times may alter the resilience of the esophagus to protect itself from physiological reflux, and this effectively can provide the foothold for either the initiation or perpetuation of acid injury.

REFERENCES

1. Orlando RC. Reflux esophagitis. In: Yamada T, Alpers DH, Laine L, Owyang C, Powell DW, eds. Textbook of Gastroenterology. Philadelphia: Lippincott Williams & Wilkins, 1999:1235–1263.
2. Helm JF, Dodds WJ, Pelc LR, Palmer DW, Hogan WJ, Teeter BC. Effect of esophageal emptying and saliva on clearance of acid from the esophagus. N Engl J Med 1984; 310:284.
3. Dent J, Dodds WJ, Friedman RH, Sekiguci T, Hogan WJ, Arndorfer RC, Petrie DJ. Mechanism of gastroesophageal reflux in recumbent asymptomatic subjects. J Clin Invest 1980; 65:256.
4. Lichter I, Muir RC. The pattern of swallowing during sleep. Electroencephalogr Clin Neurophysiol 1975; 38:427.
5. Schneyer LH, Schneyer LH, Pigman W, Hanahan L, Gilmore RW. Rate of flow of human parotid, sublingual and submaxillary secretions during sleep. J Dent Res 1956; 35:109.
6. Orlando RC. Pathophysiology of gastroesophageal reflux disease: esophageal epithelial resistance. In: Castell DO, Richter JE, eds. The Esophagus. Philadelphia: Lippincott Williams & Wilkins, 1999:409–420.
7. Salo JA, Lehto VP, Kivilaakso E. Morphologic alterations in experimental esophagitis: light microscopic and scanning and transmission electron microscopic study. Dig Dis Sci 1983; 28:440.
8. Lillemoe KD, Johnson LF, Harmon JW. Alkaline esophagitis: a comparison of the ability of components of gastroduodenal contents to injure the rabbit esophagus. Gastroenterology 1983; 85:621.

9. Lillemoe KD, Johnson LF, Harmon JW. Role of the components of the gastroduodenal contents in experimental acid esophagitis. Surgery 1982; 92:276.
10. Redo SF, Bames WA, de la Sierra CA. Perfusion of the canine esophagus with secretions of upper gastrointestinal tract. Ann Surg 1959; 149:556.
11. Safaie-Shirazi S, DenBesten L, Zike WL. Effect of bile salts on the ionic permeability of the esophageal mucosa and their role in the production of esophagitis. Gastroenterology 1975; 68:728.
12. Salo J, Kivilaakso E. Role of luminal H^+ in the pathogenesis of experimental esophagitis. Surgery 1982; 92:61.
13. Bateson MC, Hopwood D, Milne G, Boucher IAD. Oesophageal epithelial ultrastructure after incubation with gastrointestinal fluids and their components. J Pathol 1981; 133:33.
14. Schweitzer EJ, Bass B, Batzri S, Harmon J. Bile acid accumulation by rabbit esophageal mucosa. Dig Dis Sci 1986; 31:1105.
15. Bernstein LM, Baker LA. A clinical test for esophagitis. Gastroenterology 1958; 34:760.
16. Flemstrom G, Garner A. Gastroduodenal HCO_3-transport: characteristics and proposed role in acidity regulation and mucosal protection. Am J Physiol 1982; 242: G183.
17. Allen A, Garner A. Mucus and bicarbonate secretion in the stomach and their possible role in mucosal protection. Gut 1980; 21:249.
18. Quigley EMM, Turnberg LA. pH of the microclimate lining human gastric and duodenal mucosa in vivo. Studies in control subjects and in duodenal ulcer patients. Gastroenterology 1987; 92:1876.
19. Abdulnour-Nakhoul S, Nakhoul NL, Orlando RC. Lumen-to-surface pH gradients in opossum and rabbit esophagi: role of submucosal glands. Am J Physiol 2000; 278:G113–G120.
20. Dixon J, Pearson JP, Griffin MS, Welfare M, Dettmar PW, Allen A. Mucus gel barrier absent in normal oesophagus but present in Barrett's oesophagus. Gastroenterology 1999; 116:A149.
21. Hamilton BH, Orlando RC. In vivo alkaline secretion by mammalian esophagus. Gastroenterology 1989; 97:640.
22. Powell DW. Barrier function of epithelia. Am J Physiol 1981; 241:G275.
23. Orlando RC. Why is the high grade inhibition of gastric acid secretion afforded by proton pump inhibitors often required for healing of reflux esophagitis? An epithelial perspective. Am J Gastroenterol 1996; 91:1692.
24. Al Yassin T, Toner PG. Fine structure of squamous epithelium and submucosal glands of human esophagus. J Anat 1977; 123:705.
25. Elias PM, McNutt NS, Friend DS. Membrane alterations during codification of mammalian squamous epithelia: a freeze-fracture, tracer and thin-section study. Anat Rec 1977; 189:577.
26. Orlando RC, Lacy ER, Tobey NA, Cowart K. Barriers to paracellular permeability in rabbit esophageal epithelium. Gastroenterology 1992; 102:910.
27. Khalbuss WE, Marousis CG, Subramanyam M, Orlando RC. Effect of HCl on transmembrane potentials and intracellular pH in rabbit esophageal epithelium. Gastroenterology 1995; 108:662–672.

28. Tobey NA, Caymaz-Bor C, Hosseini SS, Awayda MS, Orlando RC. Effect of luminal acidity on the apical membrane Na channel in rabbit esophageal epithelium (abstr). Gastroenterology 2000. In press.
29. Diamond JM. Channels in epithelial cell membranes and junctions. Fed Proc 1978; 37:2639.
30. Moreno JH, Diamond JM. Discrimination of monovalent inorganic cations by "tight" junctions of gallbladder epithelium. J Membr Biol 1974; 15:277.
31. Hopwood D, Logan KR, Coghill G, Bouchier IAD. Histochemical studies of mucosubstances and lipids in normal human oesophageal epithelium. Histochem J 1977; 9:153.
32. Christie KN, Thomas C, Xue L, Lucocq JM, Hopwood D. Carbonic anhydrase isoenzymes I, II, III and IV are present in human esophageal epithelium. J Histochem Cytochem 1997; 45:35.
33. Tobey NA, Reddy SP, Keku TO, Cragoe EJ Jr, Orlando RC. Studies of pHi in rabbit esophageal basal and squamous epithelial cells in culture. Gastroenterology 1992; 103:830.
34. Tobey NA, Reddy SP, Khalbuss WE, Silvers SM, Cragoe EJ Jr, Orlando RC. Na^+-dependent and -independent Cl^-/HCO_3-exchangers in cultured rabbit esophageal epithelial cells. Gastroenterology 1993; 104:185.
35. Layden TJ, Schmidt L, Agnone L, Lisitza P, Brewer J, Goldstein JL. Rabbit esophageal cell cytoplasmic pH regulation: role of Na^+-H^+ antiport and Na^+-dependent HCO_3 transport systems. Am J Physiol 1992; 263(3 pt 1):G407.
36. Bass BL, Schweitzer EJ, Harmon JW, Kraimer J. H^+ back diffusion interferes with intrinsic reactive regulation of esophageal mucosal blood flow. Surgery 1984; 96: 404.
37. Feldman MJ, Morris GP, Dinda PK, Paterson WG. Mast cells mediate acid-induced augmentation of opossum esophageal blood flow via histamine and nitric oxide. Gastroenterology 1996; 110:121.
38. Tobey NA, Powell DW, Schreiner VJ, Orlando RC. Serosal bicarbonate protects against acid injury to rabbit esophagus. Gastroenterology 1989; 96:1466.
39. Carney CN, Orlando RC, Powell DW, Dotson MM. Morphologic alterations in early acid-induced epithelial injury of the rabbit esophagus. Lab Invest 1981; 45:198.
40. Orlando RC, Bryson JC, Powell DW. Mechanisms of HCl injury in rabbit esophageal epithelium. Am J Physiol 1984; 246:G718.
41. Orlando RC, Powell DW, Carney CN. Pathophysiology of acute acid injury in rabbit esophageal epithelium. J Clin Invest 1981; 68:286.
42. Tobey NA, Caymaz-Bor C, Hosseini SS, Awayda MS, Orlando RC. Circuit analysis of cell membrane and junctional resistances in healthy and acid-damaged rabbit esophageal epithelium. Gastroenterology 1999; 116:A334.
43. Tobey NA, Reddy SP, Keku TO, Cragoe EJ Jr, Orlando RC. Mechanisms of HCl-induced lowering of pH I in rabbit esophageal epithelial cells. Gastroenterology 1993; 105:1035.
44. Tobey NA, Koves G, Orlando RC. Identification of Na/H exchange in human esophageal epithelial cells grown in primary culture. Am J Gastroenterol 1998; 93:2075.
45. Tobey NA, Koves G, Orlando RC. HCl-induced cell edema in primary cultured rabbit esophageal epithelium. Gastroenterology 1997; 112:847.

46. Tobey NA, Cragoe, EJ Jr, Orlando RC. HCl-induced cell edema in rabbit esophageal epithelium: a bumetanide-sensitive process. Gastroenterology 1995; 109:414.
47. Khalbuss WE, Alkiek R, Marousis CG, Orlando RC. K conductance in rabbit esophageal epithelium. Am J Physiol 1993; 265 (Gastrointest Liver Physiol 28):G28.
48. Lemasters JJ. Mechanisms of hepatic toxicity. V. Necapoptosis and the mitochondrial permeability transition: shared pathways to necrosis and apoptosis. Am J Physiol 1999; 276 (Gastrointest Liver Physiol 39):G1.
49. Bennett MW, O'Connell J, O'Sullivan GC, Roche D, Brady C, Collins JK, Shanahan F. Fas ligand and Fas receptor are coexpressed in normal human esophageal epithelium: a potential mechanism of apoptotic epithelial turnover. Dis Esoph 1999; 12: 90.
50. Silen W. Gastric mucosal defense and repair. In: Johnson LR, Christensen J, Jacobson ED, Jackson MJ, Walsh JH, eds. Physiology of the Gastrointestinal Tract. Vol 2, 2nd ed. New York: Raven Press, 1987:1055.
51. Feil W, Wenzl E, Vattay P, Starlinger M, Sogukoglu, Schiessel R. Repair of rabbit duodenal mucosa after acid injury in vivo and in vitro. Gastroenterology 1987; 92: 1973.
52. Bell B, Almy TP, Lipkin M. Cell proliferation kinetics in the gastrointestinal tract of man. III. Cell renewal in esophagus, stomach and jejunum of a patient with treated pernicious anemia. J Natl Cancer Inst 1967; 38:615.
53. Leblond CP, Greuiich RC, Pereira JPM. Relationship of cell formation and cell migration in the renewal of stratified squamous epithelia. In: Montagna W, Billingham RE, eds. Advances in Biology of Skin. Vol 5. Wound Healing. New York: Pergamon Press, 1974:39.
54. DeBacker A, Haentjens P, Willems G. Hydrochloric acid: a trigger of cell proliferation in the esophagus of dogs. Dig Dis Sci 1985; 30:884.
55. Livstone EM, Sheahan DG, Behar J. Studies of esophageal epithelial cell proliferation in patients with reflux esophagitis. Gastroenterology 1977; 73:1315.
56. Naya MJ, Pereboom D, Ortego J, Alda JO, Lanas A. Superoxide anions produced by inflammatory cells play an important part in the pathogenesis of acid and pepsin induced oesophagitis in rabbits. Gut 1997; 40:175.
57. Orlando RC, Powell DW. Studies of esophageal epithelial electrolyte transport and potential difference in man. In: Allen A, Flemström G, Garner A, et al., eds. Mechanisms of Mucosal Protection in the Upper Gastrointestinal Tract. New York: Raven Press, 1984:75.
58. Orlando RC, Powell DW, Bryson JC, Kinard HB III, Carney CN, Jones JD, Bozymski EM. Esophageal potential difference measurements in esophageal disease. Gastroenterology 1982; 83:1026.
59. Tobey NA, Carson JL, Alkiek RA, Orlando RC. Dilated intercellular spaces: a morphological feature of acid reflux-damaged human esophageal epithelium. Gastroenterology 1996; 111:1200.
60. Rodrigo J, Hernandez DJ, Vidal MA, Pedrosa JA. Vegetative innervation of the esophagus. III. Intraepithelial endings. Acta Anat 1975; 92:242.
61. Parkman HP, Reynolds JC, Elfman KS, Ogorek CP. Calcitonin gene-related peptide: a sensory and motor neurotransmitter in the feline lower esophageal sphincter. Regul Pept 1989; 25:131.

62. Lou Y-P, Lundberg JM. Inhibition of low pH evoked activation of airway sensory nerves by casazepine, a novel capsaicin-receptor antagonist. Biochem Biophys Res Commun 1992; 189:537.
63. Lloyd DA, Borda IT. Food-induced heartburn: effect of osmolality. Gastroenterology 1981; 80:740.
64. Rodriguez-Stanley S, Robinson M, Earnest DL, Greenwood-Van Meerveld B, Miner PB. Esophageal hypersensitivity may be a major cause of heartburn. Am J Gastroenterol 1999; 94:628.
65. Ismail-Beigi F, Horton PF, Pope CE II, Histological consequences of gastroesophageal reflux in man. Gastroenterology 1970; 58:163.
66. Tobey NA, Hosseini SS, Orlando RC. Nonerosive acid injury increases esophageal permeability to luminal EGF (abstr). Gastroenterology 2000. In press.
67. Schlesinger PK, Donahue PE, Schmid B, Layden TJ. Limitations of 24 hour intraesophageal pH monitoring in the hospital setting. Gastroenterology 1985; 89: 797.
68. Cucchiara S, Staiano A, Casali LG, Boccieri A, Paone FM. Value of the 24 hour intraoesophageal pH monitoring in children. Gut 1990; 31:129.
69. Masclee AAM, DeBest ACAM, DeGraaf R, Cluysenaer OJJ, Jansen JBMJ. Ambulatory 24-hour pH-metry in the diagnosis of gastroesophageal reflux disease. Scand J Gastroenterol 1990; 25:225.
70. Hirschowitz BI. A critical analysis, with appropriate controls of gastric acid and pepsin secretion in clinical esophagitis. Gastroenterology 1991; 101:1149.
71. Orlando RC, Bryson JC, Powell DW. Effect of cigarette smoke on esophageal epithelium of the rabbit. Gastroenterology 1986; 91:1536.
72. Chung RSK, Johnson GM, Denbesten L. Effect of sodium taurocholate and ethanol on hydrogen ion absorption in rabbit esophagus. Am J Dig Dis 1977; 22:582.
73. Lanas A, Sousa FL, Esteva F, Ortego J, Blas J, Sainz R. Aspirin (ASA) renders the esophageal mucosa more permeable to acid and pepsin in rabbits. Gastroenterology 1993; 104:A129.
74. Long JD, Marten E, Tobey NA, Orlando RC. Luminal hypertonicity and the susceptibility of rabbit esophagus to acid injury. Dis Esoph 1998; 11:94.
75. Tobey NA, Sikka D, Marten E, Caymaz-Bor C, Hosseini SS, Orlando RC. Effect of heat stress on rabbit esophageal epithelium. Am J Physiol 1999; 276 (Gastrointest Liver Physiol 39):G1322.
76. Pursnani KG, Mohiuddin MA, Geisinger KR, Weinbaum G, Katzka DA, Castell DO. Experimental study of acid burden and acute oesophagitis. Br J Surg 1998; 85: 677.

7

Esophageal Complications (Other Than Barrett's) of Gastroesophageal Reflux Disease

Nicholas J. Shaheen and Eugene M. Bozymski
University of North Carolina, Chapel Hill, North Carolina

Because of the ubiquity of gastroesophageal reflux disease (GERD), multiple esophageal complications of the disease are commonly encountered by the practicing gastroenterologist. Among the esophageal complications of GERD are stricture, hemorrhage, ulceration, and possibly Schatzki's ring. Columnar-lined lower esophagus, also known as Barrett's esophagus, another esophageal complication of GERD, is considered in another chapter.

Following brief discussions of hemorrhage and ulceration, this chapter will focus primarily on esophageal strictures. The epidemiology, pathogenesis, clinical presentation, diagnosis, and management of strictures will be considered.

ULCERATION

Most disruption of esophageal epithelium occurs in the setting of erosive esophagitis. Deep ulcers in the squamous epithelium are rarely encountered in reflux disease. If deep ulcers are seen in the esophagus, the differential diagnosis is broad and includes those entities listed in Table 1. Most of these causes can be excluded by taking a careful history. Many nonpeptic causes of esophageal ulceration are especially prevalent in immunocompromised hosts, making assessment of human immunodeficiency virus (HIV) status a useful investigation following the discovery of such a lesion. Indeed, in our experience, esophageal ulceration has been the first indication of HIV positivity in some patients.

Table 1 Differential Diagnosis of Esophageal Ulcers

Infectious
Viral
Cytomegalovirus
Herpes simplex
Human immunodeficiency virus
Bacterial
Tuberculosis
Atypical mycobacteria
Other
Fungal
Reflux-induced
Barrett's ulcer
Non-Barrett's ulcer
Mechanical
Mallory-Weiss tear
Cameron's ulcer
Iatrogenic
Nasogastric tube–induced
Postsclerotherapy or variceal ligation
Pill-induced
Radiation-induced
Graft-vs.-host disease
Neoplastic
Benign
Leiomyoma
Lipoma
Malignant
Adenocarcinoma
Squamous cell carcinoma
Lymphoma
Sarcoma
Nonesophageal primary
Idiopathic
Bullous pemphigoid
Epidermolysis bullosa dystrophica
Crohn's disease
Sarcoid
Behçet's disease

The most common presenting symptom of esophageal ulceration is odynophagia; however, dysphagia, anorexia, and chest pain are also commonly encountered. Because the endoscopic appearance of an esophageal ulcer may be similar for different pathogenic mechanisms, biopsies for pathological analysis are often essential. Additionally, depending on the patient's profile and the appearance of the lesion, cultures for viral organisms, fungi, atypical mycobacteria, or other pathogens may be appropriate (1,2). In patients with reflux-induced ulceration and Barrett's esophagus, attention should be paid to whether the ulceration occurs in the area epithelialized by columnar cells. These ''Barrett's ulcers'' are sometimes resistant to medical therapy, and may be an independent risk factor for dysplasia or adenocarcinoma of the esophagus (3,4). Perforation of a Barrett's ulcer is an unusual, but well-documented indication for esophageal resection (3,5,6). Pill-induced ulcerations are associated with multiple different medications, with tetracycline, NSAIDs, and potassium supplements among the most common offenders (7).

HEMORRHAGE

Although erosive esophagitis has been reported in up to 20% of patients undergoing endoscopy for reflux symptoms (8), the incidence of hemodynamically significant hemorrhage secondary to reflux-induced mucosal damage is quite low. Most reported series of patients presenting with acute upper-gastrointestinal bleeding show the proportion of patients suffering from hemorrhage from erosive esophagitis to be 10% or less of the total (9,10). Conversely, the overall rate of hemorrhage from any esophageal source is generally greater than 30% in these series, with esophageal variceal bleeding, and Mallory-Weiss tears responsible in the majority of patients. Certain patient groups may be at increased risk for hemorrhage from erosive esophagitis. These include the elderly, those with chronic renal insufficiency, and those taking anticoagulants or NSAIDs (11).

Ulceration associated with a hiatal hernia (''Cameron's'' ulcer) is an underrecognized etiology of upper gastrointestinal hemorrhage (12). This lesion is thought to be secondary to local ischemic effects in the gastric wall at the level of the diaphragm. While not secondary to GERD per se, the frequent association of a hiatal hernia with GERD symptoms makes this diagnosis a consideration in GERD patients presenting with upper gastrointestinal bleeding. This lesion is commonly overlooked, and may be responsible for an increased incidence of iron deficiency anemia in patients with large hiatal hernias (13,14).

SCHATZKI'S RING

Schatzki's ring occurs at the junction between the squamous esophageal and columnar gastric mucosa. The upper surface of Schatzki's ring is lined by squamous

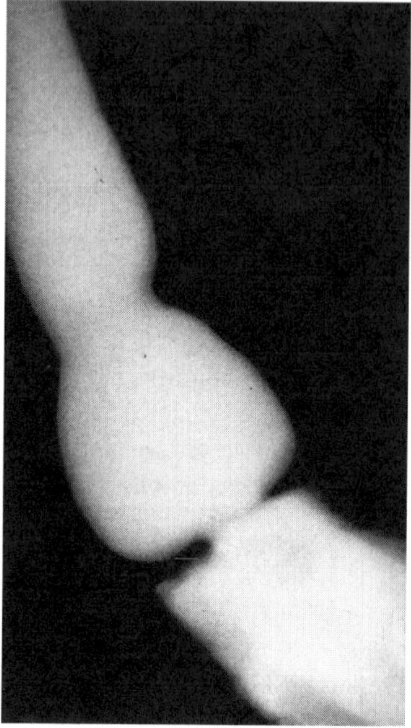

Figure 1 Radiographic view of a Schatzki's ring. (From Ref. 85, used with permission.)

mucosa, while the lower surface is covered by columnar epithelium (15). The ring is usually quite thin, measuring less than 5 mm in most radiographic views (Fig. 1). Pronounced invagination of the ring into the esophageal lumen is a common cause of dysphagia (Fig. 2).

The etiology of Schatzki's ring is unclear. It may be a congenital variant of normal. However, there is some evidence that GERD may be more prevalent in those with a Schatzki's ring (16). Given that many patients with symptomatic rings have no GERD symptoms, and most GERD patients do not have rings, any association between the two, while interesting, remains speculative.

ESOPHAGEAL PEPTIC STRICTURES

Epidemiology

Approximately 10% of patients receiving medical attention for GERD will develop strictures (17). Reliable prognostic factors for stricture development among those patients with GERD do not exist. The severity of GERD only weakly corre-

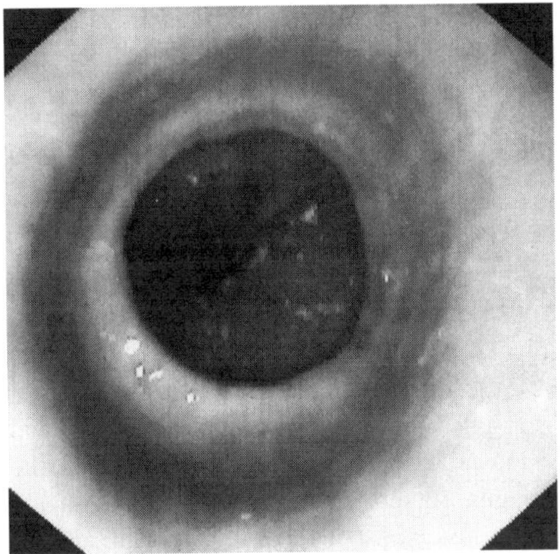

Figure 2 Endoscopic view of a Schatzki's ring, a common cause of dysphagia.

lates with the propensity to form strictures. The incidence of peptic strictures does increase with age, perhaps reflecting the cumulative insult of decades of reflux disease (18). Other risk factors for stricture formation among those with GERD include Caucasian race and male sex (19,20). Additionally, those conditions in which NSAID use is common have been shown to be associated with the formation of esophageal stricture (21).

Pathogenesis

The pathogenesis of peptic strictures, like the pathogenesis of GERD, appears to be multifactorial. While the factors leading one individual with reflux disease to stricture and another to heal without complication are not clear, several observations shed light on the etiology of strictures in reflux disease (22). GERD patients with strictures appear to be less sensitive to intraesophageal acid than GERD patients without strictures (23). Also, while low resting lower esophageal sphincter (LES) pressures are not consistently seen in patients with uncomplicated GERD, patients with peptic strictures generally do have lower resting LES pressures than either typical GERD patients or controls (24,25). In fact, a resting LES pressure of less than 8 mmHg is highly predictive of stricture formation in GERD patients. Next, the presence of a hiatal hernia is more common in those GERD patients with strictures than those without (26). Finally, patients with strictures appear to have decreased amplitude and frequency of esophageal peristalsis, leading to reduced acid clearance (20). This concept is supported by data showing that those patients who develop strictures have higher levels of gastric acid exposure on 24-h pH monitoring than those with uncomplicated GERD. Other host factors, such as differences in fibrogenesis or gastric acid hypersecretion in stricture formers, have been postulated but not proven.

Stricture formation appears to take place in several stages. In response to early reflux episodes, mucosal edema and muscular spasm occur. The histological picture at this stage may include basal cell hyperplasia and infiltration of the mucosa with eosinophils. These conditions are usually reversible with vigorous acid suppression (27). Continued exposure to pathological levels of gastric acid leads to ulceration, with reactive fibrosis. As this fibrotic reaction extends into the muscularis propria, the muscular and neural elements responsible for peristalsis are damaged, impairing the clearance mechanisms of the esophagus and leading to increased dwell times of the refluxate within the esophagus. In the ongoing struggle to repair the esophagus, increasing amounts of collagen are deposited, which over time result in the loss of esophageal luminal caliber and stricture formation.

Presentation

While the majority of patients with peptic strictures will have a history of GERD symptoms predating their presentation, approximately one in three patients with strictures will have had no previous history of reflux symptoms (27). This phenomenon has been attributed to the decrease in sensitivity to esophageal acid described above. The majority of patients presenting with peptic strictures have dysphagia with solids as a presenting symptom; however, odynophagia and food impaction are also common presentations. Localization of the level of obstruction by the patient's symptoms may be accurate in the majority of cases; however, in a significant subset of patients, the sensation of dysphagia will not correspond to the level of the obstruction (28).

Diagnosis

Approximately 70% of strictures result from chronic reflux. The differential diagnosis of peptic strictures is broad (Table 2). Most nonpeptic causes of esophageal stricture can be ruled out by history. Neoplastic strictures, especially adenocarcinomas arising near the gastroesophageal junction, can be difficult to differentiate from benign peptic strictures, making multiple biopsies of such lesions essential at endoscopy.

Two diagnostic tests are commonly used in the evaluation of dysphagia. The first is esophageal contrast radiography (Fig. 3). This modality is sensitive for detecting mild, early, and/or subtle strictures (29). Stricture morphology is easily assessed, and distal portions of the stricture sometimes not accessible by

Table 2 Differential Diagnosis of Esophageal Strictures

Ingestion of caustic substances
Alkali
Acid
Iatrogenic
Radiation therapy
Photodynamic therapy
Variceal sclerotherapy or banding
Chronic graft-vs.-host disease
Postoperative
Pill-induced
Chronic nasogastric tube–induced
Idiopathic diseases
Epidermolysis bullosa dystrophica
Tylosis
Pemphigus
Bullous pemphigoid
Scleroderma
Esophageal webs or strictures
Eosinophilic esophagitis
Crohn's disease
Sarcoidosis
Acid peptic
Barrett's associated
Non–Barrett's associated
Neoplasia
Adenocarcinoma
Squamous cell carcinoma
Nonepithelial tumors
Infectious
Syphilis
Candida
Herpes simplex
Cytomegalovirus
Tuberculosis

endoscopy may be visualized. Also, digestion of a tablet or solid may enhance the sensitivity of this examination for detecting abnormalities associated with dysphagia (30,31). The second, often complementary examination is upper endoscopy. Upper endoscopy has the advantage of being both a therapeutic and diagnostic maneuver (see below). Additionally, tissue samples can be taken to

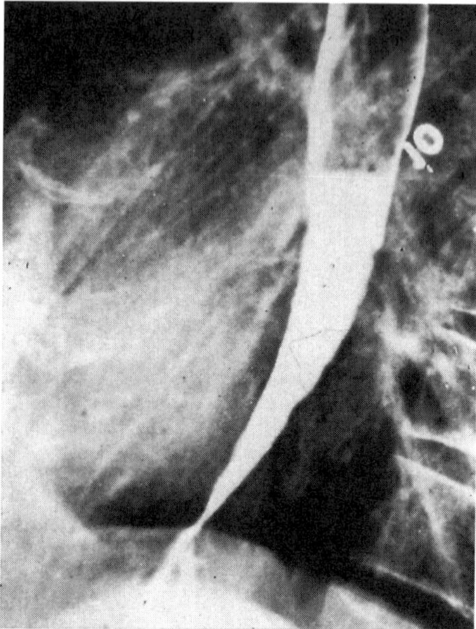

Figure 3 Barium radiograph of an esophageal stricture. (From Ref. 85, used with permission.)

rule out malignancy. However, in tight strictures (Fig. 4, a and b), passage of even a neonatal or pediatric endoscope is impossible.

While it has been suggested that barium esophagram is the examination of choice for the evaluation of dysphagia (32), many clinicians will proceed directly to upper endoscopy. This may be especially appropriate in the older patient with weight loss, where the pretest probability of significant disease is high, and either a therapeutic intervention or tissue sampling is likely (33). If this diagnostic strategy is to be followed, the clinician may occasionally be faced with a peptic stricture that will not allow passage of the endoscope, and whose distal morphology is unknown. Without knowledge of the morphology of the stricture, it may be wise to defer dilatation until a barium esophogram has been obtained.

Management

Medical

While esophageal dilatation has long been the cornerstone on which the therapy for peptic strictures rests, increasing amounts of data suggest that pharmacologi-

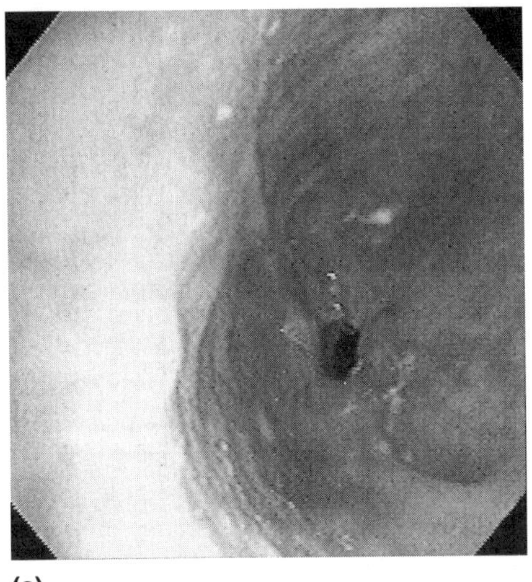

(a)

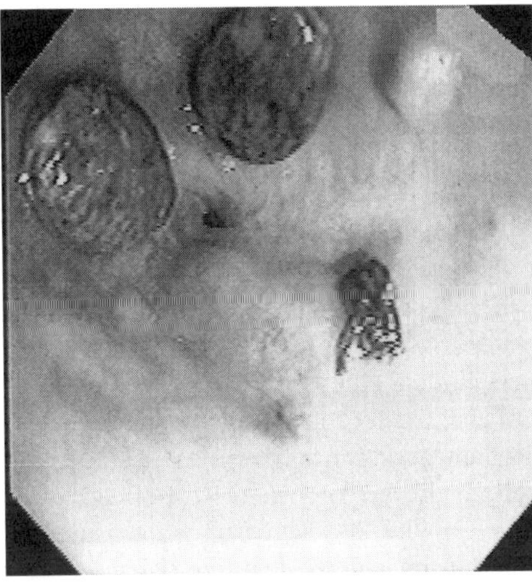

(b)

Figure 4 (a and b) Endoscopic views of tight strictures. Note the watermelon seeds in (b) for scale. (From Ref. 85, used with permission.)

cal interventions in patients with peptic strictures positively impact their course. This is logical for several reasons. First, decreasing the active inflammation of the esophagus may actually increase luminal caliber by decreasing mucosal edema. Second, acid suppression may slow or halt the ongoing mucosal insult, resulting in improved luminal caliber in the long term. Finally, the sensation of dysphagia is not dependent on luminal caliber alone. Data show that the degree of mucosal inflammation present is actually more predictive of the degree of dysphagia that patients with strictures experience than is the luminal diameter (34).

The frequency of dilatations necessary to insure adequate luminal caliber is the most commonly used yardstick in the medical literature to assess the effect of pharmacological interventions on peptic strictures. This measure is suboptimal for several reasons. It may hide physician-specific differences in the practice of dilatation, such as the threshold of dysphagia necessary to prompt dilatation. Also, it fails to recognize specific subgroups of patient profiles based on the pathophysiological mechanisms outlined above. For instance, salutary effects in patients with early strictures amenable to acid suppression may well be hidden by a lack of effect in older, more established fibrotic strictures. Next, the perception of dysphagia, as well as the psychological distress it causes, may vary dramatically from patient to patient. Finally, when compared to historical or nonmedicated controls, the placebo effect of the medication itself may actually delay the patient's request for dilatation, regardless of any physiological effect of the medication. Other measures, such as dysphagia scores and endoscopic evaluation of mucosal damage, have been used to supplement this outcome measure.

Data regarding the effect of rigorous acid suppression support its routine use in patients with peptic strictures. While early data reporting the use of H_2-receptor antagonists on patients with strictures failed to show any decreased need for dilatation (35,36), several investigators have demonstrated that proton pump inhibitors (PPIs) positively impact their clinical course. PPIs decrease the need for recurrent dilatation, speed healing of coexistent esophagitis, and improve dysphagia more effectively than H_2-receptor antagonists or placebo (37–41). Despite the higher cost of PPIs, these medications are actually more cost-effective for managing patients with peptic strictures, owing to decreased ''downstream'' costs (42). For these reasons, PPIs should be considered first-line pharmacological therapy for patients with peptic stricture.

Dilatation

The mainstay of medical management of established peptic strictures is esophageal dilatation. Dilatation is a centuries-old practice. Initial descriptions of dilatation date to the 16th century, when wax candles were used to perform dilatation. In fact, the term ''bougienage'' originates from the Algerian town of Bouginhay, the capital of the wax candle trade in the Middle Ages (43). Blunt-tipped mercury dilators were first used in 1915 by the British surgeon Arthur Hurst. His design was later modified by Maloney to include a tapered end to allow passage through tight strictures. In 1951, an over-the-wire method of dilatation utilizing oval metal dilators, termed "olives," was developed by Eder and Peustow. This system could be monitored fluoroscopically, but has become obsolete with the advent of more recent over-the-wire methods for dilatation.

Three types of esophageal dilatation systems are presently commonly used in the United States. These include blunt or tapered mercury-filled bougies, over-the-wire polyvinyl graduated-sized bougies, and through-the-scope (TTS) balloon dilators. Following is a brief description of each system, as well as the techniques involved in using it.

Mercury-Filled Bougienage. Despite the advent of more sophisticated systems for esophageal dilatation, mercury-filled bougienage remains a popular and commonly used method for achieving esophageal dilatation. The reasons for this are several. First and foremost is simplicity. Mercury-filled bougienage requires no fluoroscopy, or guidewires. Because these adjunct measures are not necessary, costs are relatively low. Also, because mercury-filled bougies have been available for so long, many clinicians are very experienced and confident with their use.

Two types of mercury-filled bougies are commonly used in the United States. The first is the Hurst dilator, which is a relatively blunt-tipped instrument, and the second is the Maloney dilator, which has a tapered end (Fig. 5). The technique involved in using both systems is the same. Some previous assessment

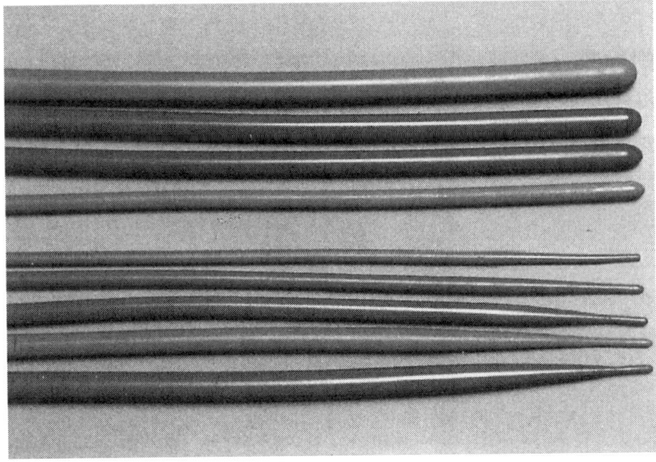

Figure 5 Hurst (above) and Maloney dilators. (From Ref. 85, used with permission.)

of stricture caliber, by either barium radiograph or endoscopy, is essential. The patient is placed in the sitting or left lateral decubitus position. The initial dilator size should be approximately the same size as the tightest diameter of the stricture. Topical pharyngeal anesthesia and lubrication are applied. Systemic sedation is not essential, but is sometimes helpful in the anxious patient. The head is slightly hyperextended. Held like a pencil in the dominant hand, the dilator is slid into the posterior pharynx over the dorsal surface of the first and second fingers of the nondominant hand (Fig. 6). The patient is asked to swallow, and the dilator is smoothly slid into the esophagus when the upper-esophageal sphincter relaxes. The deepest penetration of the dilator should be such that the dilator's maximal diameter goes several centimeters past the most distal extent of the stricture. This is especially important when performing dilatation with a Maloney dilator, since resistance can be encountered with the tapered tip well before the maximal diameter of the dilator is through the stricture. This procedure is repeated with gradually increasing sizes of dilators.

The optimal number of dilatations performed at a single sitting is not clear, and varies based on the morphology of the stricture, the tolerance of the patient, and the amount of resistance encountered. A useful empirical guideline is that no more than three dilatations to resistance in any single session is advisable (the so-called "rule of three"). While the rule of three may be useful, it must be

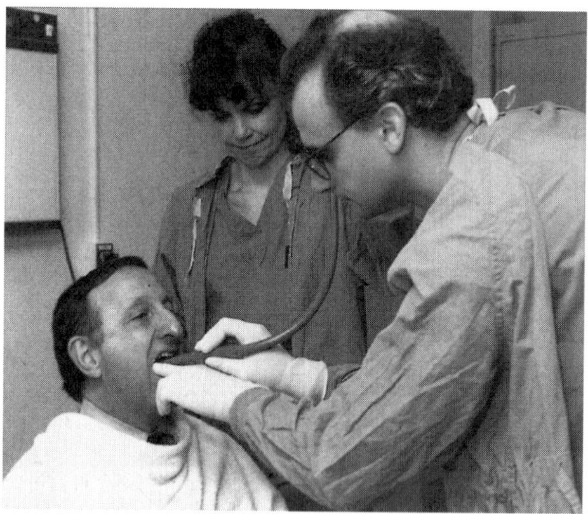

Figure 6 Appropriate technique for insertion of a Hurst dilator with the patient in the upright position. (From Ref. 85, used with permission.)

stressed that any time undue force is necessary to pass a dilator, it is inadvisable to continue with larger dilators. The goal of dilatation is to accomplish a luminal diameter of 45–60 Fr (15–20 mm). At this diameter, most patients are free of dysphagia (44). This goal can usually be accomplished in less than three sittings. Objective criteria, such as the passage of a barium tablet of 12-mm diameter, may represent a superior goal for dilatation (45).

Mercury-filled dilators are especially useful in several situations. Patients who have well-characterized, short, simple strictures are good candidates for mercury-filled bougienage. Also, those with Schatzki's rings or congenital webs respond well to a single passage of a large (>50 Fr) dilator. Most patients with Schatzki's ring will be asymptomatic after this therapy (46). These dilators are less useful in tortuous strictures or very tight strictures. Especially in tight strictures, these dilators may impact on the shoulder of the stricture, coil in the proximal esophagus, and never traverse the stricture zone. Mercury-filled dilators should not be used in strictures associated with adjacent esophageal pseudodiverticula (Fig. 7), where a wire- or endoscopically guided technique provides more reliable dilatation.

While success rates of greater than 85% in relieving dysphagia are commonly reported, there is some suggestion in the literature that the performance of mercury-filled bougienage with fluoroscopic guidance might improve outcomes

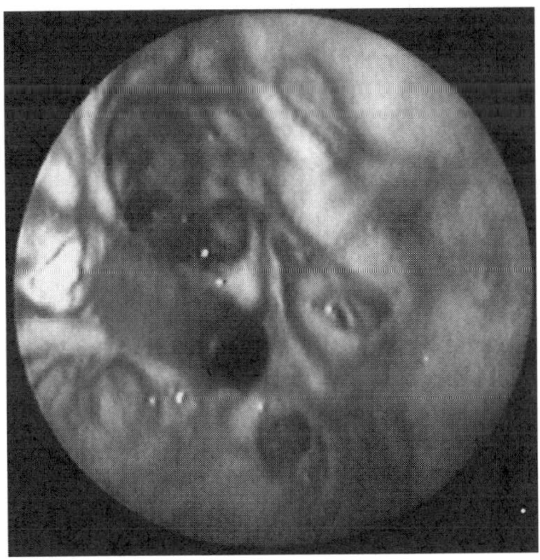

Figure 7 Stricture with pseudodiverticulae. Dilatation of this stricture with mercury bougienage may place the patient at increased risk of perforation.

(47,48). However, the markedly increased cost per session this entails, as well as the mandatory radiation exposure, makes mercury-filled bougienage less attractive. Additionally, dilatation without fluoroscopy appears safe for the vast majority of patients (49). Redilatation rates vary markedly among patients, but as many as 40% of patients will require only one dilatation for symptom relief (50,51). Some patients may need weekly sessions for several months to ensure adequate luminal caliber, and others may need maintenance dilatations to avoid recurrent dysphagia or food impactions. Predictors of the need for recurrent dilatation include fibrous strictures, a maximal dilator size of less than 44 Fr, and more than two initial sessions to relieve dysphagia (50).

Self-Dilatation with Mercury-Filled Dilators

In patients who require frequent regular dilatations of benign peptic strictures to remain symptom-free, self-dilatation with a mercury-filled dilator can be effective and convenient. The limited data available on this practice suggest that it is safe in selected, motivated patients (52). If this course is to be attempted, proper instruction in technique, as well as follow-up to assure that complications have not occurred, is essential (53). Also, the age and condition of the dilator(s) need to be monitored to avert cracking or spillage of mercury.

Polyvinyl Over-the-Wire Dilators. Two commercially available polyvinyl over-the-wire dilators exist in the United States, the Savary dilating system (Wilson Cook) and the American Endoscopy dilating system (Bard) (Fig. 8). They

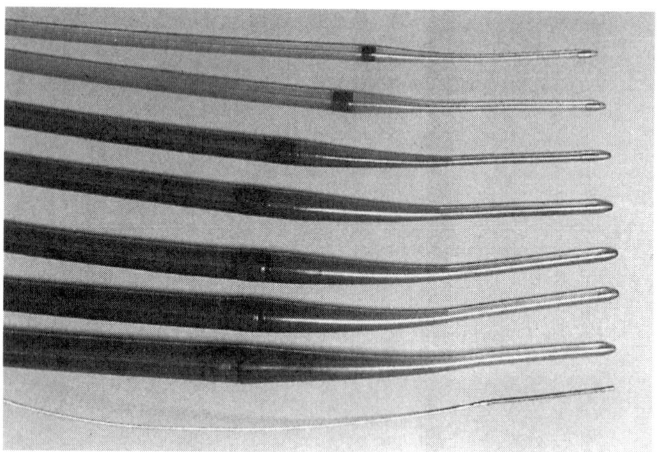

Figure 8 Savary dilators, with guidewire. (From Ref. 85, used with permission.)

differ slightly in the shape of the dilator and the design of the guidewire. Additionally, the Savary system has only a radiopaque band at the point where the dilator reaches its widest diameter, while the American Endoscopy system is impregnated along the entire dilator with barium sulfate for easier fluoroscopic visualization. The techniques involved in dilating with both systems are the same.

Before performing any procedure, one must make sure that the mouthpiece will allow passage of the largest dilator to be used. First, routine endoscopy with either a standard upper endoscope or, in the case of tight or angulated strictures, a pediatric or neonatal endoscope is performed. The diameter of the narrowest portion of the stricture is assessed, using the known diameter of the endoscope as a guideline. Next, the guidewire is placed. The spring-tipped end of the wire is placed through the scope and, under direct visualization, advanced until the tip of the wire lies along the greater curve of the stomach in the antrum. The scope is then ''traded out,'' or exchanged, with the guidewire being advanced through the scope 4 or 5 cm for every 4 or 5 cm of scope withdrawn. If this is done correctly, the scope can be completely withdrawn leaving approximately 60 cm of wire in the patient. Careful note should be made of the wire markings at the patient's teeth, so that after each dilatation, minimal wire migration either forward or backward can be assured.

Next, the dilators are passed. To do this, an assistant fixes the wire in space such that it does not advance with the advancing dilator. Again, the patient's neck is slightly hyperextended to allow easier passage of the dilator through the cervical area. After the wire is lubricated with silicone, the stiff end of the wire is inserted into the hollow tip of the dilator. With the dilator held like a pencil in the dominant hand, it is passed over the wire, with the assistant applying gentle traction on the wire to avoid advancement of the wire with the dilator. The dilator should be inserted until the maximal diameter of the dilator is completely through the stricture zone. For strictures that are either tight or tortuous, correct dilator placement is best ascertained by use of fluoroscopy. The dilator is then withdrawn, while the wire is forwarded through it. When the dilator is removed, the position of the wire as measured by the markings on it should be within 5 cm of the initial starting point. If significant wire migration has occurred, especially outward, removal of the wire and reinsertion of the endoscope may be necessary to properly replace the wire. Do not try to reinsert the endoscope over the wire, as doing so will almost certainly cause damage to the inner channel of the scope. If reinsertion of an endoscope over a guidewire is unavoidable, a plastic ERCP catheter can be inserted into the working channel of the scope to protect it as the wire is put through the scope in a retrograde fashion.

As with mercury-filled bougies, the rule of three is a useful guideline as to how many wire-guided dilators to pass. On the final dilatation, both the wire and the final bougie are removed simultaneously. If significant resistance to passage of the dilator is met, the operator should reassess the wire position, as back-migration of the wire may cause the tip of the dilator to impact on the spring end.

Through-the-Scope (TTS) Balloons. TTS balloons provide effective dilatation of esophageal strictures (Fig. 9). Polyethylene balloons ranging from 4 to 18 mm are available, though sizes 9–18 mm are most commonly used in the esophagus. Balloon lengths range from 5 to 8.5 cm. While data exist demonstrating adequate relief of dysphagia and low complication rates with TTS dilatation (54,55), this method is less commonly used by practicing gastroenterologists. This may be because of the associated costs of the single-use balloon catheters, or because the technology is newer than either over-the-wire methods or mercury-filled bougienage.

Like over-the-wire dilatation, TTS dilatation is usually prefaced by a standard endoscopic examination. Endoscopes with working channels of 3.2 or

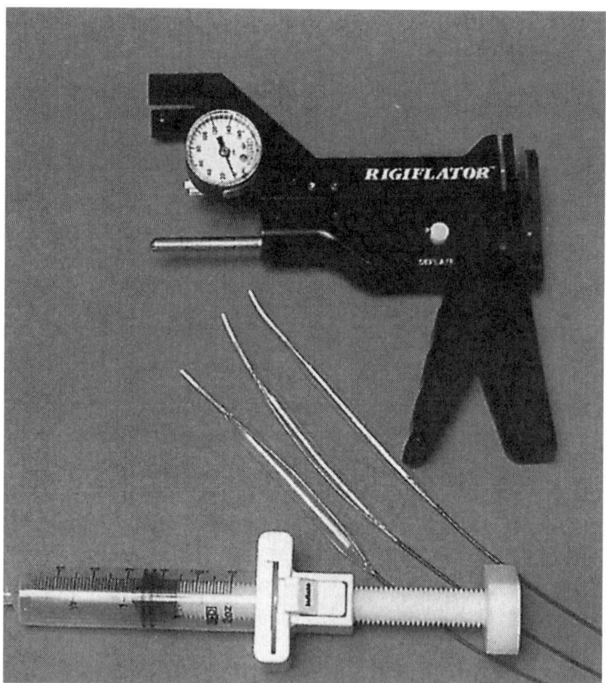

Figure 9 Through-the-scope (TTS) balloons of various sizes. The fluid-filled syringe, when inserted into the gun device, provides water insufflation of the balloon at controlled pressures. (From Ref. 85, used with permission.)

greater mm should be used. Approximation of stricture diameter is made during this examination. Also, assessment of stricture morphology is made, so that appropriate balloon selection can be made. In situations where the stricture is too narrow to allow passage of even a small-caliber scope, a barium study will help delineate stricture morphology.

After the examination, the balloon is inserted through the scope. Prior to insertion of the balloon, it should be checked outside the patient for patency. Most balloons have a lifespan of 5–10 uses if handled carefully. We generally use water to expand the balloons; however, dilute contrast may also be used in situations where fluoroscopy may also be performed.

Balloon selection is important. A long, uncomplicated stricture may respond well to dilatation using a single long balloon. On the other hand, it may be advisable to dilate a long, angulated stricture in segments with a shorter balloon to minimize the chance of perforation. The tip of the balloon is coated with silicon for easier passage. The balloon is then passed through the scope and across the portion of the stricture to be dilated. The rim of the plastic catheter shaft must be visualized prior to any inflation of the balloon, to assure that the entire balloon has exited the scope. The balloon is then slowly inflated. Usually, as the balloon is inflated, there is a cephalad migration, because the proximal portion of the balloon fills first, causing the balloon to ''back out'' of the stricture zone. For this reason, frequent repositioning of the balloon may be necessary during inflation. No balloon should ever be inflated across a stricture without knowledge of the morphology of the stricture, as inflation of a long, rigid balloon in a sharply angulated stricture may cause perforation by the distal balloon. Balloons are inflated to their maximal dilating pressures, and held in place for 2 min (Fig. 10). This may be repeated 2–3 times; however, if fluoroscopy shows obliteration of the waist of a stricture, dilatation is successful and little is to be gained by additional inflations. After inflation, complete deflation of the balloon must be achieved prior to withdrawal through the scope.

TTS balloons exert only radial, not shearing, force. Therefore, investigators hoped that more aggressive dilatation of strictures might be possible, since damage to the tissues might be less (56). Unfortunately, attempts to dilate tight strictures to adequate diameters in a single session with TTS balloons appear to be ill-advised (57). Like over-the-wire and mercury-filled dilatations, the most prudent approach to tight strictures is serial sessions. These sessions can combine dilating modalities, for example, using TTS for an initially very tight stricture, with over-the-wire or mercury-filled dilatations for later sessions.

Complications of Dilatation

Potential complications of dilatation of peptic strictures include those inherent to the dilatation, and, in the case of TTS or over-the-wire dilatations, those inher-

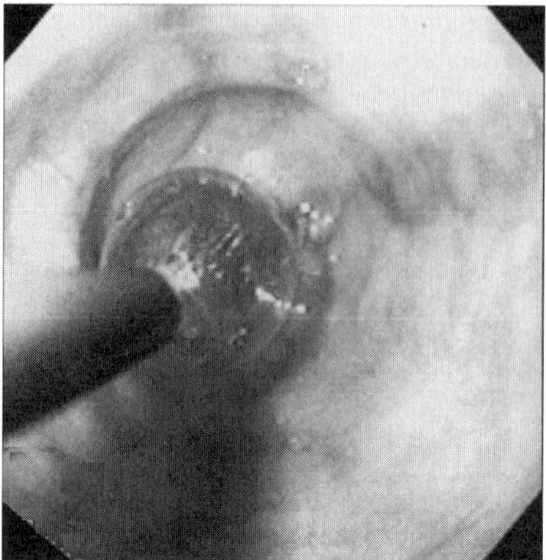

Figure 10 TTS balloon inflated across an esophageal stricture. (From Ref. 85, used with permission.)

ent in the endoscopy as well. The main risks of esophageal dilatation include perforation, bleeding, and bacteremia. The risks of endoscopy include bleeding, perforation, aspiration, and sedation-related complications. In addition to the risk of bleeding, which appears to be marginally increased in patients with strictures, the risks of endoscopy appear to be similar to those of other patients undergoing diagnostic upper endoscopy.

Esophageal perforation is the most morbid complication of esophageal dilatation. In most published series, the rate of perforation is low, usually less than 4 per 1000 procedures (58–62). In patients who do suffer perforation, it may be the cervical esophagus, not the stricture zone, in which the perforation occurs. This is especially true in series utilizing the Eder-Puestow olives. Among the current commonly used methods of dilatation, perforation rates appear to be similar. Although routine use of fluoroscopy has been suggested to lower the risk of perforation, no randomized studies have demonstrated lesser risk. In fact, investigators using only endoscopy as an adjunct to dilatation have reported acceptably low complication rates (62). Risk factors for perforation have been assessed in several series, and include long strictures, very tight strictures, large hiatal hernias, and angulation within the stricture zone (57,63). Although plain radiography demonstrating subcutaneous emphysema or air in the mediastinum may suggest the diagnosis, postprocedure esophageal perforations are best demonstrated by contrast radiography using nonbarium contrast agents. Multiple views in different patient positions may be required to demonstrate small leaks. Surgical consultation is essential, but many perforations can be managed medically with good outcomes.

Bleeding requiring blood transfusion occurs in about 5 in 1000 patients. Bleeding may occur from the dilated stricture zone itself, or from mucosa above the stricture zone that was abraded by the shearing force of a push dilator. Repeat endoscopy with injection of epinephrine or saline may halt bleeding and allow reepithelialization. Bleeding requiring operative intervention is rare.

Many patients undergoing dilatation experience transient bacteremia (64). In the vast majority of patients, this is of no consequence. However, there have been reported cases of serious infectious complications, including endocarditis, meningitis, and brain abscess (61,65–67). Although there are few data to support their use, antibiotics are often given to patients with prosthetic heart valves, a history of endocarditis, or other high-risk profiles, to decrease the chance of infectious complications after dilatation.

Stricture Recurrence After Dilatation

Most studies report that greater than 50% of patients undergoing dilatation of peptic strictures to goal diameters will have recurrence of dysphagia necessitating repeat dilatation (50,51,68). This appears to be true regardless of the system used in the initial dilatation. Moreover, the number of recurrences of stricturing appears to predict the likelihood of future stricturing. For example, in one reported cohort, if a patient experienced two recurrences of peptic stricturing requiring dilatation, chances were 94% that a third episode of stricturing requiring dilatation would occur (50). Other predictors of the need for frequent dilatations include weight loss and the lack of the sensation of heartburn (69).

Comparative Studies Between Dilating Systems

Conclusive, prospective, randomized comparative studies of the currently utilized dilating systems have not been performed. Given the low rate of major complications with all of the current systems, thousands of patients might be necessary to show significant differences between the systems. One study comparing TTS balloons to Savary dilators in treating benign esophageal strictures showed no difference in complication rates or success rates between the two systems (54). This study did suggest, however, that the need for long-term recurrent dilatation may be lower in those patients treated with TTS balloons. A second study comparing balloons to Savary dilators again showed no difference in safety. In this study, however, those undergoing dilatation with Savary dilators required fewer subsequent dilatations and had larger esophageal diameters 1 year after the initial dilatation (55). Given the conflicted nature of the data, at present no firm recommendation for one system over the other can be made. Investigators have demonstrated equal efficacy, lower complication rates, and greater patient comfort with Savary dilators compared to Eder-Puestow olives (70), prompting the abandonment of the latter system by most clinicians.

Stenting of Benign Esophageal Strictures

In patients with strictures unresponsive to attempts at dilatation, esophageal stenting has been proposed as an alternative to surgery. This procedure may be especially attractive in those patients who are elderly or those whose multiple comorbid conditions make surgery prohibitive (71). Several groups have now reported their initial experience with the placement of expandable metal stents in benign esophageal strictures (72–74). While these reports feature high patency rates, the unclear long-term consequences of stenting in benign esophageal disease make this option inadvisable for the patient with a considerable life expectancy. Despite the relative infancy of expandable metallic stents, multiple reports of stent migration, occlusion by overgrowth of hyperplastic tissue at the ends of the stent, and other problems exist (74,75).

Surgical Management of Strictures

Indications

Clearly, the best management of esophageal strictures is early and adequate medical therapy to avert their development. The role of surgery in peptic strictures has changed with both the advent of laparoscopic surgical procedures and the development of better acid suppression. In patients with an esophagus of normal length and a stricture responsive to dilatation, the indications for surgery are similar to those of the general GERD population. In these patients, a standard laparoscopic antireflux procedure is generally the procedure of choice. As with all GERD patients, preoperative esophageal manometry demonstrating good motility is essential. When surgical antireflux procedures are performed in a patient with a stricture, postoperative rates of dysphagia may be higher than in the general GERD population (76). For this reason, some have advocated the Belsey partial fundoplication in this group (77). In general, results of surgical fundoplication in stricture patients appear as good as those of the general GERD population.

In the patient with a fibrotic shortened esophagus and a stricture amenable to dilatation, an esophageal lengthening procedure coupled with an antireflux procedure may give good relief of symptoms and control of GERD without an esophageal resection. Standard antireflux procedures often fail in this patient population because inadequate lengths of the distal esophagus can be mobilized, and the fundoplication is under tension. Two procedures, the Collis-Belsey gastroplasty and the Collis-Nissen gastroplasty, have been reported to provide good results in this patient population (78,79). In both of these procedures, the high cardia is tubularized and serves as an elongation of the esophagus. The fundoplication then occurs around this length of tubularized cardia. Results of these procedures are good in 50–80% of cases.

In patients with strictures unresponsive to recurrent dilatation, esophageal resection may be necessary. In these situations, interposition of other luminal organs such as colon or jejunum may be performed (80–82), or mobilization of the stomach, with esophagogastric anastamosis in the chest. Gastric interposition combined with pyloroplasty is the most commonly performed procedure, because it requires only one anastamosis. Published results with this procedure show good or excellent function in 70% of patients, and an operative mortality of <5% (83). In young patients, left colonic interposition has been advocated (84). Although this procedure is more technically demanding and has a higher operative mortality rate, its long-term functional results may be superior to those of gastric or jejunal interposition.

Limited data exist on the use of laparoscopic surgical procedures in the patient with peptic esophageal stricture. Although earlier investigators felt that esophageal stricture might be a contraindication to the laparoscopic approach because of inability to mobilize the esophagus and fully assess the stricture, more recent work reports high rates of success of the laparoscopic Nissen fundoplication in patients with strictures. Reports of success with laparoscopic esophageal lengthening and resection procedures exist, but definitive studies of their safety and efficacy are necessary.

CONCLUSION

Esophageal complications of GERD, including stricture, ulceration, and Barrett's esophagus, are commonly encountered by the practicing gastroenterologist. Our main goal in treating patients with reflux disease is to prevent complications with a rigorous antireflux program. Significant improvements in the management of stricture patients include wire-guided and through-the-scope dilating systems, as reviewed above. Maintenance of patients with peptic strictures on chronic acid inhibition with proton pump inhibitors improves symptoms, and decreases the need for recurrent esophageal dilatation. Despite these improvements in management, a small portion of patients will go on to require surgery. The choice of the surgical procedure depends on the characteristics of the patient and the stricture, as well as the experience of the surgeon.

REFERENCES

1. Wilcox CM, Straub RF, Schwartz DA. Prospective endoscopic characterization of cytomegalovirus esophagitis in AIDS. Gastrointest Endosc 1994; 40:481–484.

2. Wilcox CM, Schwartz DA. Endoscopic characterization of idiopathic esophageal ulceration associated with human immunodeficiency virus infection. J Clin Gastroenterol 1993; 16:251–256.
3. Pearson FG, Cooper JD, Patterson GA, Prakash D. Peptic ulcer in acquired columnar-lined esophagus: results of surgical treatment. Ann Thorac Surg 1987; 43:241–244.
4. Komorowski RA, Hogan WJ, Chausow DD. Barrett's ulcer: the clinical significance today. Am J Gastroenterol 1996; 91:2310–2313.
5. Altorki NK, Skinner DB, Segalin A, Stephens JK, Ferguson MK, Little AG. Indications for esophagectomy in nonmalignant Barrett's esophagus: a 10-year experience. Ann Thorac Surg 1990; 49:724–726.
6. Cappell MS, Sciales C, Biempica L. Esophageal perforation at a Barrett's ulcer. J Clin Gastroenterol 1989; 11:663–666.
7. Kikendall JW. Pill-induced esophageal injury. Gastroenterol Clin North Am 1991; 20:835–846.
8. Spechler SJ. Epidemiology and natural history of gastro-oesophageal reflux disease. Digestion 1992; 51(suppl 1):24–29.
9. Wara P. Incidence, diagnosis, and natural course of upper gastrointestinal hemorrhage. Prognostic value of clinical factors and endoscopy. Scand J Gastroenterol 1987; 137(suppl):26–27.
10. Sugawa C, Steffes CP, Nakamura R, Sferra JJ, Sferra CS, Sugimura Y, et al. Upper GI bleeding in an urban hospital. Etiology, recurrence, and prognosis. Ann Surg 1990; 212:521–526.
11. Zimmerman J, Shohat V, Tsvang E, Arnon R, Safadi R, Wengrower D. Esophagitis is a major cause of upper gastrointestinal hemorrhage in the elderly. Scand J Gastroenterol 1997; 32:906–909.
12. Weston AP. Hiatal hernia with cameron ulcers and erosions (review). Gastrointest Endosc Clin North Am 1996; 6:671–679.
13. Cameron AJ, Higgins JA. Linear gastric erosion. A lesion associated with large diaphragmatic hernia and chronic blood loss anemia. Gastroenterology 1986; 91: 338–342.
14. Cameron AJ. Incidence of iron deficiency anemia in patients with large diaphragmatic hernia. A controlled study. Mayo Clin Proc 1976; 51:767–769.
15. DeVault KR. Lower esophageal (Schatzki's) ring: pathogenesis, diagnosis and therapy. Dig Dis 1996; 14:323–329.
16. Marshall JB, Kretschmar JM, Diaz-Arias AA. Gastroesophageal reflux as a pathogenic factor in the development of symptomatic lower esophageal rings. Arch Intern Med 1990; 150:1669–1672.
17. Marks RD, Shukla M. Diagnosis and management of peptic esophageal strictures. Gastroenterologist 1996; 4:223–237.
18. Sonnenberg A, Massey BT, Jacobsen SJ. Hospital discharges resulting from esophagitis among Medicare beneficiaries. Dig Dis Sci 1994; 39:183–188.
19. el-Serag HB, Sonnenberg A. Associations between different forms of gastro-oesophageal reflux disease. Gut 1997; 41:594–599.
20. Marks RD, Shukla M. Diagnosis and management of peptic esophageal strictures. Gastroenterologist 1996; 4:223–237.

21. el-Serag HB, Sonnenberg A. Association of esophagitis and esophageal strictures with diseases treated with nonsteroidal anti-inflammatory drugs. Am J Gastroenterol 1997; 92:52–56.
22. Cioffi U, Rosso L, De Simone M. Gastroesophageal reflux disease. Pathogenesis, symptoms and complications. Panminerva Med 1998; 40:132–138.
23. Winwood PJ, Mavrogiannis CC, Smith CL. Reduced sensitivity to intra-oesophageal acid in patients with reflux-induced strictures. Scand J Gastroenterol 1993; 28:109–112.
24. Parkman HP, Fisher RS. Contributing role of motility abnormalities in the pathogenesis of gastroesophageal reflux disease. Dig Dis 1997; 15(suppl 1):40–52.
25. Parkman HP, Fisher RS. Contributing role of motility abnormalities in the pathogenesis of gastroesophageal reflux disease. Dig Dis 1997; 15(suppl 1):40–52.
26. Bell NJ, Burget D, Howden CW, Wilkinson J, Hunt RH. Appropriate acid suppression for the management of gastro-oesophageal reflux disease. Digestion 1992; 51(suppl 1):59–67.
27. Jaspersen D, Schwacha H, Schorr W, Brennenstuhl M, Raschka C, Hammar CH. Omeprazole in the treatment of patients with complicated gastro-oesophageal reflux disease. J Gastroenterol Hepatol 1996; 11:900–902.
28. Wilcox CM, Alexander LN, Clark WS. Localization of an obstructing esophageal lesion. Is the patient accurate? Dig Dis Sci 1995; 40:2192–2196.
29. Halpert RD, Feczko PJ, Spickler EM, Ackerman LV. Radiological assessment of dysphagia with endoscopic correlation. Radiology 1985; 157:599–602.
30. Ghahremani GG, Weingardt JP, Curtin KR, Yaghmai V. Detection of occult esophageal narrowing with a barium tablet during chest radiography. Clin Imaging 1996; 20:184–190.
31. van Westen D, Ekberg O. Solid bolus swallowing in the radiologic evaluation of dysphagia. Acta Radiol 1993; 34:372–375.
32. Castell DO. Approach to the patient with dysphagia. In: Yamada T, ed. Textbook of Gastroenterology, 2nd ed. Philadelphia: JB Lippincott, 1995:638–648.
33. Gupta SD, Petrus LV, Gibbins FJ, Dellipiani AW. Endoscopic evaluation of dysphagia in the elderly. Age Ageing 1987; 16:159–164.
34. Dakkak M, Hoare RC, Maslin SC, Bennett JR. Oesophagitis is as important as oesophageal stricture diameter in determining dysphagia. Gut 1993; 34:152–155.
35. Ferguson R, Dronfield MW, Atkinson M. Cimetidine in treatment of reflux oesophagitis with peptic stricture. Br Med J 1979; 2:472–474.
36. Starlinger M, Appel WH, Schemper M, Schiessel R. Long-term treatment of peptic esophageal stenosis with dilatation and cimetidine: factors influencing clinical result. Eur Surg Res 1985; 17:207–214.
37. Smith PM, Kerr GD, Cockel R, Ross BA, Bate CM, Brown P, et al. A comparison of omeprazole and ranitidine in the prevention of recurrence of benign esophageal stricture. Restore Investigator Group. Gastroenterology 1994; 107:1312–1318.
38. Colin-Jones DG. The role and limitations of H2-receptor antagonists in the treatment of gastro-oesophageal reflux disease. Aliment Pharmacol Ther 1995; 9(suppl 1):9–14.
39. Klinkenberg-Knol EC, Festen HP, Meuwissen SG. Pharmacological management of gastro-oesophageal reflux disease. Drugs 1995; 49:695–710.

40. Freston JW, Malagelada JR, Petersen H, McCloy RF. Critical issues in the management of gastroesophageal reflux disease. Eur J Gastroenterol Hepatol 1995; 7:577–586.
41. Swarbrick ET, Gough AL, Foster CS, Christian J, Garrett AD, Langworthy CH, et al. Prevention of recurrence of oesophageal stricture, a comparison of lansoprazole and high-dose ranitidine. Eur J Gastroenterol Hepatol 1996; 8:431–438.
42. Marks RD, Richter JE, Rizzo J, Koehler RE, Spenney JG, Mills TP, et al. Omeprazole versus H2-receptor antagonists in treating patients with peptic stricture and esophagitis. Gastroenterology 1994; 106:907–915.
43. Earlam R, Cunha-Melo JR. Benign oesophageal strictures: historical and technical aspects of dilatation. Br J Surg 1981; 68:829–836.
44. Swaroop VS, Desai DC, Mohandas KM, Dhir V, Dave UR, Gulla RI, et al. Dilation of esophageal strictures induced by radiation therapy for cancer of the esophagus. Gastrointest Endosc 1994; 40:311–315.
45. Saeed ZA, Ramirez FC, Hepps KS, Cole RA, Schneider FE, Ferro PS, et al. An objective end point for dilation improves outcome of peptic esophageal strictures: a prospective randomized trial. Gastrointest Endosc 1997; 45:354–359.
46. Eckardt VF, Kanzler G, Willems D. Single dilation of symptomatic Schatzki rings. A prospective evaluation of its effectiveness. Dig Dis Sci 1992; 37:577–582.
47. Tucker LE. The importance of fluoroscopic guidance for Maloney dilation. Am J Gastroenterol 1992; 87:1709–1711.
48. McClave SA, Brady PG, Wright RA, Goldschmid S, Minocha A. Does fluoroscopic guidance for Maloney esophageal dilation impact on the clinical endpoint of therapy: relief of dysphagia and achievement of luminal patency? Gastrointest Endosc 1996; 43:93–97.
49. Ho SB, Cass O, Katsman RJ, Lipschultz EM, Metzger RJ, Onstad GR, et al. Fluoroscopy is not necessary for Maloney dilation of chronic esophageal strictures. Gastrointest Endosc 1995; 41:11–14.
50. Glick ME. Clinical course of esophageal stricture managed by bougienage. Dig Dis Sci 1982; 27:884–888.
51. Patterson DJ, Graham DY, Smith JL, Schwartz JT, Alpert E, Lanza FL, et al. Natural history of benign esophageal stricture treated by dilatation. Gastroenterology 1983; 85:346–350.
52. Grobe JL, Kozarek RA, Sanowski RA. Self-bougienage in the treatment of benign esophageal stricture. J Clin Gastroenterol 1984; 6:109–112.
53. Heiser MC. Esophageal self-dilatation: interdisciplinary responsibilities for a comprehensive treatment plan. Gastroenterol Nurs 1990; 12:246–249.
54. Saeed ZA, Winchester CB, Ferro PS, Michaletz PA, Schwartz JT, Graham DY. Prospective randomized comparison of polyvinyl bougies and through-the-scope balloons for dilation of peptic strictures of the esophagus. Gastrointest Endosc 1995; 41:189–195.
55. Cox JG, Winter RK, Maslin SC, Dakkak M, Jones R, Buckton GK, et al. Balloon or bougie for dilatation of benign esophageal stricture? Dig Dis Sci 1994; 39:776–781.
56. McLean GK, LeVeen RF. Shear stress in the performance of esophageal dilation: comparison of balloon dilation and bougienage. Radiology 1989; 172:983–986.

57. Kozarek RA. Hydrostatic balloon dilation of gastrointestinal stenoses: a national survey. Gastrointest Endosc 1986; 32:15–19.
58. Silvis SE, Nebel O, Rogers G, Sugawa C, Mandelstam P. Endoscopic complications. Results of the 1974 American Society for Gastrointestinal Endoscopy Survey. JAMA 1976; 235:928–930.
59. Marks RD, Richter JE. Peptic strictures of the esophagus. Am J Gastroenterol 1993; 88:1160–1173.
60. Dumon JF, Meric B, Sivak MVJ, Fleischer D. A new method of esophageal dilation using Savary-Gilliard bougies. Gastrointest Endosc 1985; 31:379–382.
61. Clouse RE. Complications of endoscopic gastrointestinal dilation techniques. Gastrointest Endosc Clin North Am 1996; 6:323–341.
62. Marshall JB, Afridi SA, King PD, Barthel JS, Butt JH. Esophageal dilation with polyvinyl (American) dilators over a marked guidewire: practice and safety at one center over a 5-yr period. Am J Gastroenterol 1996; 91:1503–1506.
63. Kozarek RA. Esophageal dilation and prostheses. Endosc Rev 1987; 4:9–14.
64. Nelson DB, Sanderson SJ, Azar MM. Bacteremia with esophageal dilation. Gastrointest Endosc 1999; 48:563–567.
65. Coles EF, Reed WW, Tighe JF, Jr. Bacterial meningitis occurring after esophageal dilation in an otherwise healthy patient. Gastrointest Endosc 1992; 38:384–385.
66. Ersahin Y, Mutluer S, Cakir Y. Multiple brain abscesses following esophageal dilation. Childs Nerv Syst 1995; 11:351–353.
67. Harp DL, Schlitt M, Williams JP, Shamoun JM. Brain abscess following dilatation of esophageal stricture. Clin Imaging 1989; 13:140–141.
68. Wesdorp IC, Bartelsman JF, den Hartog J, Huibregtse K, Tytgat GN. Results of conservative treatment of benign esophageal strictures: a follow-up study in 100 patients. Gastroenterology 1982; 82:487–493.
69. Agnew SR, Pandya SP, Reynolds RP, Preiksaitis HG. Predictors for frequent esophageal dilations of benign peptic strictures. Dig Dis Sci 1996; 41:931–936.
70. Yamamoto H, Hughes RWJ, Schroeder KW, Viggiano TR, DiMagno EP. Treatment of benign esophageal stricture by Eder-Puestow or balloon dilators: a comparison between randomized and prospective nonrandomized trials. Mayo Clin Proc 1992; 67:228–236.
71. Foster DR. Self-expandable oesophageal stents in the management of benign peptic oesophageal strictures in the elderly. Br J Clin Pract 51:199.
72. Moores DW, Ilves R. Treatment of esophageal obstruction with covered, self-expanding esophageal Wallstents. Ann Thorac Surg 1996; 62:963–967.
73. Sheikh RA, Trudeau WL. Expandable metallic stent placement in patients with benign esophageal strictures: results of long-term follow-up. Gastrointest Endosc 1998; 48:227–229.
74. Song HY, Park SI, Do YS, Yoon HK, Sung KB, Sohn KH, et al. Expandable metallic stent placement in patients with benign esophageal strictures: results of long-term follow-up. Radiology 1997; 203:131–136.
75. Hramiec JE, O'Shea MA, Quinlan RM. Expandable metallic esophageal stents in benign disease: a cause for concern. Surg Laparosc Endosc 1998; 8:40–43.
76. Ellis FHJ, Garabedian M, Gibb SP. Fundoplication for gastroesophageal reflux. Indications, surgical technique, and manometric results. Arch Surg 1973; 107:186–192.

77. Skinner DB. Benign esophageal strictures. Adv Surg 1976; 10:177–196.
78. Richardson JD, Richardson RL. Collis-Nissen gastroplasty for shortened esophagus: long-term evaluation. Ann Surg 1998; 227:735–740.
79. Beggs FD, Salama FD, Knowles KR. Management of benign oesophageal stricture by total fundoplication gastroplasty. J R Coll Surg Edinb 1995; 40:305–307.
80. Mansour KA, Bryan FC, Carlson GW. Bowel interposition for esophageal replacement: twenty-five year experience. Ann Thorac Surg 1997; 64:752–756.
81. Picchio M, Lombardi A, Zolovkins A, Della CU, Paolini A, Fegiz G, et al. Jejunal interposition for peptic stenosis of the esophagus following esophagomyotomy for achalasia. Int Surg 1997; 82:198–200.
82. Thomas P, Fuentes P, Giudicelli R, Reboud E. Colon interposition for esophageal replacement: current indications and long-term function. Ann Thorac Surg 1997; 64:757–764.
83. Orringer MB, Marshall B, Stirling MC. Transhiatal esophagectomy for benign and malignant disease. J Thorac Cardiovasc Surg 1993; 105:265–276.
84. Ahmad SA, Sylvester KG, Hebra A, Davidoff AM, McClane S, Stafford PW, et al. Esophageal replacement using the colon: is it a good choice? J Ped Surg 1996; 31: 1026–1030.
85. Meyers RL, Bozymski EM. Therapeutic Esophageal Endoscopy. In: Orlando RC, ed. Gastroenterology and Hepatology. Philadelphia, PA: Churchill-Livingstone, 1997: 10.1–10.18.

8
Barrett's Esophagus

Stuart Jon Spechler
Dallas Veterans Affairs Medical Center, Dallas, Texas

DEFINITION AND DIAGNOSIS

Barrett's esophagus is the condition in which an abnormal columnar epithelium replaces the stratified squamous epithelium that normally lines the distal esophagus (1). The condition is a sequela of chronic gastroesophageal reflux disease (GERD) in most, if not all, cases. On histological examination, the columnar lining of Barrett's esophagus usually is an incomplete form of intestinal metaplasia that may have features of small intestinal, colonic, and gastric epithelia (Fig. 1) (2). This metaplastic lining has been called specialized columnar epithelium or specialized intestinal metaplasia, and it appears to be more resistant to reflux-induced injury than the native squamous mucosa (3). Unfortunately, the metaplastic cells of Barrett's esophagus are predisposed to develop genetic changes that lead to malignancy. Indeed, GERD and Barrett's esophagus are the major recognized risk factors for esophageal adenocarcinoma (1,4).

The diagnosis of Barrett's esophagus usually is suspected on endoscopic examination when an abnormal mucosa is seen lining the distal esophagus. The diagnosis is confirmed when biopsy specimens of the abnormal mucosa reveal specialized intestinal metaplasia. Although these diagnostic steps may seem straightforward, there has been intense controversy recently regarding the diagnostic criteria for Barrett's esophagus (5). The deceptively simple, conceptual definition of the disorder as the condition in which an abnormal columnar epithelium replaces squamous epithelium in the distal esophagus does not translate easily into practical diagnostic criteria for two reasons: (1) It is difficult to identify the precise point at which the esophagus ends and the stomach begins (i.e., the anatomical gastroesophageal junction), and (2) normal, gastric-type columnar ep-

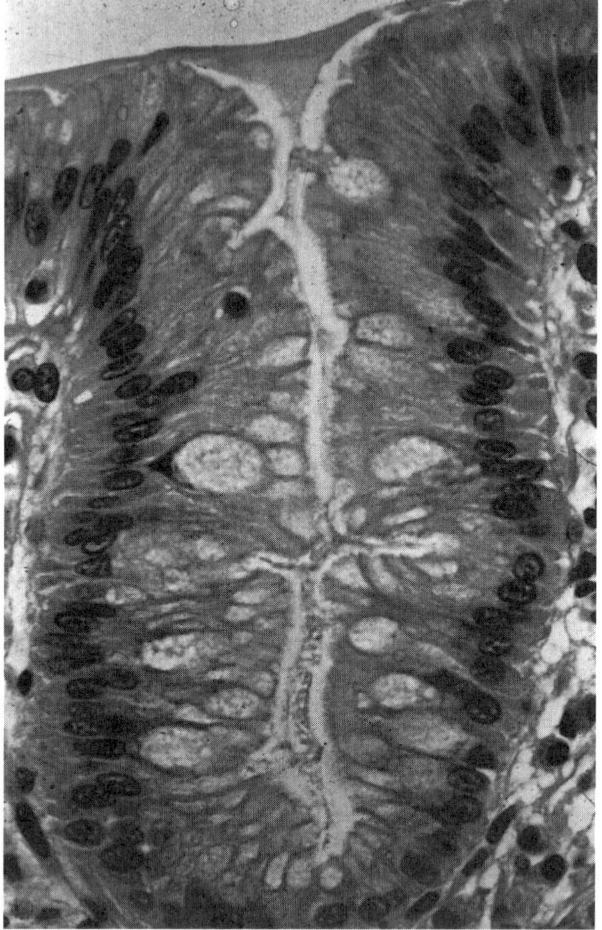

Figure 1 High-magnification photomicrograph of specialized intestinal metaplasia in Barrett's esophagus. Note that there are gastric surface-type cells, intestinal-type goblet cells, and cells that resemble intestinal absorptive cells with a rudimentary brush border. (From the Clinical Teaching Project of the American Gastroenterological Association.)

ithelium (grossly indistinguishable from the metaplastic epithelium of Barrett's esophagus) might line a short segment of the distal esophagus in normal individuals (6). These two factors make it difficult for the endoscopist to determine whether short segments of columnar epithelium that appear to line the distal esophagus in fact line the esophagus and not the proximal stomach (the gastric

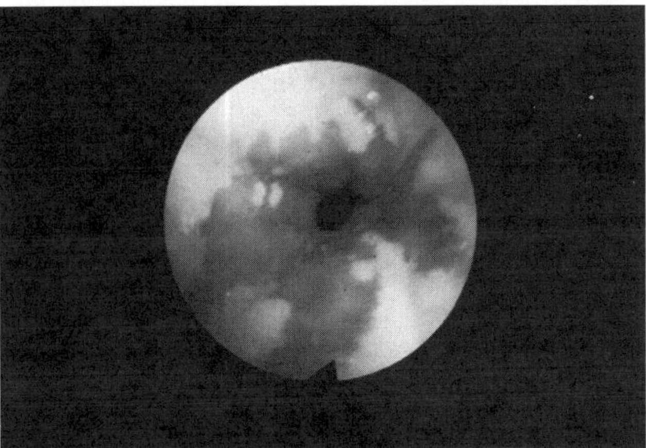

Figure 2 Endoscopic photograph showing the characteristic appearance of traditional Barrett's esophagus, with long segments of columnar epithelium extending well above the gastroesophageal junction. (From the Clinical Teaching Project of the American Gastroenterological Association.)

cardia), and whether the columnar epithelium is abnormal irrespective of its location.

The gastroesophageal junction has been defined variably by anatomical, radiological, physiological, and endoscopic features, and the location of the junction identified by these various approaches may differ by several centimeters or more (7). Columnar epithelium, with its reddish color and velvet-like texture, usually can be distinguished readily from the pale, glossy squamous epithelium of the esophagus on endoscopic examination (8). Therefore, Barrett's esophagus is identified easily when the endoscopist sees long segments of columnar epithelium that extend up from the stomach to reach the middle and proximal esophagus (Fig. 2). As noted above, diagnostic difficulties arise for patients who have short segments of columnar epithelium that appear to be confined to the most distal esophagus. Without precise landmarks for the gastroesophageal junction, one cannot ascertain whether these short segments of columnar epithelium in fact line the distal esophagus, or whether they line a segment of the gastric cardia that the endoscopist has mistakenly identified as esophagus. In an attempt to avoid making false-positive diagnoses of Barrett's esophagus in this situation, early investigators established arbitrary criteria for the extent of esophageal columnar lining necessary to include patients in their studies. Published diagnostic criteria varied considerably, ranging from as few as 2 cm to as many as 5 cm of esophageal columnar lining (1). These criteria that were based on arbitrary measurements, designed by and for investigators, became embraced by clinicians who adopted the investigative criteria into their clinical practices. By adherence to these diagnostic criteria, clinicians limited the problem of false-positive diagnoses of Barrett's esophagus, but failed to recognize short segments of metaplastic epithelium in the distal esophagus.

In a seminal study in which manometric techniques were used to ensure that biopsy specimens were obtained above the lower esophageal sphincter (i.e., in the esophagus and not the gastric cardia), three types of columnar epithelia were identified in Barrett's esophagus (9): (1) specialized columnar epithelium (specialized intestinal metaplasia), (2) gastric fundic-type epithelium with oxyntic glands containing chief and parietal cells, and (3) junctional-type epithelium comprised almost exclusively of mucus-secreting cells. The latter two epithelial types can be indistinguishable from the normal lining of the gastric fundus and cardia. The histological demonstration of these gastric epithelial types in biopsy specimens obtained endoscopically from the gastroesophageal junction region does not establish a diagnosis of Barrett's esophagus because there is no way to prove that these epithelia were acquired through the process of metaplasia. In contrast, specialized intestinal metaplasia with its prominent goblet cells (which are not found normally in either esophagus or stomach) is clearly metaplastic.

In an attempt to eliminate diagnostic difficulties, some authorities have proposed that the diagnosis of Barrett's esophagus should be based solely on the presence of specialized intestinal metaplasia, not on any specific extent of esophageal columnar lining (10). Unfortunately, even this approach does not obviate diagnostic problems. Without precise criteria for the anatomical gastroesophageal junction, it is difficult to determine whether the specialized intestinal metaplasia found in this region is esophageal or gastric in origin. Perhaps the major problem with defining Barrett's esophagus solely by the presence of specialized intestinal metaplasia relates to the frequency with which short segments of this metaplastic epithelium can be found in the gastroesophageal junction region. In 1994, investigators in Boston reported that they found short, inconspicuous segments of specialized intestinal metaplasia in the region of the gastroesophageal junction in 18% of patients in a general endoscopy unit, many of whom had no signs or symptoms of GERD (11). A number of subsequent studies have confirmed these observations (Table 1) (12,13). The risks for developing cancer and GERD complications have not yet been defined for patients with short segments of specialized intestinal metaplasia in the region of the gastroesophageal junction. To distinguish this condition from traditional (''long-segment'') Barrett's esophagus that clearly is associated with cancer and severe GERD, some authorities have proposed terms like ''short-segment Barrett's esophagus'' for patients who have fewer than 3 cm of specialized intestinal metaplasia lining the distal esophagus (Table 2) (14,15). Others have suggested that the artificial term ''Barrett's esophagus'' should be eliminated altogether, and that the condition

Table 1 Frequency of Intestinal Metaplasia in the Gastroesophageal Junction Region

Study author	Country	No. of patients	Frequency of metaplasia (%)
Johnston	U.S.	170	9
Voutilainen	Finland	1019	10
Hirota	U.S.	889	13
Spechler	U.S.	142	18
Chalasani	U.S.	87	18
Trudgill	U.K.	120	18
Nandurkar	Australia	158	36
Overall		2585	14

Table 2 Proposed Classification for Columnar-Lined Esophagus

Long-segment Barrett's esophagus (intestinal metaplasia ≥3 cm)
Short-segment Barrett's esophagus (intestinal metaplasia <3 cm)
Gastric cardia intestinal metaplasia

Source: Ref. 15.

Table 3 Proposed Classification for Columnar-Lined Esophagus

Columnar-lined esophagus *with* specialized intestinal metaplasia
Columnar-lined esophagus *without* specialized intestinal metaplasia
Specialized intestinal metaplasia at the GE junction

Source: Ref. 1.

should be called simply ''columnar-lined esophagus'' with or without specialized intestinal metaplasia (Table 3) (1).

Although the debate over terminology still rages, it is clear that recognition of a columnar-lined esophagus requires precise criteria by which to delimit the esophagus and the stomach. Figure 3 shows endoscopically recognizable landmarks that can be used to identify structures at the gastroesophageal junction. The squamocolumnar junction (SCJ, or Z-line) is the visible line formed by the juxtaposition of pale, glossy squamous epithelium and red, velvet-like columnar

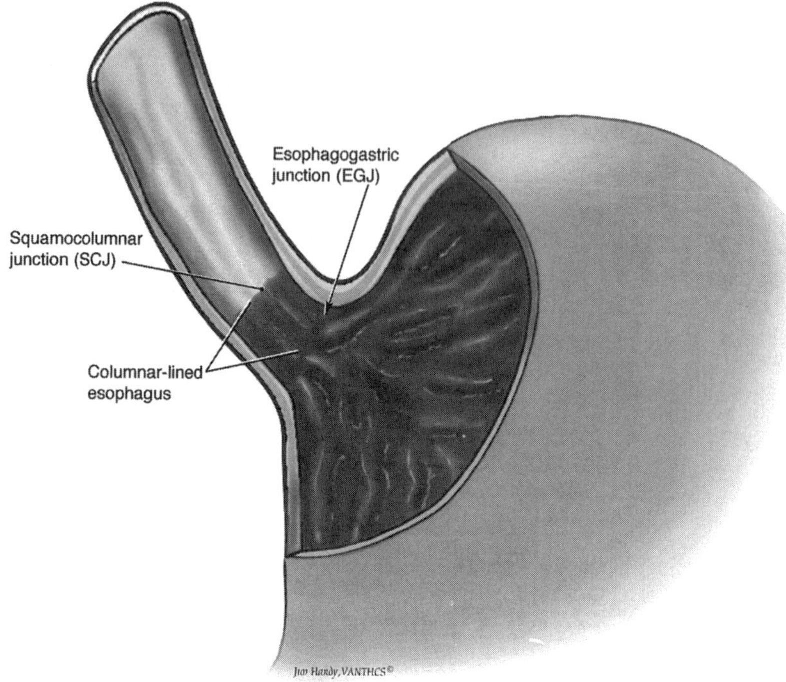

Figure 3 Landmarks at the gastroesophageal junction region. The squamocolumnar junction (SCJ, or Z-line) is the visible line formed by the juxtaposition of squamous and columnar epithelia. The gastroesophageal junction (GEJ) is the imaginary line at which the esophagus ends and the stomach begins. The GEJ corresponds to the most proximal extent of the gastric folds, and marks the proximal extent of the gastric cardia. When the SCJ is located proximal to the GEJ, there is a columnar-lined segment of esophagus. (From Ref. 18.)

mucosa. The gastroesophageal junction (GEJ) is the imaginary line at which the esophagus ends and the stomach begins anatomically. The GEJ has been defined by endoscopists, somewhat arbitrarily, as the level of the most proximal extent of the gastric folds (16). In normal individuals, the proximal extent of the gastric folds generally corresponds to the point at which the tubular esophagus flares to become the sack-shaped stomach in the region of the lower esophageal sphincter. In patients with hiatal hernias whose lower esophageal sphincters are weak and in whom there may be no clear-cut flare at the GEJ, the proximal margin of the gastric folds is determined when the distal esophagus is minimally inflated with air because overinflation obscures this landmark (15). When the SCJ is located

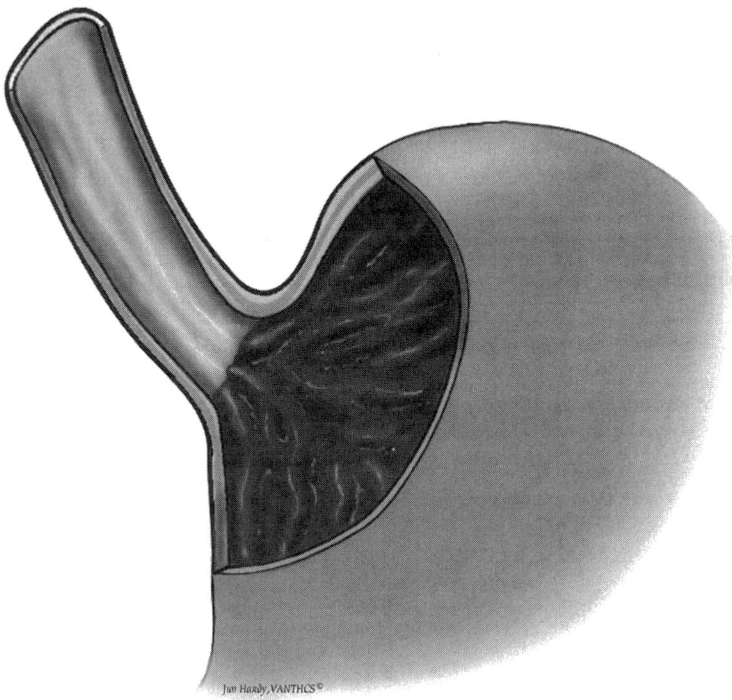

Figure 4 The SCJ and GEJ coincide. In this situation, the entire esophagus is lined by squamous epithelium. (From Ref. 18.)

proximal to the gastroesophageal junction, there is a columnar-lined segment of esophagus. When the SCJ and the GEJ coincide (Fig. 4), the entire esophagus is lined by squamous epithelium. There is no reported description of an SCJ located distal to the GEJ. The gastric cardia, by definition, starts at the GEJ. There are no endoscopic landmarks that define the distal extent of the gastric cardia.

PATHOGENESIS OF INTESTINAL METAPLASIA

Intestinal metaplasia is associated with adenocarcinoma both in the esophagus and in the stomach (1,17). For patients with short segments of intestinal metaplasia in the region of the GEJ, the issue of whether the metaplastic epithelium arose from esophageal or gastric tissue has practical significance only if there are important pathogenetic and clinical features that depend on the metaplasia's site of origin. If intestinal metaplasia has the same pathogenesis and predisposition to cancer regardless of its location, then debates over terminology (e.g., short-segment Barrett's esophagus vs. intestinal metaplasia of the gastric cardia) can be considered trivial, semantic arguments. However, if there are substantial clinical differences between esophageal and gastric intestinal metaplasia, then it is important for clinicians to distinguish between the conditions. Much evidence suggests that there are indeed fundamental differences between gastric and esophageal forms of intestinal metaplasia (18).

In the body and antrum of the stomach, *Helicobacter pylori* infection is strongly associated with the development of intestinal metaplasia and cancer (17,19). The International Agency for Research on Cancer has deemed *H. pylori* a group I carcinogen (a definite cause of gastric cancer in humans) (20), and the recent demonstration that infection with *H. pylori* induces the development of intestinal metaplasia and gastric cancer in Mongolian gerbils provides compelling evidence of a pathogenetic role for *H. pylori* in these conditions (21). The gastric pathway to carcinogenesis proposed by Correa and others is shown in Figure 5 (22). Strains of *H. pylori* that have a CagA gene (associated with cytotoxin expression) can cause a particularly severe form of gastritis that is especially predisposed to progress to cancer (23).

GERD is an important risk factor for esophageal adenocarcinoma (4), pre-

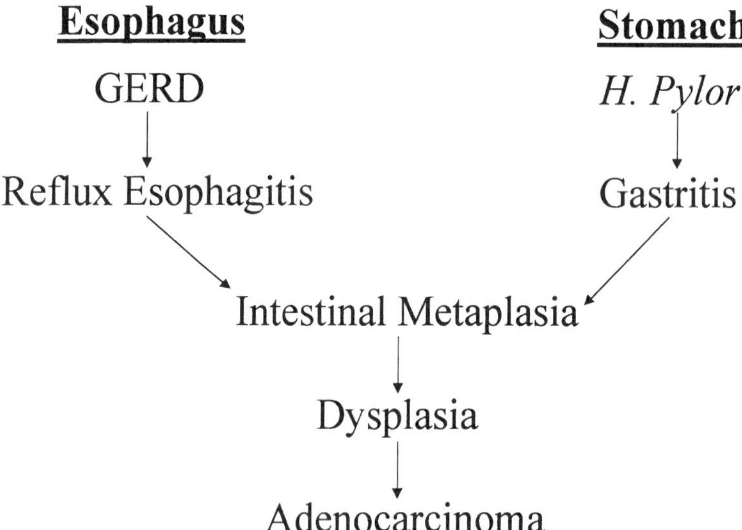

Figure 5 Proposed carcinogenetic pathways in the esophagus and stomach. Note that the development of intestinal metaplasia is a key feature of carcinogenesis for both organs.

sumably because GERD leads to the development of intestinal metaplasia in the esophagus (Fig. 5). GERD causes reflux esophagitis and, in some individuals, the damaged esophageal epithelium heals through the process of intestinal metaplasia. As in the stomach, the development of intestinal metaplasia precedes the development of neoplasia in the esophagus. In contrast to the stomach, infection with *H. pylori* does not appear to play a direct role in the pathogenesis of esophageal inflammation and metaplasia. A number of studies on this issue have found no positive association between gastric infection with *H. pylori* and either reflux esophagitis or Barrett's esophagus (24–31). Indeed, recent reports have suggested that gastric infection with *H. pylori* actually may *protect* the esophagus by preventing the development of reflux esophagitis and Barrett's esophagus (32,33). Also, recent studies have found a significant negative association between esophageal adenocarcinoma and *H. pylori* infections, particularly for infections with CagA-positive strains (34–36). For example, Vicari et al. found CagA positivity in 11 of 26 (42%) control subjects who were infected with *H. pylori*, but in none of seven infected patients who had dysplasia or adenocarcinoma in Barrett's esophagus (36). Graham and Yamaoka have proposed that *H. pylori* infections that cause severe pangastritis also cause a decrease in gastric acid production that may protect against GERD (37). Regardless of the mechanisms involved, evidence suggests that *H. pylori* infection is a risk factor for intestinal metaplasia in the distal stomach but not in the esophagus, whereas GERD is the major risk factor for intestinal metaplasia in the esophagus.

In addition to pathogenetic differences, there are data to suggest that certain morphological histochemical, and clinical features of intestinal metaplasia in the esophagus differ from those of intestinal metaplasia in the stomach. Several schemes have been proposed for the classification of gastric intestinal metaplasia (38–40). These schemes focus on how "complete" the metaplasia is (i.e., how strongly the epithelium resembles that of the normal small intestine) and, if the metaplasia is incomplete, on whether the mucus-secreting cells contain colonic-type sulfomucins that stain with high iron-diamine. Complete, or type I intestinal metaplasia is comprised largely of (1) absorptive cells that do not secrete mucus and that have a well-defined brush border containing distinctive small intestinal enzymes such as alkaline phosphatase, aminopeptidase, and disaccharidases; (2) numerous goblet cells containing sialomucins that stain with Alcian blue; and (3) occasional Paneth cells. Incomplete forms of intestinal metaplasia have few or no absorptive cells and generally are devoid of Paneth cells. In incomplete intestinal metaplasia, the predominant cell type is a columnar "intermediate" cell that secretes mucus. Incomplete forms of intestinal metaplasia also contain numerous goblet cells that secrete sialomucins, sulfomucins, or both. The intestinal metaplasia is categorized as type II if the intermediate cells secrete neutral mucins (as do normal gastric surface cells) and acid sialomucins, and as type III if the intermediate cells secrete predominantly acid sulfomucins. Type I is the predominant form of intestinal metaplasia found in the stomach, both in benign conditions and in patients with gastric cancer (40,41). Type III intestinal metaplasia is the least common form in the stomach, but the one most strongly associated with gastric cancer (17,42,43).

Although the intestinal metaplasia found in Barrett's esophagus can be morphologically indistinguishable from that in the stomach, it has not been a common practice for investigators to characterize intestinal metaplasia in the esophagus according to type. However, studies that have focused on the morphology and mucin histochemistry of Barrett's esophagus suggest that the characteristic specialized intestinal metaplasia is usually incomplete (type II or III) (44–46). In addition, specialized intestinal metaplasia has been found to react with a monoclonal antibody (called $7E_{12}H_{12}$ or MAb DAS-1) raised against colonic epithelial cells (47).

Morphological studies of Barrett's esophagus using scanning electron microscopy have revealed distinctive features of esophageal intestinal metaplasia. In biopsy specimens taken from the SCJ of patients with Barrett's esophagus, Shields et al. found a peculiar hybrid cell that had both microvilli (a feature of columnar cells) and intercellular ridges (a feature of squamous cells) on its surface (48). Another line of evidence that there are fundamental differences between esophageal and gastric intestinal metaplasia comes from recent studies showing that the cytokeratin staining pattern of intestinal metaplasia in the esophagus may differ from that of intestinal metaplasia in the stomach. Cytokeratins are a family of at least 20 structural proteins that are found in the cytoplasm of epithelial cells. Ormsby et al. recently identified unique patterns of staining for two cytokeratins (cytokeratins 7 and 20) in biopsy specimens of intestinal metaplasia from the esophagus and stomach (49). Salo et al. found that intestinal metaplasia in Barrett's esophagus showed immunoreactivity for cytokeratin 13 (a cytokeratin normally found in squamous epithelium) (50), and Boch et al. found immunoreactivity for both squamous and glandular cytokeratin markers in esophageal columnar epithelium that exhibited the phenomenon of multilayering (51). These observations suggest that esophageal columnar metaplasia might arise from squamous precursor cells that are not present in the stomach. Table 4 summarizes some of the major differences between intestinal metaplasia in the stomach and esophagus. If one accepts the premise that there are important differences in the metaplasia found in these two organs, then it is important for investigators who take biopsy specimens in the region of the gastroesophageal junction to ascertain whether those specimens are taken from the distal esophagus or from the gastric cardia.

CLINICAL FEATURES OF BARRETT'S ESOPHAGUS

Most studies on the clinical features of Barrett's esophagus were conducted before 1994 (when the frequency of short-segment disease was first recognized)

Table 4 Features of Intestinal Metaplasia (IM) in the Esophagus and Stomach

	IM in stomach	IM in esophagus
H. pylori association	Positive	Negative
GERD association	No	Yes
Usual type of metaplasia	Complete	Incomplete
"Barrett's" CK7/20 pattern	No	Yes

and, consequently, are comprised almost exclusively of patients with traditional, long-segment disease. The conclusions of these studies may not be applicable to patients who have short segments of intestinal metaplasia in the region of the GEJ.

Traditional Barrett's esophagus usually is discovered in middle-aged and older adults, although the condition has been described in children as young as age 5 (52,53). Children with Barrett's esophagus often have comorbid disorders such as neurological diseases or cystic fibrosis (53). In adults, the average age at the time of diagnosis of Barrett's esophagus is approximately 55 years, and the condition is not usually associated with comorbid disorders (other than GERD). White males predominate in most series. For unknown reasons, Barrett's esophagus rarely affects black individuals. Most patients are seen initially for symptoms of the underlying GERD such as heartburn, regurgitation, and dysphagia. The metaplastic epithelium itself causes no symptoms, and even may be less pain-sensitive to noxious stimuli such as acid than the native squamous mucosa (54).

Among patients who have endoscopic examinations for symptoms of GERD, traditional Barrett's esophagus can be found in approximately 10% (55). A study of 701 patients with GERD symptoms evaluated by gastroenterologists in community practices showed that the likelihood of finding Barrett's esophagus on endoscopy increased with the duration of GERD symptoms (56). For patients who had symptoms for less than 1 year, only 4% had Barrett's esophagus, whereas for those with more than 10 years of GERD symptoms, endoscopy showed Barrett's esophagus in 21%. For many patients with Barrett's esophagus, however, symptoms of GERD are either absent or judged too trivial to warrant endoscopic evaluation. These cases are not recognized unless endoscopy is performed for other reasons. There are data suggesting that more than 90% of individuals with Barrett's esophagus in the general population do not seek medical attention for esophageal symptoms, and therefore most cases go unrecognized (57). Among patients seen by physicians, however, the GERD associated with traditional Barrett's esophagus often is severe and complicated by esophageal ulceration, stricture, and hemorrhage. In contrast, patients with short-segment Barrett's esophagus often have no signs or symptoms of GERD (12).

GERD IN PATIENTS WITH BARRETT'S ESOPHAGUS

Patients with traditional Barrett's esophagus have been shown to have a number of physiological abnormalities that might contribute to the severity of GERD. Some patients exhibit hypersecretion of gastric acid, for example, and may require high doses of antisecretory drugs to effect esophageal healing (58,59). Some patients have duodenogastric reflux and, consequently, bile and pancreatic juice may be present in the stomach (60). With these abnormalities, the gastric contents available for reflux may be exceptionally caustic, containing high concentrations of acid, bile, and pancreatic secretions. Manometric study of the Barrett esophagus often reveals extreme hypotension of the lower esophageal sphincter (an important barrier to gastroesophageal reflux), and therefore these patients are exceptionally predisposed to reflux (61). Poor esophageal contractility also has been described, a phenomenon that may delay the clearance of noxious material from the esophagus (62). Some patients have diminished esophageal pain sensitivity, and consequently the reflux of caustic material into the Barrett esophagus may not cause heartburn (54). Without heartburn, patients may have no warning that they are experiencing gastroesophageal reflux and little incentive to comply with antireflux therapy. Finally, decreased salivary secretion of epidermal growth factor, a peptide that enhances the healing of peptic ulceration, has been reported in some patients with Barrett's esophagus (63). Decreased salivary secretion of this growth factor might delay the healing of the reflux-damaged esophagus. In summary, patients with Barrett's esophagus may be exceptionally predisposed to the reflux of unusually caustic gastric material into the esophagus. Such reflux might not elicit pain, the esophagus may be unable to clear the noxious material effectively, and healing of the resulting esophageal injury may be delayed. In view of this substantial predisposition to reflux esophagitis, it is not surprising that patients with traditional Barrett's esophagus often have severe GERD complicated by esophageal ulceration, stricture, and bleeding.

The physiological abnormalities that predispose to the severe GERD that characterizes traditional Barrett's esophagus have not been described in patients with short-segment disease. As mentioned, many of the latter patients have no signs or symptoms of GERD whatsoever. Some data suggest that the length of metaplastic mucosa in Barrett's esophagus may be related to the duration of esophageal acid exposure as measured by 24-h pH monitoring (64). Thus, patients with short-segment Barrett's esophagus may have 24-h esophageal acid exposure values that are normal or only minimally increased.

Given the propensity for severe GERD in patients with traditional Barrett's esophagus, one might assume that metaplasia should progress in extent over the years as columnar epithelium replaces more and more squamous epithelium that is damaged by ongoing reflux. Such progression is observed infrequently, however, and Barrett's esophagus appears to develop to its full extent relatively quickly in most cases. For example, Cameron and Lomboy reviewed the records of 377 patients found to have Barrett's esophagus at the Mayo Clinic between 1976 and 1989 (65). When these patients were grouped according to age, the length of esophagus lined by columnar epithelium was not found to differ significantly among the various age groups (i.e., 20-year-old patients had a segment of columnar-lined esophagus similar in length to that of the 80-year-olds). Furthermore, no significant change in the extent of metaplastic epithelium was found among 101 patients who had follow-up endoscopic examinations performed after a mean interval of 3.2 years. It is not known why Barrett's esophagus usually does not progress in extent despite ongoing GERD.

CANCER RISK IN BARRETT'S ESOPHAGUS

Through the 1960s, the vast majority of esophageal cancers in the United States were squamous cell carcinomas (66). Adenocarcinoma of the esophagus was considered such an uncommon tumor that some authorities questioned its very existence. Over the past two decades, however, the frequency of adenocarcinoma of the esophagus has nearly quadrupled (66–69). Today, adenocarcinomas comprise approximately 50% of all esophageal malignancies in this country. GERD and Barrett's esophagus are the major recognized risk factors for these lethal tumors (1,4). For patients with traditional Barrett's esophagus, the reported incidence of esophageal adenocarcinoma has ranged from 0.2% to as high as 2.1% per year (70). A recent meta-analysis of six prospective studies has suggested that the mean annual incidence of esophageal cancer in this condition is approximately 1% (Table 5) (71). All reports on cancer incidence in patients with Barrett's

Table 5 Prospective Studies on Cancer Incidence in Barrett's Esophagus

Study author	No. of patients	Follow-up (patient-yrs)	Cases of cancer	Annual cancer incidence (%)
Hammeeteman	50	260	5	1.9
Bonelli	71	110	2	1.8
Robertson	56	224	4	1.8
Miros	81	289	3	1.0
Iftikhar	102	462	4	0.8
Drewitz	170	834	4	0.5
Total	530	2179	21	1.0

Source: Data from Ref. 71.

esophagus have concluded that the risk of developing esophageal cancer is increased at least 30-fold above that of the general population. Esophageal adenocarcinoma remains a relatively uncommon tumor in the general population, however, despite the dramatic increase in its frequency over the past 20 years. In 1995, for example, it was estimated that there were only approximately 6000 new cases of esophageal adenocarcinoma in the United States (72). Even a 30-fold increase in this low incidence rate represents a small risk for an individual patient, and esophageal cancer appears to be an uncommon cause of death for patients with Barrett's esophagus (73). Two groups of investigators have found that the actuarial survival of their patients with endoscopically obvious Barrett's esophagus (whose mean age was greater than 55 years) did not differ significantly from that of age- and sex-matched control subjects in the general population (74,75). Many of these older patients succumbed to other diseases before developing adenocarcinoma in their Barrett's esophagus.

The results of studies on cancer risk for patients with endoscopically obvious Barrett's esophagus may not be applicable to the ''silent majority'' of patients who have inconspicuous, short segments of intestinal metaplasia at the GEJ. For the latter patients, the risk of developing esophageal cancer is not known. Considering the large number of such individuals and the relative infrequency of cancers in this location, it would appear that the risk imposed by short segments of intestinal metaplasia at the GEJ is small (76). Carcinogenesis in metaplastic cells is judged to proceed through a series of genetic mutations that activate oncogenes and disable tumor suppressor genes (77). The risk for acquiring such mutations might increase as the number of predisposed cells increases and, therefore, patients with long segments of intestinal metaplasia would be expected to have a higher risk for cancer development than those with short segments. Data from several studies support this contention (73,78,79). Assume, for the sake of argument, that a patient with a long segment of specialized intestinal metaplasia is 10 times more likely to develop adenocarcinoma than a patient with a short segment of this epithelium. Short-segment disease in the general population appears to be more than 10 times as frequent as long-segment disease (11). Despite the higher individual risk of cancer development imposed by long segments of intestinal metaplasia, adenocarcinomas of the GEJ will be seen more frequently in patients with short-segment disease simply because there are so many more of them in the general population. The precise risk of malignancy for patients with short-segment Barrett's esophagus or intestinal metaplasia of the gastric cardia remains to be determined.

DYSPLASIA IN BARRETT'S ESOPHAGUS

Carcinogenesis in the metaplastic cells of Barrett's esophagus begins with genetic alterations that activate proto-oncogenes (e.g., c-erbB-2), disable tumor suppres-

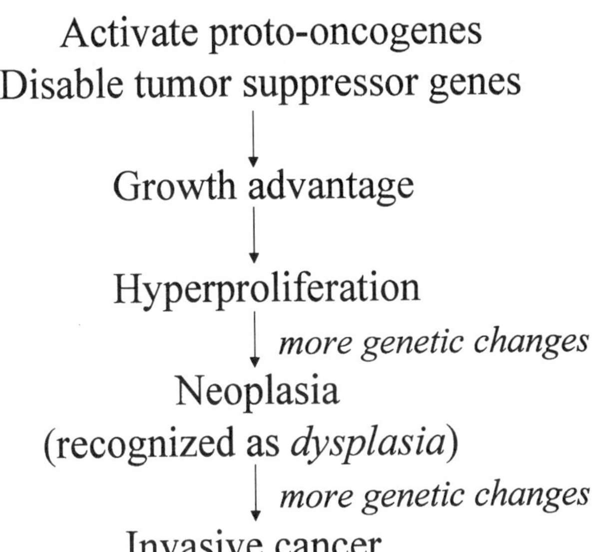

Figure 6 Proposed carcinogenetic pathway in the metaplastic epithelium of Barrett's esophagus.

sor genes (e.g., p53), or both (Fig. 6) (77,80). These mutations endow the cells with certain growth advantages, and the advantaged cells hyperproliferate. During hyperproliferation, the cells acquire more genetic changes that eventuate in autonomous cell growth (neoplasia). When enough DNA abnormalities accumulate, a clone of malignant cells emerge that have the ability to invade adjacent tissues and to proliferate in unnatural locations. Before the cells acquire enough DNA damage to become frankly malignant, the earlier genetic alterations often cause histological changes that can be recognized by the pathologist as dysplasia. Dysplastic cells are neoplastic, but not necessarily malignant. In dysplasia, the neoplastic cells remain confined within the basement membranes of the glands from which they arose (81). The dysplastic changes are graded as low-grade or high-grade depending upon the degree of alterations in nuclear morphology and glandular architecture. Endoscopic surveillance for cancer in Barrett's esophagus is performed primarily to seek high-grade dysplasia, with the rationale that removal of the dysplastic epithelium should prevent the progression to invasive malignancy (82).

Biopsy sampling error is a major problem that limits the utility of dysplasia as a biomarker for malignancy in Barrett's esophagus. Among patients who have esophageal resections performed because endoscopic examination reveals high-grade dysplasia, approximately one-third have been found to have an inapparent malignancy in the resected specimen that was missed due to biopsy sampling error (83). Sampling error can be reduced by increasing the number of biopsy specimens obtained during the endoscopic examination. For example, Levine et al. reported that they could differentiate high-grade dysplasia from early adenocarcinoma in Barrett's esophagus by adherence to a very rigorous endoscopic biopsy protocol wherein the esophagus was sampled extensively (84). They obtained four-quadrant biopsy specimens using ''jumbo'' biopsy forceps at 2-cm intervals throughout the columnar-lined esophagus, and took many additional samples from sites of known dysplasia. After preoperative evaluation by this protocol, none of seven patients who had an esophageal resection for high-grade dysplasia in Barrett's epithelium was found to have invasive cancer in the resected esophagus. For each of those seven patients, however, an average of 99 preoperative biopsy specimens were available for review. In one patient, 185 biopsy specimens were obtained during five preoperative endoscopies from a segment of columnar epithelium that spanned only 3 cm. This extensive sampling undoubtedly minimized the problem of biopsy sampling error. In an earlier study from the same group, four patients were described who had high-grade dysplasia associated with intramucosal carcinoma in Barrett's esophagus (85). In one patient, the intramucosal cancer was found in only one of 154 biopsy specimens. This, and other observations, led the investigators to conclude that ''there is no doubt that some intramucosal carcinomas accompanying high-grade dysplasia will be missed by endoscopic biopsies.''

The use of jumbo biopsy forceps has not been shown to influence the problem of biopsy sampling error. In one recent study, 38 patients with high-grade dysplasia in Barrett's esophagus had preoperative evaluation with four-quadrant biopsy specimens taken at intervals of every 2 cm (the so-called Seattle biopsy protocol) (86). In 16 patients in whom the preoperative specimens were obtained with standard biopsy forceps, invasive cancer was found in the resected specimen in 6 (38%). In 12 patients in whom the specimens were taken with jumbo forceps, invasive cancer was found in four (33%). Thus, the use of jumbo forceps did not significantly increase the cancer detection rate, and the sampling error rate was substantial. Extensive biopsy sampling can reduce, but cannot eliminate, the problem of biopsy sampling error in Barrett's esophagus.

Although high-grade dysplasia in Barrett's esophagus is widely regarded as the precursor of invasive cancer, the natural history of this lesion is not well defined. Some studies suggest that high-grade dysplasia progresses to malignancy often and rapidly. For example, Hameeteman et al. described eight patients with high-grade dysplasia in Barrett's esophagus, five of whom developed adenocarcinoma within 1 year of the discovery of high-grade dysplasia (87). However, there are reports of patients in whom high-grade dysplasia persisted for years with no apparent progression to carcinoma (88). In the aforementioned study by Levine et al., seven of 29 patients (24%) with high-grade dysplasia were found to progress to invasive cancer during a follow-up period of 2–46 months (84). A preliminary report of a large series of patients with Barrett's esophagus followed at the Hines VA Hospital described 69 patients who had high-grade dysplasia and no evidence of invasive cancer on initial endoscopic evaluation (89). Only 10 (14.5%) of these patients developed adenocarcinoma during a mean follow-up period of 3.8 years. The reasons underlying the disparate results of these studies are not clear. Thus, the precise rate at which patients with high-grade dysplasia develop invasive cancer remains poorly defined.

Interobserver variation in the grading of dysplasia in Barrett's esophagus is another factor that limits the utility of this histological finding as a biomarker for malignancy. In one study in which eight expert morphologists were asked to grade dysplastic changes in Barrett's esophagus, interobserver agreement rates of 85% and 87% were found for the diagnoses of high-grade dysplasia and intramucosal carcinoma, respectively (90). When differentiating low-grade dysplasia from reactive epithelial changes caused by reflux esophagitis, the interobserver agreement was unacceptably poor. Thus, there can be substantial variation among expert pathologists in the grading of dysplastic changes in Barrett's esophagus.

ALTERNATIVE BIOMARKERS FOR MALIGNANCY IN BARRETT'S ESOPHAGUS

Noting the above-mentioned shortcomings of dysplasia as a biomarker for the malignant potential of Barrett's esophagus, investigators have sought alternative biomarkers as summarized in Table 6. Much attention has focused on the p53 tumor-suppressor gene that is located on the short arm of chromosome 17 (allele 17p). Expression of mutated p53 protein and deletion of a normal 17p allele have been reported for a number of human malignancies including cancers of the lung,

Table 6 Proposed Biomarkers for Malignancy in Barrett's Esophagus

Ornithine decarboxylase
Carcinoembryonic antigen (CEA)
Mucus abnormalities
Flow cytometry—aneuploidy
Flow cytometry—abnormal cellular proliferation
Chromosomal abnormalities (allelic imbalance in 3q,4q,5q,6q,9p,10q,12p,12q,17q,18q)
Oncogenes (c-Ha-ras, c-erb-B)
Tumor suppressor genes (p53)
Growth regulatory factors (EGF, TGF-α, EGF-R)
Cell proliferation markers—proliferating cell nuclear antigen, Ki67

breast, and colon. In these tumors, carcinogenesis appears to involve mutation of one p53 gene with deletion of the 17p allele that harbors a normal p53 gene (a phenomenon, called loss of heterozygosity, that is characteristic of tumor suppressor genes). Allelic deletions of 17p have been found in the majority of cancers in Barrett's esophagus (91,92). Furthermore, enhanced expression of p53 protein (presumably a mutated protein) by the metaplastic epithelium adjacent to the cancers has been found in one-half to two-thirds of cases (91,93–95). In patients with no apparent adenocarcinoma, immunohistochemical staining for p53 has been shown to correlate with the histological finding of dysplasia (96,97), and p53 abnormalities can be found occasionally in metaplastic mucosa with no histological signs of dysplasia (97–99). One recent report has even described the finding of antibodies to p53 in the serum of 11 of 33 patients with esophageal carcinoma and in three of 36 patients with benign Barrett's esophagus (100).

DNA abnormalities in Barrett's esophagus can be recognized by flow cytometry, a technique in which cell nuclei prepared from tissue specimens are treated with a fluorescent dye that binds to DNA (97,101,102). The treated nuclei are passed through a flow cytometer wherein the DNA-bound dye is excited by laser irradiation, and an estimate of DNA content is obtained by measuring the intensity of fluorescent light emitted. Flow cytometry can identify aneuploid cell populations (cells with an abnormal amount of DNA), and can provide information on the proportion of diploid cells (cells in the G_0/G_1 phase of the cell cycle that contain two copies of each chromosome) and tetraploid cells (cells in the G_2/M phase that contain four copies of each chromosome) in the sampled tissue. In a prospective study, Reid et al. found flow-cytometric abnormalities (aneuploidy or increased G_2/tetraploid populations) in biopsy specimens of Barrett's mucosa obtained during the initial endoscopic evaluation for 13 of 62 patients (101). During a mean follow-up period of 34 months, nine of the 13 patients with flow-cytometric abnormalities on initial evaluation developed high-grade dysplasia, adenocarcinoma, or both. In contrast, none of the 49 patients without flow-cytometric abnormalities developed high-grade dysplasia or cancer. During the apparent progression from dysplasia to adenocarcinoma, flow cytometry frequently showed multiple aneuploid populations of cells. No patient in this series progressed to invasive cancer without first exhibiting high-grade dysplasia on histological examination, however.

The studies mentioned above suggest that flow-cytometric and p53 abnormalities may be earlier and more specific markers for cancer development than the histological finding of dysplasia. Nevertheless, these markers do not yet provide sufficient additional information to justify their routine application in clinical practice (99,103). Indeed, none of the biomarkers listed in Table 6 provides such information. Despite the problems, the finding of dysplasia remains the most appropriate biomarker for the clinical evaluation of patients with Barrett's esophagus.

ENDOSCOPIC TECHNIQUES TO IDENTIFY DYSPLASIA

During endoscopic surveillance for patients with Barrett's esophagus, clinicians usually rely on the results of random biopsy sampling to detect early neoplasia in the metaplastic epithelium. Several techniques have been proposed to improve the yield of surveillance endoscopy by enabling the endoscopist to identify areas of abnormal tissue during the endoscopic examination. These techniques include chromoendoscopy, endosonography, optical coherence tomography, and fluorescence detection techniques.

Chromoendoscopy involves the perendoscopic application of vital dyes to the esophagus to enhance the detection of metaplastic and dysplastic epithelia. Studies on chromoendoscopy for Barrett's esophagus have evaluated Lugol's iodine (which stains the squamous epithelium black) (104), toluidine blue (105) and methylene blue (which stain intestinal metaplasia blue) (106), and indigo carmine (which highlights mucosal surface features) (107). Magnification endoscopy also has been used to identify the villous surface pattern of intestinal metaplasia (107). These studies are interesting, but limited in extent, and none has shown that chromoendoscopy provides sufficient additional information to justify its routine application in clinical practice.

Endoscopic ultrasonography has been used for the evaluation of tumors and dysplasia in Barrett's esophagus. The transducer is applied directly to the wall of the esophagus, enabling the use of high-frequency ultrasonic waves (e.g., 12 or 20 MHz) that can provide detailed images of the wall of the esophagus and its adjacent structures. For cancer surveillance purposes, endoscopic ultrasonography conceivably could demonstrate mucosal thickening indicative of dysplasia or early cancer. Preliminary studies addressing the role of endosonography in the evaluation of dysplasia in the columnar lined esophagus have been disappointing. In one study, for example, nine patients who eventually had esophageal resections for high-grade dysplasia in Barrett's esophagus all had preoperative endosonography (108). Endosonography correctly staged the disease in only four of the nine cases. In three patients the disease was overstaged, whereas the disease was understaged in two patients. Both of the latter patients had early cancer in the resected esophagus even though endosonography revealed no abnormality suggestive of malignancy. At present, the use of endoscopic ultrasonography for surveillance of Barrett's esophagus does not appear to be justified.

Optical coherence tomography (OCT) is an experimental imaging technique that can provide high-resolution cross-sectional imaging of the esophageal mucosa (109). The technique is similar in application and principle to ultrasonography, but OCT uses infrared light rather than ultrasonic waves for imaging. Image formation in OCT depends on variations in the reflectance of light from different tissue layers. OCT does not require direct contact between the optical fiber and the tissue, and the spatial resolution of the OCT image is up to 10 times higher than that of endosonography. Studies are needed to determine whether OCT will have a role in the management of Barrett's esophagus.

Fluorescence endoscopy is an exciting new technique that may enable the endoscopist to identify areas of dysplasia for biopsy sampling during the endoscopic examination (110). Different cells contain variable amounts of endogenous fluorophores, substances like NADH and porphyrins that can absorb laser light and re-emit it as fluorescent light with wavelengths and intensities that can be measured by fluorescence spectroscopy. For some tissues, the fluorescence spectra induced by laser irradiation are sufficiently characteristic to distinguish normal from neoplastic epithelia. Panjehpour et al. used laser-induced fluorescence spectroscopy (LIFS) to study 36 patients who had a columnar-lined esophagus with specialized intestinal metaplasia (111). An excellent correlation was observed between fluorescence spectral abnormalities and the finding of high-grade (but not low-grade) dysplasia on histological examination. One major drawback to the use of LIFS is the time and effort required to sample large areas of mucosa with these pinpoint ''optical biopsies.'' Laser-induced fluorescence endoscopy (LIFE) is a technique that uses real-time fluorescence imaging to study large areas of the mucosal surface. Preliminary experience with LIFE suggests that the technique can identify dysplastic lesions in Barrett's esophagus that are not apparent by conventional (white light) endoscopy (112,113).

Expensive, sophisticated instruments are needed to interpret the spectral properties of the faint fluorescent light emitted by endogenous fluorophores. Stronger fluorescent signals that are far easier to measure can be obtained by administering an exogenous fluorophore that is concentrated selectively in neoplastic tissue (111–113). Exogenous fluorophores that have been used in this fashion include hematoporphyrin derivatives and 5-aminolevulinic acid, a substance that is metabolized by cells into the potent fluorophore protoporphyrin IX. More studies are needed before fluorescence endoscopy using either endogenous or exogenous fluorophores can be recommended for widespread clinical application.

TREATMENT

The management of patients with Barrett's esophagus involves four major components: (1) treatment of the associated GERD, (2) prescription of endoscopic surveillance to detect dysplasia, (3) treatment of dysplasia, and (4) consideration of experimental techniques for ablating the metaplastic mucosa. All of these components of patient management are controversial because no study clearly documents the benefit of GERD treatment, endoscopic surveillance, dysplasia therapies, and mucosal ablation in preventing the development of adenocarcinoma.

Treatment of GERD in Barrett's Esophagus

The goals of GERD treatment for patients with Barrett's esophagus might include the following: (1) control of GERD symptoms, (2) prevention of GERD complications (e.g., esophageal stricture), (3) prevention of the extension of metaplastic epithelium up the esophagus, (4) induction of the regression of the metaplastic epithelium already present, and (5) prevention of the progression from metaplasia to malignancy. Modern antireflux therapies, both medical and surgical, have been shown to be highly effective for controlling GERD symptoms in patients with Barrett's esophagus (114,115). However, very few published data support the efficacy of any GERD treatment in accomplishing the latter four goals.

The mainstay of modern medical therapy for severe GERD is aggressive suppression of gastric acid through the administration of proton pump inhibitors (PPIs) (4). For patients with established peptic esophageal strictures, PPI therapy both improves dysphagia and decreases the need for subsequent esophageal dilations (117,118). Few reports have documented the development of peptic strictures in patients known to have uncomplicated GERD, however, and no study has established that any form of antireflux therapy prevents the formation of these strictures (119). Although it seems logical to assume that aggressive GERD treatment prevents GERD complications, there are few published data to support this notion. As mentioned above, esophageal metaplasia usually does not progress in extent, even in the absence of PPI therapy (65). Thus, there is little support for the notion that aggressive antireflux therapy is needed to prevent the progression in extent of Barrett's esophagus.

Metaplasia is a potentially reversible process if the responsible pathogenetic factors can be controlled (120). Unfortunately, control of GERD (the factor judged to be responsible for metaplasia in Barrett's esophagus) rarely, if ever, results in the complete reversal of the metaplastic epithelium (121). Partial regression of Barrett's esophagus (with the appearance of islands of squamous epithelium within the metaplastic columnar lining) is observed frequently in patients treated with PPIs or antireflux surgery, but the importance of this phenomenon is not known (121). In a prospective study, Sharma et al. obtained 39 biopsy specimens from squamous islands in 22 patients with Barrett's esophagus, most of whom had been treated with PPIs (122). Intestinal metaplasia underlying squamous epithelium was found in 15 of the 39 specimens (39%), suggesting that the partial regression of metaplasia induced by PPI therapy might have little effect in decreasing the cancer risk.

The notion that control of acid reflux prevents the progression from metaplasia to malignancy in Barrett's esophagus is based largely on circumstantial evidence. GERD appears to cause Barrett's esophagus, and GERD is clearly a strong risk factor for esophageal adenocarcinoma (4). However, it is not clear whether GERD predisposes to malignancy by causing the initial metaplasia, by promoting the transition from metaplasia to neoplasia, or both. Chronic reflux esophagitis might predispose to cancer by damaging metaplastic epithelial cells, thereby increasing their proliferation. While few would argue that GERD treatment is indicated for the treatment of reflux esophagitis, no study has established that any form of antireflux therapy reduces the risk of cancer in Barrett's esophagus.

Fitzgerald et al. found that biopsy specimens of Barrett's esophagus maintained in organ culture exhibited cellular hyperproliferation when exposed to short pulses (1 h in duration) of acid (Fig. 7) (123). This observation suggests that the episodic acid reflux that occurs frequently in patients with Barrett's esophagus might stimulate cellular hyperproliferation and thereby promote carcinogenesis. Although this study indirectly supports the notion that elimination of acid reflux might prevent carcinogenesis in Barrett's esophagus, conventional medical therapy for GERD does not eliminate episodes of acid reflux in most patients. Indeed, recent studies have shown that approximately 70% of individuals (normal subjects as well as patients with GERD and Barrett's esophagus) who are treated with a PPI twice a day experience nocturnal gastric acid breakthrough (defined as a gastric pH <4 for >1 h at night), and that brief episodes of acid reflux occur frequently during these breakthrough periods (124,125). Furthermore, patients with Barrett's esophagus often exhibit pathological levels of acid reflux, even during therapy with PPIs in doses that completely eliminate GERD symptoms

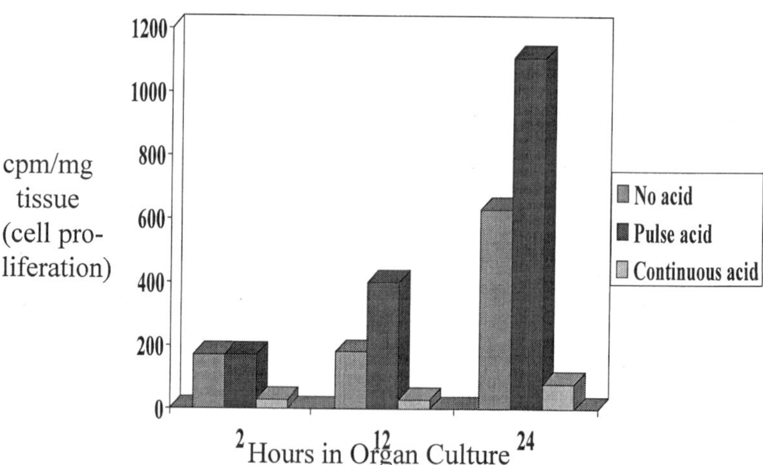

Figure 7 Effects of acid exposure on cellular proliferation in Barrett's esophagus organ cultures. (Data from Ref. 123.)

and signs (126,127). Clearly, conventional medical therapy for GERD does not abolish acid reflux in most patients with Barrett's esophagus.

Nocturnal acid breakthrough can be eliminated in most patients on PPI therapy by the addition of a histamine H_2-receptor blocker at bedtime (128). Thus, with polypharmacy that includes PPIs and histamine H_2-receptor blockers, it is possible to abolish acid reflux in patients with Barrett's esophagus. Nevertheless, this therapy should not be recommended routinely for the following reasons: (1) Perfect control of acid reflux clearly is not necessary to effect the healing of reflux esophagitis in most patients. Indeed, elimination of the symptoms and signs of GERD can be achieved in most patients who are treated with a PPI taken in conventional dosage (i.e., only once each day) (129). (2) The evidence to support the notion that complete elimination of acid reflux reduces the cancer risk in Barrett's esophagus is indirect and weak at best. It may not be appropriate to extrapolate the results of studies performed in the artificial environment of organ culture to the clinical situation. Furthermore, there are some experimental data to suggest that elimination of acid reflux may not be desirable. In an experimental model of esophageal adenocarcinoma involving rats treated with a carcinogen, for example, exposure of the esophagus to acidic gastric juice *protected* against the development of cancer (130). (3) Complete elimination of acid reflux would entail considerable inconvenience and expense, both for the multiple medications required and for the esophageal pH monitoring studies necessary to document the efficacy of therapy in controlling acid reflux. Available data support only the administration of medications in dosages that will eliminate the symptoms and endoscopic signs of GERD for patients with Barrett's esophagus. More aggressive therapy is based on unproved speculation. The general guidelines established for the medical treatment of GERD (116) seem applicable, irrespective of the presence of Barrett's esophagus.

Endoscopic Surveillance

The recommendation for endoscopic surveillance in Barrett's esophagus is based on a number of unproved and controversial assumptions including: (1) the assumption that Barrett's esophagus adversely influences survival, and (2) the assumption that endoscopic surveillance can reliably detect early, curable neoplasia in the columnar-lined esophagus. As discussed above, no study has yet demonstrated that Barrett's esophagus adversely influences survival. Endoscopic surveillance clearly can detect early neoplasia in Barrett's esophagus, but the reliability of surveillance for detecting curable neoplasia has not been established. For example, one study compared the outcome for 58 patients who first presented to the hospital with symptoms of esophageal cancer (in whom Barrett's esophagus was discovered incidentally during evaluation of the malignancy) with that for 19 patients known to have Barrett's esophagus who had cancers discovered during endoscopic surveillance (131). The patients whose cancers were discovered during surveillance had tumors in an earlier stage of development than those who presented to the hospital with cancer symptoms. The 5-year actuarial survival in the surveillance group (62%) also was significantly better than that in the patients who presented with cancer (20%, $p = 0.007$). More recently, these investigators reviewed their experience with endoscopic surveillance for patients with Barrett's esophagus and concluded that the outcome compared favorably to that of the common practice of mammographic surveillance for breast cancer (132). These retrospective studies do not prove that endoscopic surveillance reduces the mortality from esophageal cancer, but they do show that surveillance can detect some early, curable esophageal neoplasms in patients known to have Barrett's esophagus. Unfortunately, the studies also show that some patients develop advanced cancers in Barrett's esophagus despite their participation in an endoscopic surveillance program. Thus, the efficacy of surveillance in decreasing morbidity and mortality from esophageal cancer remains unclear.

The efficacy of endoscopic surveillance for Barrett's esophagus is likely to remain unclear for a long time. Although this issue might be resolved by a prospective study in which patients are randomly assigned to receive surveillance or no surveillance, the logistical and ethical issues imposed by such a study are daunting. Even if one ignores the substantial ethical and practical issues involved in convincing patients to accept randomization to the no-surveillance arm of the trial, it has been estimated that the study would require 5000 patients to be followed for 10 years in order to show a significant effect for surveillance in decreasing cancer mortality (assuming a cancer incidence rate of approximately 1% per year) (133). It is highly unlikely that the results of such a study will be available in the near future.

In the absence of definitive studies, some investigators have used computer models to estimate the value of endoscopic surveillance. For example, Provenzale et al. explored the value of different endoscopic surveillance strategies using a Markov model to construct a computer cohort simulation of 10,000 patients with Barrett's esophagus (133). The model was highly sensitive to the value chosen for the incidence of cancer in Barrett's esophagus. Using data from this study, Figure 8 shows the optimal endoscopic surveillance intervals if the goal is to maximize quality-adjusted life expectancy. Notice how the cancer incidence rate affects the surveillance recommendations. If the annual cancer incidence rate is below 0.5%, then no endoscopic surveillance at all is the preferred strategy, whereas yearly endoscopy is the preferred strategy when cancer incidence exceeds 2.0%. As shown in Table 5, reported cancer incidence rates in prospective studies on Barrett's esophagus range between 0.5% and 1.9%. Applying the computer model, therefore, preferred endoscopic surveillance strategies could range from no surveillance at all to yearly endoscopy depending on which estimate

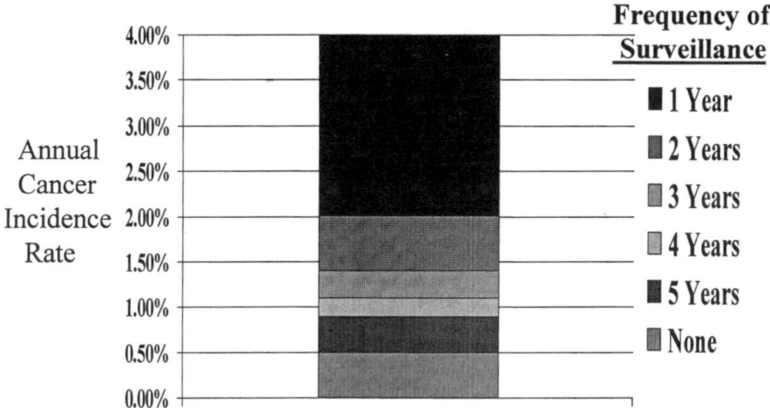

Figure 8 Estimated optimal endoscopic surveillance intervals if the goal is to maximize quality-adjusted life expectancy. Note how the cancer incidence rate affects the surveillance recommendations. (Data from Ref. 133.)

for cancer incidence is chosen. The choice of preferred surveillance strategy is exquisitely sensitive to tiny differences in cancer incidence, and all available estimates of that incidence are imprecise.

Ablative Therapies for Dysplasia and Metaplasia

As discussed above, high-grade dysplasia in Barrett's esophagus is judged to be the precursor of invasive cancer. Esophageal resection is the only therapy that clearly interrupts the progression from dysplasia to malignancy in this condition, but the role of esophageal resection in the management of patients with high-grade dysplasia is disputed (134). Some authorities advocate intensive endoscopic surveillance for patients found to have high-grade dysplasia, and withhold esophageal resection until surveillance demonstrates invasive cancer. Others favor an aggressive approach, and recommend esophageal resection (unless precluded by advanced age or comorbidity) for all patients found to have high-grade dysplasia in Barrett's esophagus (135). The arguments for and against esophageal resection for high-grade dysplasia in Barrett's esophagus are summarized in Tables 7 and 8. In the absence of definitive studies on this issue, the controversy will continue.

Recently, endoscopic ablation therapy has been proposed as a safer and easier alternative to esophageal resection for patients with high-grade dysplasia in Barrett's esophagus (136). A number of recent studies have shown that it is possible to ablate the metaplastic columnar lining in Barrett's esophagus endoscopically using thermal or photochemical energy (Table 9) (137). When acid

Table 7 Arguments Against Esophageal Resection for High-Grade Dysplasia in Barrett's Esophagus

High-grade dysplasia may not invariably progress to invasive cancer.
Regression of high-grade dysplasia has been observed occasionally.
Rigorous endoscopic surveillance may detect early, curable cancer.
Mortality for esophageal resection is in the range of 4–10%.
Esophageal resection often causes substantial morbidity.

Table 8 Arguments Favoring Esophageal Resection for High-Grade Dysplasia in Barrett's Esophagus

~1/3 of patients with high-grade dysplasia already have invasive cancer.
Exclusion of cancer requires extensive biopsy sampling.
Progression to cancer occurs frequently and may be rapid.
Efficacy of surveillance in detecting curable cancers is not clear.
Established esophageal cancers often are not curable.

Table 9 Modalities for Ablating Barrett's Esophagus

Thermal energy
Laser (argon, Nd:YAG, KTP)
Multipolar electrocoagulation
Argon beam plasma coagulation
Photochemical energy
Photodynamic therapy

reflux is controlled with PPIs or fundoplication, the ablated columnar epithelium heals with the regeneration of squamous epithelium. The relative merits of the various endoscopic ablation methods listed in Table 9 are disputed, and it is not yet clear which is the ''best'' form of ablative therapy for Barrett's esophagus. When choosing among the available modalities, however, there appears to be a trade-off between the completeness of mucosal ablation and the frequency of complications. Modalities that induce relatively superficial mucosal injury (e.g., argon laser) cause few complications, but often leave residual foci of metaplastic epithelium behind. Conversely, modalities that can cause deep injury (e.g., Nd:YAG laser) appear to be more effective at eliminating metaplastic mucosa, but the rate of complications such as esophageal perforation and stricture formation is high.

Much attention has focused on photodynamic therapy (PDT) in which patients are given a systemic dose of a light-activated drug (e.g., a porphyrin) that is taken up by the metaplastic columnar cells. Using a low-power laser, the esophagus is irradiated endoscopically with laser light (usually red laser light at a wavelength of 630 nm) that activates the porphyrin. The activated porphyrin can transfer its energy to oxygen, thereby producing singlet oxygen that is toxic to cells. Thus, any cell that concentrates the photosensitizer is destroyed when the drug is activated by exposure to laser light. In Barrett's esophagus, the porphyrin photosensitizer is concentrated by both neoplastic and nonneoplastic cells. Therefore, PDT can ablate dysplastic cells, malignant cells, and nonneoplastic cells that line the esophagus.

There is published experience on two photosensitizing agents used for primary PDT in Barrett's esophagus: porfimer sodium and 5-aminolevulinic acid (5-ALA) (136). Porfimer sodium, a mixture of hematoporphyrins, must be administered intravenously and produces skin photosensitivity that can last for months. The endoscopic application of laser light must be delayed approximately 2–3 days after the porfimer sodium is given, and PDT with this agent frequently is complicated by esophageal stricture formation. 5-ALA normally is produced endogenously as part of the heme biosynthetic pathway. The exogenous administration of large quantities of 5-ALA results in the intracellular accumulation of protoporphyrin IX, a potent photosensitizer that is the immediate precursor of heme. Unlike porfimer sodium, 5-ALA can be administered orally, laser light can be applied only 4–6 h later, skin photosensitivity lasts days rather than months, and esophageal stricture formation occurs infrequently. Unfortunately, 5-ALA does not appear to be as effective as porfimer sodium for eradicating dysplasia in Barrett's esophagus (138). The published experience with PDT in Barrett's esophagus is limited, and comparisons among studies are confounded by differences in the photosensitizing agent used (porfimer sodium or 5-ALA), the dose of the agent given (porfimer sodium dose range 1.5–2 mg/kg), the wavelength of laser light irradiated (630 nm or 635 nm), the dose of light energy administered (range 100–300 J/cm), and the type of endoscopic delivery system employed (naked diffuser or centering balloon) (139–144).

Recently, Overholt et al. published the results of PDT with porfimer sodium for 100 patients who had either superficial cancer or dysplasia in Barrett's esophagus. The patients were followed for a mean duration of 19 months (range 4–84 months) (144). For 13 patients with superficial cancers, PDT appeared to eliminate the malignancy in 10 cases (77%). Following PDT for 73 patients with high-grade dysplasia, there was no evidence of dysplasia on follow-up endoscopy in 56 cases (77%). For 14 patients with low-grade dysplasia, PDT resulted in apparent eradication of dysplasia in 13 cases (93%). Unfortunately, the rate of side effects and complications was high. Most patients experienced minor problems with photosensitivity, whereas four of the 100 patients experienced substantial problems when they exposed themselves to direct sunlight. Most patients experienced chest pain and dysphagia of mild-to-moderate severity for 5–7 days after the laser treatment, and many required treatment with intravenous fluids to maintain hydration during that period. Small, clinically inapparent pleural effusions also developed in most patients, a phenomenon suggesting that PDT often causes transmural injury to the esophagus. Three patients developed atrial fibrillation after PDT, all of whom were treated successfully without sequelae. Perhaps most worrisome was the high rate of esophageal stricture formation. Thirty-four patients (34%) developed esophageal strictures that required one or more sessions of dilation therapy. This high rate of stricture formation also suggests that PDT inflicts deep esophageal injury.

To reduce the rate of PDT complications, Laukka and Wang tried ''low-dose'' PDT (porfimer sodium 1.5 mg/kg, 175 J/cm light energy) in five patients who had dysplasia in Barrett's esophagus (140). All patients experienced partial regression of columnar metaplasia following PDT (24% mean decrease in overall length of columnar epithelium), but dysplasia persisted in all five cases. Two groups have reported the results of PDT using 5-ALA in Barrett's esophagus (142,143). Barr et al. treated five patients with high-grade dysplasia (142). No evidence of dysplasia was found in any patient on endoscopic examinations performed during follow-up periods ranging from 26 to 44 months, but biopsy specimens taken in treated areas revealed residual foci of columnar metaplasia buried under squamous epithelium in two of the five patients. Gossner et al. used PDT with 5-ALA to treat 22 patients with superficial cancers and 10 patients with high-grade dysplasia in Barrett's esophagus (143). During a mean follow-up period of 9.9 months, no residual cancer was found in 17 of 22 patients (77%), and high-grade dysplasia appeared to have been eradicated in all 10 cases. Cancers with a thickness of >2 mm were not eliminated by PDT with ALA. The treatment caused only minor side effects including short-lived nausea, mild photosensitivity, and minor elevations in serum aminotransferase levels. No patients developed esophageal strictures. All patients had residual metaplastic columnar epithelium in the esophagus, however.

Although these reports document the feasibility of ablating metaplastic columnar epithelium in the esophagus with PDT, they do not establish the benefit of the technique. PDT with porfimer sodium is an expensive treatment that entails substantial risk and inconvenience. The use of 5-ALA instead of porfimer sodium results in fewer complications, but the depth of injury induced by PDT with 5-ALA may be too shallow to eradicate metaplastic mucosa reliably. When interpreting the results of studies on PDT, furthermore, it is important to consider the substantial problem of biopsy sampling error. Patients found to have high-grade dysplasia in Barrett's esophagus often harbor inapparent foci of invasive cancer that are missed due to biopsy sampling error (83). Without histological examination of the resected esophagus or very long durations of follow-up, it is not possible to verify the claims of available reports that dysplasia and cancer in Barrett's esophagus were "eliminated" by PDT. These claims were based on random biopsy sampling of the treated esophagus, and such sampling is subject to considerable error (7). Some of the patients who appeared to be cured in fact may still be harboring inapparent foci of cancer or dysplasia that might eventually cause illness. The progression from dysplasia to cancer in Barrett's esophagus may be slow (88), and reports from China have documented that untreated, early esophageal cancers can remain asymptomatic for 5 years or more (145). Thus, it is inappropriate to conclude on the basis of random biopsy specimens obtained within months of PDT that cancer and dysplasia have been eradicated. Also, PDT usually does not eliminate all of the metaplastic epithelium in the esophagus. Residual foci of metaplasia remain in most patients, and some of these foci may be buried under a superficial layer of squamous epithelium where they are invisible to the endoscopist. Failure to obliterate all of the metaplastic epithelium might leave patients at high risk for malignancy, and the inability to detect metaplasia hidden by the overgrowth of squamous epithelium might compromise surveillance programs. No study yet has established that PDT has any effect on the risk for cancer development in Barrett's esophagus.

Presumably, patients treated with PDT will require lifelong antireflux therapy with potent antisecretory agents like proton pump inhibitors or with fundoplication to prevent the return of reflux esophagitis and columnar metaplasia. One report has described the results of Nd:YAG laser photoablation of Barrett's esophagus in a 43-year-old man with long-standing reflux esophagitis (146). An endoscopic examination performed 6 weeks after treatment revealed no endoscopic or histological signs of metaplastic epithelium. However, a follow-up endoscopic examination at 14 weeks showed that metaplastic mucosa had returned despite ongoing treatment with omeprazole in a dose of 20 mg daily. This report suggests that columnar metaplasia in the esophagus is both reversible and revertible. Clearly, even patients treated successfully with PDT will require regular endoscopic surveillance to ensure that metaplastic epithelium has not returned and to monitor for neoplasia.

At present, to recommend PDT of Barrett's esophagus for clinical purposes is to endorse an expensive and potentially hazardous therapy that usually does not obliterate all of the metaplastic mucosa, that has no proved efficacy in reducing cancer risk, that will likely require antireflux surgery or antisecretory drugs administered lifelong in high doses to prevent recurrence, that might produce only temporary results, and that does not obviate regular endoscopic surveillance. These considerations must temper enthusiasm for the wholesale application of this technique in clinical practice. Nevertheless, this is an exciting area for research. For patients with high-grade dysplasia or superficial cancers in Barrett's esophagus who are too old, infirm, or unwilling to assume the considerable risks of esophageal resection and reconstruction, PDT is a reasonable alternative provided the procedure is performed as part of an established study protocol.

Very few data are available to guide the clinician in managing patients found to have low-grade dysplasia in Barrett's esophagus. Histologically, it can be difficult to distinguish the changes of low-grade dysplasia from reactive changes in an epithelium that is regenerating in response to inflammatory injury. Furthermore, the natural history of low-grade dysplasia is not well described. Consequently, most authorities are reluctant to recommend an invasive and hazardous procedure like esophageal resection for patients with low-grade dysplasia in Barrett's esophagus.

MANAGEMENT RECOMMENDATIONS

As discussed, it is not clear that Barrett's esophagus adversely influences survival, or that endoscopic surveillance can reliably detect early, curable neoplasia in the columnar-lined esophagus. Nevertheless, most authorities continue to recommend regular endoscopic surveillance for patients with Barrett's esophagus. Recently, the American College of Gastroenterology recommended the following practice guidelines for cancer surveillance in this condition (147):

> Patients with Barrett's esophagus should undergo surveillance endoscopy and biopsy at an interval determined by the presence and grade of dysplasia. Gastroesophageal reflux disease should be treated aggressively prior to surveillance endoscopy to minimize confusion caused by inflammation in the interpretation of biopsy specimens. The technique of random, four-quadrant biopsies taken every 2 cm in the columnar-lined esophagus for standard histologic evaluation is recommended.
>
> For patients with no dysplasia, surveillance endoscopy is recommended at an interval of every 2 to 3 years.
>
> For patients with low-grade dysplasia, surveillance endoscopy every 6 months for the first year is recommended, followed by yearly endoscopy if the dysplasia has not progressed in severity.
>
> For patients with high-grade dysplasia, two alternatives are proposed after the diagnosis has been confirmed by an expert gastrointestinal pathologist:
>
> One alternative is intensive endoscopic surveillance until intramucosal cancer is detected. The guideline does not recommend a specific interval for such surveillance, but some investigators have studied such patients at an interval of every 3 months.
>
> The other alternative is to recommend esophageal resection, a procedure associated with substantial morbidity and mortality.

Although not specifically recommended in the practice guidelines, clinicians can consider the use of experimental ablative therapies such as photodynamic therapy for their patients with high-grade dysplasia in Barrett's esophagus, *provided the therapy is provided as part of an established, approved research protocol.* The use of ablative therapies outside of research protocols cannot be condoned at this time.

REFERENCES

1. Spechler SJ, Goyal RK. The columnar lined esophagus, intestinal metaplasia, and Norman Barrett. Gastroenterology 1996; 110:614–621.
2. Antonioli DA, Wang HH. Morphology of Barrett's esophagus and Barrett's-associated dysplasia and adenocarcinoma. Gastroenterol Clin North Am 1997; 26:495–506.
3. Spechler SJ. Laser photoablation of Barrett's epithelium: burning issues about burning tissues. Gastroenterology 1993; 104:1855–1858.
4. Lagergren J, Bergström R, Lindgren A, Nyrén O. Symptomatic gastroesophageal reflux as a risk factor for esophageal adenocarcinoma. N Engl J Med 1999; 340:825–831.
5. Spechler SJ. Short and ultrashort Barrett's esophagus: what does it mean? Semin Gastrointest Dis 1997; 8:59–67.
6. Hayward J. The lower end of the oesophagus. Thorax 1961; 16:36–41.
7. Kim SL, Waring PJ, Spechler SJ, Sampliner RE, Doos WG, Krol WF, Williford WO, and the Department of Veterans Affairs Gastroesophageal Reflux Study Group. Diagnostic inconsistencies in Barrett's esophagus. Gastroenterology 1994; 107:945–949.
8. Tytgat GNJ. Endoscopic features of the columnar-lined esophagus. Gastroenterol Clin North Am 1997; 26:507–517.
9. Paull A, Trier JS, Dalton MD, Camp RC, Loeb P, Goyal RK. The histologic spectrum of Barrett's esophagus. N Engl J Med 1976; 295:476–480.
10. Weinstein WM, Ippoliti AF. The diagnosis of Barrett's esophagus: goblets, goblets, goblets. Gastrointest Endosc 1996; 44:91–95.
11. Spechler SJ, Zeroogian JM, Antonioli DA, Wang HH, Goyal RK. Prevalence of metaplasia at the gastro-oesophageal junction. Lancet 1994; 344:1533–1536.
12. Spechler SJ. The columnar lined oesophagus: a riddle wrapped in a mystery inside an enigma. Gut 1997; 41:710–711.
13. Hirota WK, Loughney TM, Lazas DJ, Maydonovitch CL, Rholl V, Wong RKH. Specialized intestinal metaplasia, dysplasia, and cancer of the esophagus and esophagogastric junction: prevalence and clinical data. Gastroenterology 1999; 116:277–285.
14. Weston AP, Krmpotich P, Makdisi WE, Cherian R, Dixon A, McGregor DH, Banerjee SK. Short segment Barrett's esophagus: clinical and histological features, associated endoscopic findings, and association with gastric intestinal metaplasia. Am J Gastroenterol 1996; 91:981–986.

15. Sharma P, Morales TG, Sampliner RE. Short segment Barrett's esophagus—the need for standardization of the definition and of endoscopic criteria. Am J Gastroenterol 1998; 93:1033–1036.
16. McClave SA, Boyce HW Jr, Gottfried MR. Early diagnosis of columnar-lined esophagus: a new endoscopic criterion. Gastrointest Endosc 1987; 33:413–416.
17. Stemmermann GN. Intestinal metaplasia of the stomach. A status report. Cancer 1994; 74:556–564.
18. Spechler SJ. The role of gastric carditis in metaplasia and neoplasia at the gastroesophageal junction. Gastroenterology 1999; 117:218–228.
19. Asaka M, Takeda H, Sugiyama T, Kato M. What role does *Helicobacter pylori* play in gastric cancer? Gastroenterology 1997; 113:556–560.
20. Parsonnet J. *Helicobacter pylori* in the stomach—a paradox unmasked. N Engl J Med 1996; 335:278–280.
21. Watanabe T, Tada M, Nagai H, Sasaki S, Nakao M. *Helicobacter pylori* infection induces gastric cancer in Mongolian gerbils. Gastroenterology 1998; 115:642–648.
22. Correa P. *Helicobacter pylori* and gastric carcinogenesis. Am J Surg Pathol 1995; 19(suppl 1):S37–S43.
23. Parsonnet J, Friedman GD, Orentreich N, Vogelman H. Risk for gastric cancer in people with CagA positive or CagA negative *Helicobacter pylori* infection. Gut 1997; 40:297–301.
24. O'Connor HJ, Cunnane K. *Helicobacter pylori* and gastro-oesophageal reflux disease—a prospective study. Ir J Med Sci 1994; 163:369–373.
25. Liston R, Pitt MA, Banerjee AK. Reflux oesophagitis and *Helicobacter pylori* infection in elderly patients. Postgrad Med J 1996; 72:221–223.
26. Rosioru C, Glassman MS, Halata MS, Schwarz SM. Esophagitis and *Helicobacter pylori* in children: incidence and therapeutic implications. Am J Gastroenterol 1993; 88:510–513.
27. Talley NJ, Cameron AJ, Shorter RG, Zinsmeister AR, Phillips SF. *Campylobacter pylori* and Barrett's esophagus. Mayo Clin Proc 1988; 63:1176–1180.
28. Ursua I, Ramos R, Val-Bernal JF. *Helicobacter pylori* in Barrett's esophagus. Histol Histopathol 1991; 6:403–408.
29. Loffeld RJLF, Ten Tije BJ, Arends JW. Prevalence and significance of *Helicobacter pylori* in patients with Barrett's esophagus. Am J Gastroenterol 1992; 87:1598–1600.
30. Abbas Z, Hussainy AS, Ibrahim F, Jafri SM, Shaikh H, Khan AH. Barrett's oesophagus and *Helicobacter pylori*. J Gastroenterol Hepatol 1995; 10:331–333.
31. Ricaurte O, Fléjou JF, Vissuzaine C, Goldfain D, Rotenberg A, Cadiot G, Potet F. *Helicobacter pylori* infection in patients with Barrett's oesophagus: a prospective immunohistochemical study. J Clin Pathol 1996; 49:176–177.
32. Werdmuller BFM, Loffeld RJLF. *Helicobacter pylori* infection has no role in the pathogenesis of reflux esophagitis. Dig Dis Sci 1997; 42:103–105.
33. Labenz J, Blum AL, Bayerdörffer E, Meining A, Stolte M, Börsch G. Curing *Helicobacter pylori* infection in patients with duodenal ulcer may provoke reflux esophagitis. Gastroenterology 1997; 112:1442–1447.
34. Weston AP, Badr AS, Topalovski M, Cherian R, Dixon A. Prospective evaluation

of the association of gastric *H. pylori* infection with Barrett's dysplasia and Barrett's adenocarcinoma. Gastroenterology 1998; 114:A703.

35. Chow WH, Blaser MJ, Blot WJ, Gammon MD, Vaughan TL, Risch HA, Perez-Perez GI, Schoenberg JB, Stanford JL, Rotterdam H, West AB, Fraumeni JF Jr. An inverse relation between CagA+ strains of *Helicobacter pylori* infection and risk of esophageal and gastric cardia adenocarcinoma. Cancer Res 1998; 58:588–590.
36. Vicari JJ, Peek RM, Falk GW, Goldblum JR, Easley KA, Schnell J, Perez-Perez GI, Halter SA, Rice TW, Blaser MJ, Richter JE. The seroprevalence of CagA-positive *Helicobacter pylori* strains in the spectrum of gastroesophageal reflux disease. Gastroenterology 1998; 115:50–57.
37. Graham DY, Yamaoka Y. *H. pylori* and CagA: relationships with gastric cancer, duodenal ulcer, and reflux esophagitis and its complications. Helicobacter 1998; 3:145–150.
38. Matsukura N, Suzuki K, Kawachi T, Aoyagi M, Sugimura T, Kitaoka H, Numajiri H, Shirota A, Itabashi M, Hirota T. Distribution of marker enzymes and mucin in intestinal metaplasia in human stomach and relation to complete and incomplete types of intestinal metaplasia to minute gastric carcinomas. J Natl Cancer Inst 1980; 65:231–240.
39. Jass JR, Filipe MI. The mucin profiles of normal gastric mucosa, intestinal metaplasia and its variants and gastric carcinoma. Histochem J 1981; 13:931–939.
40. Filipe MI, Potet F, Bogomoletz WV, Dawson PA, Fabiani B, Chauveinc P, Fenzy A, Gazzard B, Goldfain D, Zeegen R. Incomplete sulphomucin-secreting intestinal metaplasia for gastric cancer. Preliminary data from a prospective study from three centers. Gut 1985; 26:1319–1326.
41. Craanen ME, Blok P, Dekker W, Ferwerda J, Tytgat GNJ. Subtypes of intestinal metaplasia and *Helicobacter pylori*. Gut 1992; 33:597–600.
42. Filipe MI, Munoz N, Matko I, Kato I, Pompe-Kirn V, Jutersek A, Teuchmann S, Benz M, Prijon T. Intestinal metaplasia types and the risk of gastric cancer: a cohort study in Slovenia. Int J Cancer 1994; 57:324–329.
43. Tosi P, Filipe MI, Luzi P, Miracco C, Santopietro R, Lio R, Sforza V, Barbini P. Gastric intestinal metaplasia type III cases are classified as low-grade dysplasia on the basis of morphometry. J Pathol 1993; 169:73–78.
44. Zwas F, Shields HM, Doos WG, Antonioli DA, Goldman H, Ransil BJ, Spechler SJ. Scanning electron microscopy of Barrett's epithelium and its correlation with light microscopy and mucin stains. Gastroenterology 1986; 90:1932–1941.
45. Jass JR. Mucin histochemistry of the columnar epithelium of the oesophagus: a retrospective study. J Clin Pathol 1981; 34:866–870.
46. Trier JS. Morphology of the columnar cell-lined (Barrett's) esophagus. In: Spechler SJ, Goyal RK, eds. Barrett's Esophagus: Pathophysiology, Diagnosis, and Management. New York: Elsevier Science, 1985:19–28.
47. Das KM, Prasad I, Garla S, Amenta PS. Detection of a shared colon epithelial epitope on Barrett epithelium by a novel monoclonal antibody. Ann Intern Med 1994; 120:753–756.
48. Shields HM, Zwas F, Antonioli DA, Doos WG, Kim S, Spechler SJ. Detection by scanning electron microscopy of a distinctive esophageal surface cell at the junction of squamous and Barrett's epithelium. Dig Dis Sci 1993; 38:97–108.

49. Ormsby AH, Goldblum JR, Rice TW, Richter JE, Falk GW, Vaezi MF, Gramlich TL. Cytokeratin subsets can reliably distinguish Barrett's esophagus from intestinal metaplasia of the stomach. Hum Pathol 1999; 30:288–294.
50. Salo JA, Kivilaakso EO, Kiviluoto TA, Virtanen IO. Cytokeratin profile suggests metaplastic epithelial transformation in Barrett's oesophagus. Ann Med 1996; 28: 305–309.
51. Boch JA, Shields HM, Antonioli DA, Zwas F, Sawhney RA, Trier JS. Distribution of cytokeratin markers in Barrett's specialized columnar epithelium. Gastroenterology 1997; 112:760–765.
52. Spechler SJ, Goyal RK. Barrett's esophagus. N Engl J Med 1986; 315:362–371.
53. Hassall E. Columnar-lined esophagus in children. Gastroenterol Clin North Am 1997; 26:533–548.
54. Johnson DA, Winters C, Spurling TJ, Chobanian SJ, Cattau EL Jr. Esophageal acid sensitivity in Barrett's esophagus. J Clin Gastroenterol 1987; 9:23–27.
55. Winter C Jr, Spurling TJ, Chobanian SJ, et al. Barrett's esophagus. A prevalent, occult complication of gastroesophageal reflux disease. Gastroenterology 1987; 92: 118–124.
56. Lieberman DA, Oehlke M, Helfand M. Risk factors for Barrett's esophagus in community-based practice. GORGE consortium. Gastroenterology Outcomes Research Group in Endoscopy. Am J Gastroenterol 1997; 92(8):1293–1297.
57. Cameron AJ, Zinsmeister AR, Ballard DJ, Carney JA: Prevalence of columnar-lined (Barrett's) esophagus. Comparison of population-based clinical and autopsy findings. Gastroenterology 1990; 99:918–922.
58. Collen MJ, Lewis JH, Benjamin SB. Gastric acid hypersecretion in refractory gastroesophageal reflux disease. Gastroenterology 1990; 98:654–661.
59. Mulholland MW, Reid BJ, Levine DS, Rubin CE. Elevated gastric acid secretion in patients with Barrett's metaplastic epithelium. Dig Dis Sci 1989; 34:1329–1335.
60. Gillen P, Keeling P, Byrne PJ, Healy M, O'Moore RR, Hennessy TPJ. Implication of duodenogastric reflux in the pathogenesis of Barrett's oesophagus. Br J Surg 1988; 75:540–543.
61. Iascone C, DeMeester TR, Little AG, Skinner DB. Barrett's esophagus. Functional assessment, proposed pathogenesis, and surgical therapy. Arch Surg 1983; 118: 543–549.
62. Zaninotto G, DeMeester TR, Bremner CG, Smyrk TC, Cheng SC. Esophageal function in patients with reflux-induced strictures and its relevance to surgical treatment. Ann Thorac Surg 1989; 47:362–370.
63. Gray MR, Donnelly RJ, Kingsnorth AN. Role of salivary epidermal growth factor in the pathogenesis of Barrett's columnar lined oesophagus. Br J Surg 1991; 78: 1461–1466.
64. Öberg S, DeMeester TR, Peters JH, Hagen JA, Nigro JJ, DeMeester SR, Theisen J, Campos GMR, Crookes PF. The extent of Barrett's esophagus depends on the status of the lower esophageal sphincter and degree of esophageal acid exposure. J Thorac Cardiovasc Surg 1999; 117:572–580.
65. Cameron AJ, Lomboy CT. Barrett's esophagus: age, prevalence, and extent of columnar epithelium. Gastroenterology 1992; 103:1241–1245.

66. Hesketh PJ, Clapp RW, Doos WG, Spechler SJ. The increasing frequency of adenocarcinoma of the esophagus. Cancer 1989; 64:526–530.
67. Blot WJ, Devesa SS, Kneller RW, Fraumeni JF Jr. Rising incidence of adenocarcinoma of the esophagus and gastric cardia. JAMA 1991; 265:1287–1289.
68. Blot WJ, Devesa SS, Fraumeni JF Jr. Continuing climb in rates of esophageal adenocarcinoma: an update. JAMA 1993; 270:1320.
69. Devesa SS, Blot WJ, Fraumeni JF Jr. Changing patterns in the incidence of esophageal and gastric carcinoma in the United States. Cancer 1998; 83:2049–2053.
70. Spechler SJ. The frequency of esophageal cancer in patients with Barrett's esophagus. Acta Endoscopica 1992; 22:541–544.
71. Drewitz DJ, Sampliner RE, Garewal HS. The incidence of adenocarcinoma in Barrett's esophagus: a prospective study of 170 patients followed 4.8 years. Am J Gastroenterol 1997; 92:212–215.
72. American Cancer Society. Cancer Facts and Figures—1995. Atlanta: American Cancer Society, 1995.
73. Van der Burgh A, Dees J, Hop WCJ, van Blankenstein M. Oesophageal cancer is an uncommon cause of death in patients with Barrett's oesophagus. Gut 1996; 39: 5–8.
74. Cameron AJ, Ott BJ, Payne WS. The incidence of adenocarcinoma in columnar-lined (Barrett's) esophagus. N Engl J Med 1985; 313:857–859.
75. Van der Veen AH, Dees J, Blankensteijn JD, van Blankenstein M. Adenocarcinoma in Barrett's oesophagus: an overrated risk. Gut 1989; 30:14–18.
76. Spechler SJ. Barrett's esophagus: should we brush off this ballooning problem? Gastroenterology 1997; 112:2138–2152.
77. Spechler SJ. Barrett's esophagus. Semin Oncol 1994; 21:431–437.
78. Ransom JM, Patel GK, Clift SA, Womble NE, Read RC. Extended and limited types of Barrett's esophagus in the adult. Ann Thorac Surg 1982; 33:19–27.
79. Harle IA, Finley RJ, Belsheim M, Bondy DC, Booth M, Lloyd D, McDonald JW, Sullivan S, Valberg LS, Watson WC, Frei JV, Slinger R, Troster M, Meads GE, Duff JH. Management of adenocarcinoma in a columnar-lined esophagus. Ann Thorac Surg 1985; 40:330–336.
80. Souza RF, Meltzer SJ. The molecular basis for carcinogenesis in metaplastic columnar-lined esophagus. Gastroenterol Clin North Am 1997; 26:583–597.
81. Schmidt HG, Riddell RH, Walther B, Skinner DB, Riemann JF. Dysplasia in Barrett's esophagus. J Cancer Res Clin Oncol 1985; 110:145–152.
82. Spechler SJ. Endoscopic surveillance for patients with Barrett's esophagus: does the cancer risk justify the practice? Ann Intern Med 1987; 106:902–904.
83. Spechler SJ. Complications of gastroesophageal reflux disease. In: Castell DO, ed. The Esophagus. Boston: Little, Brown, 1992:543–556.
84. Levine DS, Haggitt RC, Blount PL, Rabinovitch PS, Rusch VW, Reid BJ. An endoscopic biopsy protocol can differentiate high-grade dysplasia from early adenocarcinoma in Barrett's esophagus. Gastroenterology 1993; 105:40–50.
85. Reid BJ, Weinstein WM, Lewin KJ, Haggitt RC, VanDeventer G, DenBesten L, Rubin CE. Endoscopic biopsy can detect high-grade dysplasia or early adenocarcinoma in Barrett's esophagus without grossly recognizable neoplastic lesions. Gastroenterology 1988; 94:81–90.

86. Falk GW, Rice TW, Goldblum JR, Richter JE. Jumbo biopsy forceps protocol still misses unsuspected cancer in Barrett's esophagus with high-grade dysplasia. Gastrointest Endosc 1999; 49:170–176.
87. Hameeteman W, Tytgat GNJ, Houthoff HJ, van den Tweel JG. Barrett's esophagus: development of dysplasia and adenocarcinoma. Gastroenterology 1989; 96:1249–1256.
88. Lee RG. Dysplasia in Barrett's esophagus. A clinicopathologic study of six patients. Am J Surg Pathol 1985; 9:845–852.
89. Sontag SJ, Schnell TG, Kurucar C, O'Connell S, Levine G, Karpf J, Adelman K, Brand L, Seidel J. Barrett's high-grade dysplasia (HGD): surveillance endoscopy (EGD) once a year (yr) is sufficient in most patients (pts). Gastroenterology 1999; 116:A304–A305.
90. Reid BJ, Haggitt RC, Rubin CE, Roth G, Surawicz CM, Van Belle G, Lewin K, Weinstein WM, Antonioli DA, Goldman H, et al. Observer variation in the diagnosis of dysplasia in Barrett's esophagus. Hum Pathol 1988; 19:166–178.
91. Blount PL, Ramel S, Raskind WH, Haggitt RC, Sanchez CA, Dean PJ, Rabinovitch PS, Reid BJ. 17p allelic deletions and p53 protein overexpression in Barrett's adenocarcinomas. Cancer Res 1991; 51:5482–5486.
92. Wu TT, Watanabe T, Heitmiller R, Zahurak M, Forastiere AA, Hamilton SR. Genetic alterations in Barrett esophagus and adenocarcinomas of the esophagus and esophagogastric junction region. Am J Pathol 1998; 153:287–294.
93. Casson AG, Mukhopadhyay T, Cleary KR, Ro JY, Levin B, Roth JA. p53 gene mutations in Barrett's epithelium and esophageal cancer. Cancer Res 1991; 51: 4495–4499.
94. Ramel S, Reid BJ, Sanchez CA, et al. Evaluation of p53 protein expression in Barrett's esophagus by two-parameter flow cytometry. Gastroenterology 1992; 102: 1220–1228.
95. Schneider PM, Casson AG, Levin B, Garewal HS, Hoelscher AH, Becker K, Dittler HJ, Cleary KR, Troster M, Siewert JR, Roth JA. Mutations of p53 in Barrett's oesophagus and Barrett's cancer: a prospective study of ninety-eight cases. J Thorac Cardiovasc Surg 1996; 111:323–331.
96. Khan S, Do KA, Kuhnert P, Pillay SP, Papadimos D, Conrad R, Jass JR. Diagnostic value of p53 immunohistochemistry in Barrett's esophagus: an endoscopic study. Pathology 1998; 30:136–140.
97. Gimenez A, Minguela A, Parrilla P, Bermejo J, Perez D, Molina J, Garcia AM, Ortiz MA, Alvarez R, de Haro LM. Flow cytometric DNA analysis and p53 protein expression show a good correlation with histologic findings in patients with Barrett's esophagus. Cancer 1998; 15:83:641–651.
98. Kim R, Clarke MR, Melhem MF, Young MA, Vanbibber MM, Safatle-Ribeiro AV, Ribeiro U Jr, Reynolds JC. Expression of p53, PCNA, and C-erbB-2 in Barrett's metaplasia and adenocarcinoma. Dig Dis Sci 1997; 42:2453–2462.
99. Ireland AP, Clark GW, DeMeester TR. Barrett's esophagus. The significance of p53 in clinical practice. Ann Surg 1997; 225:17–30.
100. Cawley HM, Meltzer SJ, De Benedetti VMG, Hollstein MC, Muehlbauer KR, Liang L, Bennett WP, Souza RF, Greenwald BD, Cottrell J, Salages A, Bartsch H,

Trivers GE. Anti-p53 antibodies in patients with Barrett's esophagus or esophageal carcinoma can predate cancer diagnosis. Gastroenterology 1998; 115:19–27.

101. Reid BJ, Blount PL, Rubin CE, Levine DS, Haggitt RC, Rabinovitch PS. Flowcytometric and histological progression to malignancy in Barrett's esophagus: prospective endoscopic surveillance of a cohort. Gastroenterology 1992; 102:1212–1221.
102. Montgomery EA, Hartmann DP, Carr NJ, Holterman DA, Sobin LH, Azumi N. Barrett esophagus with dysplasia. Flow cytometric DNA analysis of routine, paraffin-embedded mucosal biopsies. Am J Clin Pathol 1996; 106:298–304.
103. Cameron AJ. Barrett's esophagus and adenocarcinoma: from the family to the gene. Gastroenterology 1992; 102:1421–1424.
104. Woolf GM, Riddell RH, Irvine EJ, Hunt RH. A study to examine agreement between endoscopy and histology for the diagnosis of columnar lined (Barrett's) esophagus. Gastrointest Endosc 1989; 35:541–544.
105. Chobanian SJ, Cattau EL Jr., Winters C Jr., Johnson DA, Van Ness MM, Miremadi A, Horwitz SL, Colcher H. In vivo staining with toluidine blue as an adjunct to the endoscopic detection of Barrett's esophagus. Gastrointest Endosc 1987; 33:99–101.
106. Canto MIF, Setrakian S, Petras RE, Blades E, Chak A, Sivak MV Jr. Methylene blue selectively stains intestinal metaplasia in Barrett's esophagus. Gastrointest Endosc 1996; 44:1–7.
107. Stevens PD, Lightdale CJ, Green PHR, Siegel LM, Garcia-Carrasquillo RJ, Rotterdam H. Combined magnification endoscopy with chromoendoscopy for the evaluation of Barrett's esophagus. Gastrointest Endosc 1994; 40:747–749.
108. Falk GW, Catalano MF, Sivak MV Jr, Rice TW, Van Dam J. Endosonography in the evaluation of patients with Barrett's esophagus and high-grade dysplasia. Gastrointest Endosc 1994; 40:297–312.
109. Kobayashi K, Izatt JA, Kulkarni MD, Willis J, Sivak MV Jr. High-resolution cross-sectional imaging of the gastrointestinal tract using optical coherence tomography: preliminary results. Gastrointest Endosc 1998; 47:515–523.
110. Stepp H, Stroka R, Baumgartner R. Fluorescence endoscopy of gastrointestinal diseases: basic principles, techniques, and clinical experience. Endoscopy 1998; 30:379–386.
111. Panjehpour M, Overholt BF, Vo-Dinh T, Haggitt RC, Edwards DH, Buckley FP III. Endoscopic fluorescence detection of high-grade dysplasia in Barrett's esophagus. Gastroenterology 1996; 111:93–101.
112. Haringsma J, Tytgat GNJ. The value of fluorescence techniques in gastrointestinal endoscopy: better than the endoscopist's eye? I: The European experience. Endoscopy 1998; 30:416–418.
113. Marcon NE, Wilson BC. The value of fluorescence techniques in gastrointestinal endoscopy: better than the endoscopist's eye? II: The North American experience. Endoscopy 1998; 30:419–421.
114. Neumann CS, Iqbal TH, Cooper BT. Long term continuous omeprazole treatment of patients with Barrett's oesophagus. Aliment Pharmacol Ther 1995; 9:451–454.
115. Spechler SJ. Comparison of medical and surgical therapy for complicated gastro-

esophageal reflux disease in veterans. Department of Veterans Affairs Gastroesophageal Reflux Disease Study Group. N Engl J Med 1992; 326:786–792.

116. DeVault KR, Castell DO, and The Practice Parameters Committee of the American College of Gastroenterology. Updated guidelines for the diagnosis and treatment of gastroesophageal reflux disease. Am J Gastroenterol 1999; 94:1434–1442.
117. Marks RD, Richter JE, Rizzo H, Koehler RE, Spenney JG, Mills TP, Champion G. Omeprazole versus H2-receptor antagonists in treating patients with peptic stricture and esophagitis. Gastroenterology 1994; 106:907–915.
118. Smith PM, Kerr GD, Cockel R, Ross BA, Bate CM, Brown P, Dronfield MW, Green JRB, Hislop WS, Theodossi A, McFarland J, Watts DA, Taylor MD, Richardson PDI, and the Restore Investigator Group. A comparison of omeprazole and ranitidine in the prevention of recurrence of benign esophageal stricture. Gastroenterology 1994; 107:1312–1318.
119. Howden CW, Castell DO, Cohen S, Freston JW, Orlando RC, Robinson M. The rationale for continuous maintenance treatment of reflux esophagitis. Arch Intern Med 1995; 155:1465–1471.
120. Spechler SJ. Laser photoablation of Barrett's epithelium: burning issues about burning tissues. Gastroenterology 1993; 104:1855–1858.
121. Sampliner RE. New treatments for Barrett's esophagus. Semin Gastrointest Dis 1997; 8:68–74.
122. Sharma P, Morales TG, Bhattacharyya A, Garewal HS, Sampliner RE. Squamous islands in Barrett's esophagus: what lies underneath? Am J Gastroenterol 1998; 93:332–335.
123. Fitzgerald RC, Omary MB, Triadafilopoulos G. Dynamic effects of acid on Barrett's esophagus. An ex vivo proliferation and differentiation model. J Clin Invest 1996; 98:2120–2128.
124. Peghini PL, Katz PO, Bracy NA, Castell DO. Nocturnal recovery of gastric acid secretion with twice-daily dosing of proton pump inhibitors. Am J Gastroenterol 1998; 93:763–767.
125. Katz PO, Anderson C, Khoury R, Castell DO. Gastro-oesophageal reflux associated with nocturnal gastric acid breakthrough on proton pump inhibitors. Aliment Pharmacol Ther 1998; 12:1231–1234.
126. Katzka DA, Castell DO. Successful elimination of reflux symptoms does not insure adequate control of acid reflux in patients with Barrett's esophagus. Am J Gastroenterol 1994; 89:989–991.
127. Ouatu-Lascar R, Triadafilopoulos G. Complete elimination of reflux symptoms does not guarantee normalization of intraesophageal acid reflux in patients with Barrett's esophagus. Am J Gastroenterol 1998; 93:711–716.
128. Peghini PL, Katz PO, Castell DO. Ranitidine controls nocturnal gastric acid breakthrough on omeprazole: a controlled study in normal subjects. Gastroenterology 1998; 115:1335–1339.
129. Castell DO, Richter JE, Robinson M, Sontag SJ, Haber MM, and the Lansoprazole Group. Efficacy and safety of lansoprazole in the treatment of erosive reflux esophagitis. Am J Gastroenterol 1996; 91:1749–1757.
130. Ireland AP, Peters JH, Smyrk TC, DeMeester TR, Clark GWB, Mirvish SS, Adrian TE. Gastric juice protects against the development of esophageal adenocarcinoma in the rat. Ann Surg 1996; 224:358–371.

131. Streitz JM Jr, Andrews CW Jr, Ellis FH Jr. Endoscopic surveillance of Barrett's esophagus. Does it help? J Thorac Cardiovasc Surg 1993; 105:383–388.
132. Streitz JM Jr, Ellis FH, Tilden RL, Erickson RV. Endoscopic surveillance of Barrett's esophagus: a cost-effectiveness comparison with mammographic surveillance for breast cancer. Am J Gastroenterol 1998; 93:911–915.
133. Provenzale D, Kemp JA, Arora S, Wong JB. A guide for surveillance of patients with Barrett's esophagus. Am J Gastroenterol 1994; 89:670–680.
134. Levine DS. Management of dysplasia in the columnar-lined esophagus. Gastroenterol Clin North Am 1997; 26:613–634.
135. Spechler SJ. Barrett's esophagus. Semin Gastrointest Dis 1996; 7:51–60.
136. Van den Boogert J, van Hillegersberg R, Siersema PD, de Bruin RW, Tilanus HW. Endoscopic ablation therapy for Barrett's esophagus with high-grade dysplasia: a review. Am J Gastroenterol 1999; 94:1153–1160.
137. Sampliner RE. Ablative therapies for the columnar-lined esophagus. Gastroenterol Clin North Am 1997; 26:685–694.
138. Nishioka NS. Drug, light, and oxygen: a dynamic combination in the clinic. Gastroenterology 1998; 114:604–606.
139. Overholt BF, Panjehpour M. Barrett's esophagus: photodynamic therapy for ablation of dysplasia, reduction of specialized mucosa, and treatment of superficial esophageal cancer. Gastrointest Endosc 1995; 42:64–70.
140. Laukka MA, Wang KK. Initial results using low-dose photodynamic therapy in the treatment of Barrett's esophagus. Gastrointest Endosc 1995; 42:59–63.
141. Overholt BF, Panjehpour M. Photodynamic therapy for Barrett's esophagus: clinical update. Am J Gastroenterol 1996; 91:1719–1723.
142. Barr H, Shepherd NA, Dix A, Roberts DJH, Tan WC, Krasner N. Eradication of high-grade dysplasia in columnar-lined (Barrett's) oesophagus by photodynamic therapy with endogenously generated protoporphyrin IX. Lancet 1996; 348:584–585.
143. Gossner L, Stolte M, Sroka R, Rick K, May A, Hahn EG, Ell C. Photodynamic ablation of high-grade dysplasia and early cancer in Barrett's esophagus by means of 5-aminolevulinic acid. Gastroenterology 1998; 114:448–455.
144. Overholt BF, Panjehpour M, Haydek JM. Photodynamic therapy for Barrett's esophagus: follow-up in 100 patients. Gastrointest Endosc 1999; 49:1–7.
145. Guanrei Y, Songliang Q, Guizen F. Natural history of early esophageal squamous carcinoma and early adenocarcinoma of the gastric cardia in the People's Republic of China. Endoscopy 1988; 20:95–98.
146. Brandt LJ, Kauvar DR. Laser-induced transient regression of Barrett's epithelium. Gastrointest Endosc 1992; 38:619–622.
147. Sampliner RE and the Practice Parameters Committee of the American College of Gastroenterology. Practice guidelines on the diagnosis, surveillance, and therapy of Barrett's esophagus. Am J Gastroenterol 1998; 93:1028–1032.

9

Extraesophageal Complications of Gastroesophageal Reflux Disease

Epidemiology, Natural History, Pathogenesis, Diagnosis, and Management

Walter J. Hogan and Reza Shaker
Medical College of Wisconsin, Milwaukee, Wisconsin

INTRODUCTION

Supraesophageal structures are not immune to the ravages of reflux disease (GERD). The role of gastroesophageal reflux in many disorders affecting contiguous anatomy positioned above the esophagus is gradually emerging from evidence obtained through clinical research and therapeutic trials.

The spectrum of supraesophageal complications of GERD has expanded in recent years and now encompasses a myriad of reported problems (Table 1). Unfortunately, a direct relationship between gastric reflux events and the majority of these suspected supraesophageal complications has been difficult to establish to date. This dilemma is further complicated by two compounding problems: patients with suspected supraesophageal complications of GERD frequently lack the characteristic features of heartburn symptoms and esophageal inflammation and the patient may have both disorders independent of each other!

Nonetheless, it is important that the clinician become aware of the possibility of GERD-associated complications and the significance of diagnosis (albeit presumptive) and subsequent treatment.

Table 1 Suspected Supraesophageal Complications of GERD

Oral cavity	Airway
Mouth ulcers/burning	Larynx/trachea
Abnormal taste	Chronic laryngitis
Halitosis	Vocal cord ulcers, granulomas, nodules
Teeth erosions	Laryngeal, subglottic stenosis
Nasal/auditory	Croup
Chronic sinusitis	Laryngospasm
Otalgia	Malignancy
Otitis	Lungs
Pharynx	Chronic cough
Pharyngitis	Asthma
Postnasal drip (throat clearing)	Aspiration pneumonia
Globus sensation	Pulmonary fibrosis
	Bronchiectasis
	Sleep apnea
Other	
SIDS	
Sandifer's Sx (torticollis)	

EPIDEMIOLOGY

GERD is one of the most common gastrointestinal disorders; U.S. population surveys, for example, suggest that up to 50% of adults, or 60 million people, have symptoms of heartburn at least once a month (1). More than one-fourth of adult Americans use antacids 3 times or more per month (2). Although nearly half of the U.S. population experiences occasional heartburn, only 4–7% complain of daily symptoms (3). This group of patients most likely represents true GERD. Interestingly, the true incidence of GERD may be underestimated because of the relatively low proportion of individuals who seek medical attention for reflux symptoms. One report found that only 5% of patients with symptoms of heartburn and regurgitation within the preceding year had visited a physician because of this problem (4).

SUPRAESOPHAGEAL COMPLICATIONS OF GERD

The majority of reports evaluating the supraesophageal complications of GERD concern its association with asthma. The prevalence of GERD among patients with asthma is frequent but this varies depending upon the study population and methods of diagnosis. Many relatively uncontrolled studies consistently report an association of symptomatic reflux in 30–90% of adults with asthma. One prospective study determined that 75% of patients with asthma have either increased frequency of reflux episodes or pathological GERD, whether or not they use bronchodilators (5). More recently, a case-control study addressing the association between asthma and acid reflux in a large population group with erosive esophagitis or stricture identified a number of disorders significantly related to esophagitis; the strongest of these was bronchial asthma (6).

SUPRAGLOTTIC DISORDERS

In a report that documented GERD by esophagogram, Esophagogastroduodenoscopy (EGD), or 24-h pH testing, refractory hoarseness was reported in 80% of patients, globus sensation in 50% of patients, and a smaller group of patients with cancer of the larynx (7). In another supporting study of a larger group of patients with laryngological disorders and suspected GERD, 24-h esophageal pH monitoring demonstrated a high percentage of acid reflux in patients with laryngeal stenosis (78%), laryngeal cancer (71%), reflux laryngitis (60%), and globus sensation (58%). Chronic cough was noted in 52% of these patients (8). Finally, a strong relationship between esophagitis and laryngeal disorders was also noted in the case-control study previously cited (6).

Abnormal acid reflux on pH testing does not assure resolution of the patient's symptoms or inflammatory process following medical or surgical treatment. Most authorities, however, feel that an abundance of epidemiological data now suggests that acid reflux represents an important risk factor for the development of supraglottic disorders.

PATHOGENESIS OF SUPRAESOPHAGEAL/GERD DISORDERS

Two different mechanisms for acid-induced supraesophageal complications have been postulated: (a) an acid-reflux-induced vagal reflex arc from the body of esophagus to the bronchopulmonary system resulting in bronchial constriction or cough (9), and (b) microaspiration of gastroesophageal reflux contents into the supraesophageal structures and bronchopulmonary system resulting in an inflammatory reaction and/or a localized reactive contractile response (10). Dual-electrode ambulatory pH monitoring studies have supported the reflex therapy. In one report, abnormal distal esophageal acid exposure was prevalent in patients with symptoms of chronic cough (50%), asthma (44%), and unexplained chest pain (54%) (11). In another report, nine of 11 asthmatic patients (82%) with demonstrable acid reflux had a good to excellent pulmonary symptom response to antireflux therapy (12). A decrease in peak expiratory flow rate (PEFR) with an increase in airway resistance was reported during intraesophageal acid perfusion in asthmatic patients with GERD (13). The mechanism was thought to be due exclusively to vagal-mediated reflex pathways rather than acid micropenetration of the airway. However, in another study of respiratory tract dynamics of 12 asthma patients with GERD utilizing forced oscillations and spirometry, no change in respiratory impedance measurement was demonstrated during intraesophageal acid perfusion. This report only points out the fact that proof-positive evidence of aerodigestive complications of GERD is controversial and often lacking (14).

The role of gastroesophageal reflux in patients with eustachian tube abnormalities, chronic sinusitis, dental erosions, and buccal ulceration is not clear. Vagal reflex mechanism interaction with these target areas seems less likely than actual acid contact arising from the esophagus below.

Regurgitation presents the opportunity for refluxed gastric contents to damage structures above the esophagus. This often is associated with chronic pulmonary fibrosis. Certainly in the situation of dental erosions, regurgitation of gastric contents appears to be the most likely cause. Detection of microaspiration is not easy to recognize or document. As an example, studies reporting 24-h pH monitoring of the esophagus and the oral cavity in a group of 14 patients with demonstrable teeth erosions demonstrated no alteration in the oral pH recording probe despite 339 esophageal acid reflux episodes (15), despite the fact that the patients were often in a prolonged supine position. On the other hand, 117 patients with GERD were evaluated for oral lesions. On both 24-h pH recording and endoscopy, 28 of these patients with the most severe reflux episodes demonstrated oral lesions (16). Another smaller group of patients with dental erosions showed significant increase in proximal (20 cm above the lower-esophageal sphincter) esophageal acid reflux (17).

Approximately 75% of asthmatics have reflux symptoms, while 80% have abnormal acid reflux (measured by pH). Sixty percent of patients have hiatal hernias, while 40% have esophageal mucosa damage from acid reflux. Although these data show that GERD is highly prevalent in asthmatics, it does not confirm GERD as a cause of asthma or asthma a cause of GERD (18).

The same controversy surrounds the laryngeal manifestations of GERD. There is a lack of consistent objective measurement of refluxate into the laryngopharynx despite a number of studies using triple-lumen pH probes to identify significant reflux episodes affecting the laryngopharynx. Part of this may be explained by the lack of sensitivity of current methodology to detect minimal acid reflux episodes or the possibility that some of the laryngopharyngeal manifestations may be due to nonacidic gastric reflux.

Recently, a technique of simultaneous placement of pH probes within the trachea and the esophagus has been performed on a small group of asthmatics (19). Four of the patients had concurrent GERD, while three other patients did not. Interestingly, five of 37 episodes of gastroesophageal reflux lasting greater than 5 min were followed by microaspiration, a decrease in the tracheal pH from 7.1 to 4.1, and a concomitant decrease in peak expiratory flow rate from 84 L/min to 8 L/min. Unfortunately, general anesthesia was required for the placement of the probes, but obviously this type of sophisticated study is necessary and larger groups of patients need to be studied before we can define the role of acid reflux in suspected supraesophageal complications of GERD. Because there are no reliable tests at present that can accurately predict which patients have GERD-related supraesophageal complications, controlled therapeutic trials may be the only method currently available that could definitively answer this question.

NATURAL HISTORY: PROTECTIVE MECHANISMS DURING SUPRAESOPHAGEAL GERD

The functional relationship between the upper airway and the gastrointestinal tract during retrograde gastrointestinal transit such as regurgitation, belching, and gastroesophageal reflux has only recently received extensive investigation.

Protective mechanisms against retrograde esophageal transit can be divided into two subgroups: (1) basal mechanisms, i.e., the lower-esophageal sphincter (LES) and the upper-esophageal sphincter (UES), with the latter maintaining a pressure gradient without a need for constant stimulation (although various stimuli may affect its function); (2) response mechanisms located primarily within the oral pharynx, which are not constantly active but can become activated upon stimulation. This stimulation is usually distension of the esophagus and/or mechanical stimulation of the pharynx. This group of response mechanisms includes secondary esophageal peristalsis (described earlier), and a number of proximal reflexes, e.g., the esophago-upper-esophageal-sphincter contractile reflex, the esophagoglottal closure reflex, and the pharyngeal (secondary) swallow.

The number of reflux episodes that reach the proximal esophagus is 25–75% of those that enter the distal esophagus in healthy as well as esophagitis patients following mealtime (20). Despite this phenomenon, very few people experience supraesophageal complications of GERD. As mentioned previously, no epidemiological studies are available on the prevalence of reflux-induced airway or aerodigestive-tract complications in esophagitis patients or the population at large. Clinical experience, however, suggests that the prevalence of these complications is relatively low compared to complications of the esophageal body as a result of GERD. This suggests an existence of potent airway defense mechanisms against esophagopharyngeal and pharyngolaryngeal reflux of gastric contents.

Basal mechanisms of lower-esophageal sphincter (LES) and UES dynamics have already been discussed along with the mechanism of secondary esophageal peristalsis. This section will be devoted to the discussion of the supraesophageal response mechanisms against gastric reflux that have been defined in the human to date.

The Esophago-UES Contractile Reflex

A number of reflexes control the function of the UES. Distension by a swallowed bolus or slow balloon inflation of the esophagus causes an increase in UES pressure and electromyographic activity of the cricopharyngeal muscle mediated by vagal afferent fibers. The proximal portion of the esophagus appears to be more sensitive than the distal portion (21). The receptors mediating this reflex may be slow-adapting mechanoreceptors of the muscular wall (22). Although, some investigators have found that slow acid infusion into the esophagus increases UES tone (23), these results have not been corroborated by more recent investigations (24). In addition, the intraluminal esophageal pH has not been found to correlate with UES tone (25).

The Esophagoglottal Closure Reflex

Gastroesophageal reflux may cause abrupt distension of the esophagus producing a circumstance favorable to esophagopharyngeal regurgitation and laryngeal aspiration of gastric contents. This is particularly true for large-volume gastroesophageal reflux episodes. Vocal cords close the opening to the trachea in response to abrupt esophageal distension (26). This reflex is postulated to be caused by stretch receptors within the body of the esophagus transmitting the impulses to the vagus nerve and to the brainstem. Vagal efferent motor fibers that traverse the recurrent laryngeal nerve and stimulate the adductor muscles of the glottis could cause this rapid closure of the vocal cords. Bilateral cervical vagotomy in the cat model abolishes this reflex (27) (Fig. 1). Reflex innervation between the digestive tract and respiratory tract has been demonstrated in the past; the esophagoglottic reflex is an example of close coordination between the two systems and during retrograde reflux of gastrointestinal contents. This reflex is postulated to be one of the airway protective mechanisms humans have against GERD. Recent studies have documented that this reflux is evoked during spontaneous gastroesophageal reflux episodes (28). Furthermore, this reflex appears to be absent or markedly decreased in about half of elderly patients greater than 70 years of age. The function of this reflex in experimental esophagitis in the cat showed that inflammation either completely abolished this reflex or caused a significant reduction in frequency of activation of this reflex (29).

Injection of water into the pharynx of humans can trigger a swallowing reflex (pharyngeal swallow). Initiation of a ''swallow'' at this site may play a

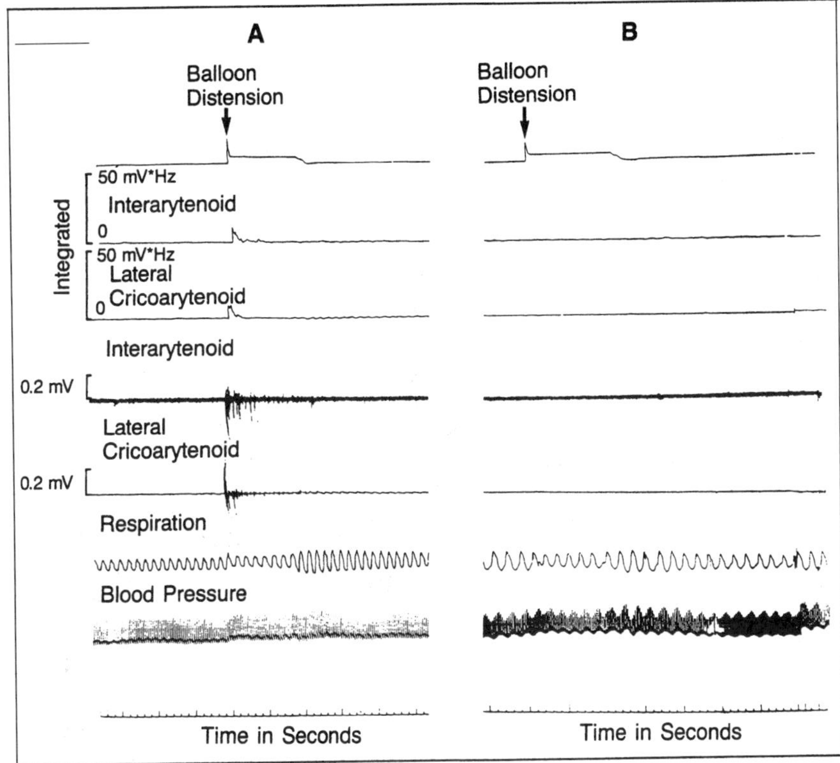

Figure 1 Example of electromyographic (EMG) recording from interarytenoid and lateral cricoarytenoid muscles during a 2.5-cm middle esophageal balloon distension before (A) and after (B) bilateral cervical vagotomy. As seen, EMG activities induced by balloon distension are completely abolished after bilateral cervical vagotomy. (From Am J Physiol 1994; 266:G147–G153.)

role in airway protection from pharyngeal reflux of gastric contents (30). Recent studies have further characterized this pharyngeal swallow and determined the threshold of volume of a liquid required to trigger this swallowing reflex in the young and elderly volunteers (31). These pharyngeal swallows triggered by direct stimulation are different from volitional or primary swallows in that they do not induce sequential contraction of the proximal tongue with the hard palate. In this regard, the pharyngeal swallow has been compared to a secondary esophageal peristalsis that bypasses the activation of the peristaltic wave from areas proximal to the point of stimulation (32). It is speculated that the pharyngeal swallow prevents aspiration by activating glottal closure, which seals off the airway and prevents aspiration during gastroesophageal reflux episodes, and that it clears the pharynx of materials that enter it during reflux episodes from the esophagus.

Water stimulation of the pharynx in humans also results in an increase in resting tone in the UES, i.e., the pharyngo-UES contractile reflex (33). It is speculated that this reflex functions as an airway protective mechanism by augmenting

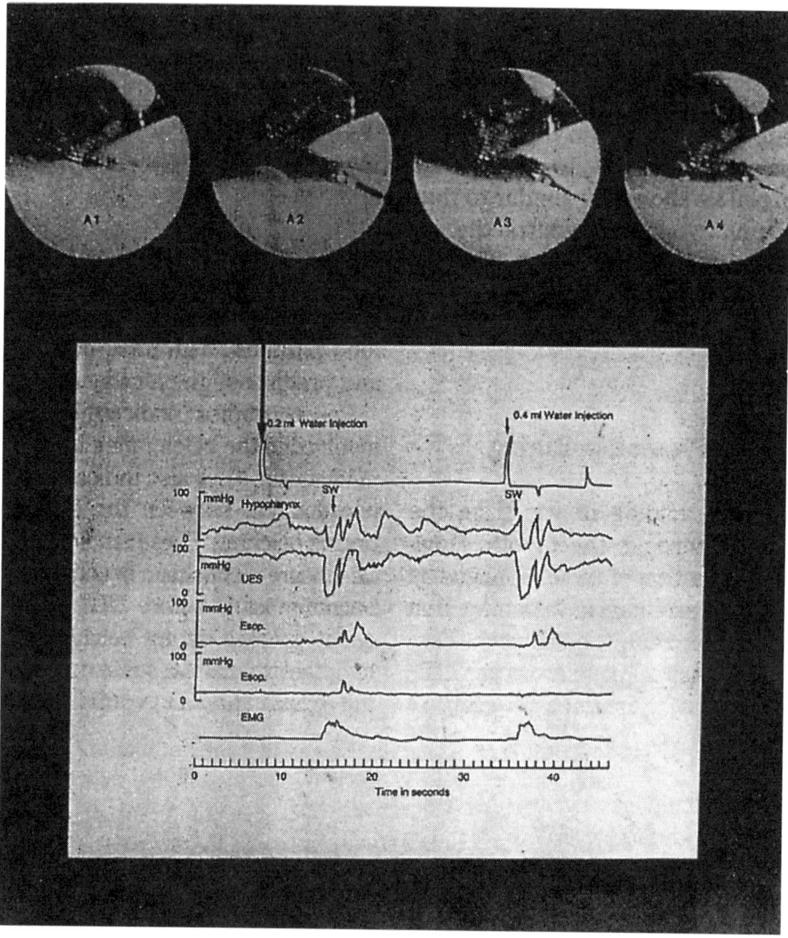

Figure 2 Example of glottal closure response to rapid pharyngeal water injection. Injection of minute amounts of 0.2 mL water into the pharynx directed posteriorly results in an abrupt closure of the vocal cords that lasts about 0.7 s. A spontaneous swallow occurs 10 s following water injection. Injection of 0.4 mL of water 15 s later results in an irrepressible (pharyngeal) swallow. (From Dysphagia 1995; 10:216–227.)

UES tone following the entry of small volumes of liquid into the pharynx, which may reduce the chance of further esophagopharyngeal reflux. Finally, when minute amounts of water are injected into the back of the pharynx, there is brief closure of the vocal cords. It is postulated that this adduction response is part of a complex protective mechanism and the threshold volume for this reflex is significantly smaller than that required to trigger an ''irrepressible'' pharyngeal swallow. The pharyngoglottal adduction reflex requires much larger volumes of liquid in the elderly to trigger this reflex (33). Figure 2 is an example of glottic closure response to rapid pharyngeal water injection.

In patients undergoing a 24-h ambulatory pH study, it is often noted that reflux events occur at the time that the patient activates the ''belch'' button on the microcomputer apparatus. Ventilation of gastric and/or esophageal gas across the UES into the pharynx may be accompanied by the entry of food particles or acid ''mist'' and predispose the airway to aspiration. Basically, investigations have indicated that the glottis is actively involved in the belch reflex by activation of its closure mechanism (34). This close relationship between the UES and glottic function during belching is demonstrated by the fact that the glottal closure mechanism is activated and the vocal cords become closed prior to UES relaxation and subsequent effacement during belching (Fig. 3). The same coordination may exist during regurgitation of material drawn into the pharynx by the venting of gastric or esophageal material.

Airway protective mechanisms have now been demonstrated and they appear to protect against antegrade aspiration. The protective mechanisms are multifactorial and involve complex interactions between the aerodigestive system. Although these mechanisms have been demonstrated in normal volunteers, for the most part, it remains to be demonstrated whether their dysfunction with suspected supraesophageal complications is a partial or major mechanism that allows gastric contents to damage structures above the esophagus proper.

DIAGNOSIS OF SUPRAESOPHAGEAL GERD

A detailed history may be very important in obtaining clues to the association of GERD and suspected supraesophageal complications. The occurrence of classic heartburn symptoms can be a significant help, but these complaints should be appropriately defined by the patient to the physician's satisfaction. The physician should not accept the complaint of ''heartburn'' without detailing the specific location and description of these symptoms. A history of regurgitation particularly at nighttime associated with cough or with symptoms suggesting aspiration is a significant clue to the possibility of supraesophageal complications of GERD. Unfortunately, this symptom complex occurs in a minority of patients. The onset of asthma in the adult particularly with nocturnal cough or wheezing or precipita-

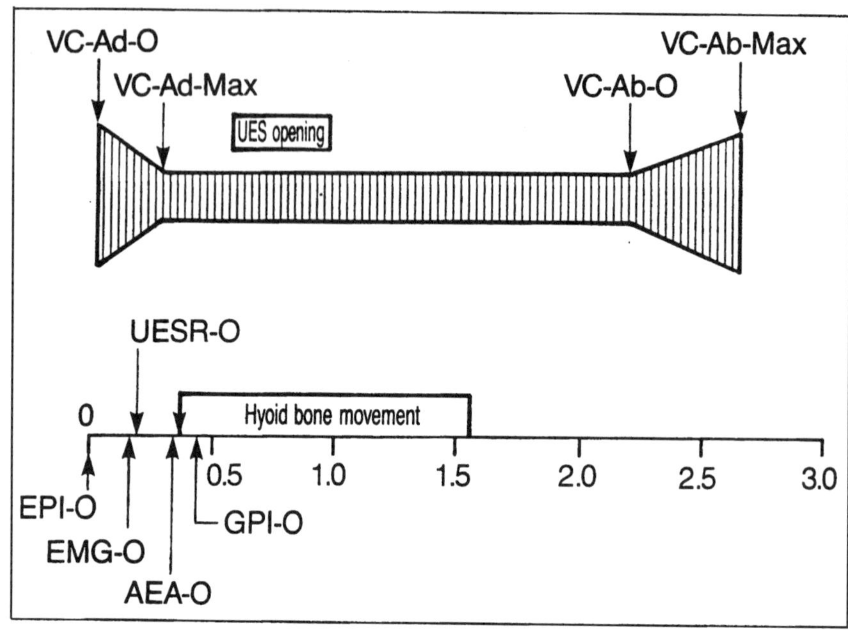

Figure 3 Temporal relationship between function of the glottis, UES, and hyoid bone and pressure phenomena of the esophagus and stomach during belching induced by intraesophageal injection of 40 mL of room air. The figure is constructed using videoendoscopic, videofluoroscopic, manometric, and electromyographic (EMG) data obtained concurrently. The belch event begins with vocal cord adduction and ends with their return to resting position. All other events, including UES opening and closure, occur while cords are fully adducted, and thereby the introitus to the trachea is closed. Fluoroscopic UES opening begins 0.35 ± 0.08 s after onset of hyoid bone movement. VC-Ad-0 = onset of vocal cord adduction; VC-Ad-Max = maximum onset of vocal cord adduction; VC-Ab-0 = onset of vocal cords opening; VC-Ab-Max = return of vocal cords to resting position; EPI-0 = onset of increase in intraesophageal pressure; AEA-0 = onset of approximation of arytenoids toward base of the epiglottis; GPI-0 = onset of increase in intragastric pressure; EMG-0 = onset of EMG signal recorded from geniohyoid, mylohyoid muscle groups; UESR-0 = onset of UES relaxation recorded manometrically. (From Am J Physiol 1992; 262:G621–G628.)

tion of bronchospasm following a large meal can be a clue suggesting the role of GERD in the patient's symptoms. In one study of a large number of patients with suspected ear, nose, and throat complications of GERD, only 43% of patients had classic symptoms of heartburn, regurgitation, or dysphagia (8). Approximately 20% of patients with chronic cough of unknown etiology will have GERD as a prime suspect (35). A history of constant throat clearing, recurrent laryngitis (particularly in the morning), halitosis, or hypersaliarrhea should alert the clinician to the possibility of supraesophageal-related acid reflux condition. Unfortunately, history alone is often unable to elicit clues suggesting acid reflux as a cause of suspected supraesophageal complications. In fact, one-third of patients with suspected bronchopulmonary manifestations of GERD have no esophageal symptoms whatsoever.

There are some clinical signs that may suggest the occurrence of acid reflux above the esophagus. The unique neck posture in Sandifer's syndrome is a clue to acid reflux disease in the infant or young child. This posture is an anatomical defense mechanism against repetitive acid reflux. The finding of idiopathic pulmonary fibrosis or recurrent noninfectious pulmonary infiltrates may be a signal to an acid reflux etiology. The presence of subglottic stenosis has been demonstrated to have a significant association with pharyngeal acid exposure (36). Recurrent mouth ulcers may be related to acid reflux disease particularly when the patient has an associated ''burning'' in the mouth, while a smooth, glazed, dished-out appearance of the dentin on the lingual surfaces of the teeth may be a clue to acid reflux as a cause of these dental erosions (37).

DIAGNOSTIC PROCEDURES THAT MAY SUPPORT THE ROLE OF GERD

Ambulatory Esophageal pH Study

Ambulatory esophageal pH monitoring is currently considered to be the best diagnostic tool available for diagnosing supraesophageal complications of GERD. This technique (described in another chapter) affords the best opportunity to document the proximal extent of acid reflux within the esophagus or the oropharynx. However, a number of controversial issues associated with this test have yet to be adequately defined, i.e., the reproducibility of the pH recording and the accuracy of ambulatory esophageal pH testing in detecting reflux events, per se. Despite these valid objections, esophageal pH monitoring is considered the ''gold standard'' by many investigators who attempt to validate the association of esophageal acid reflux with suspected supraesophageal complications.

Dual pH esophageal monitoring has become the technique of choice and is frequently used as an initial diagnostic tool by many investigators (38). The distal pH probe is located 5 cm above the LES by tradition; the proximal pH probe is usually placed 20 cm above the LES and just below the UES. A third and separate pH probe can be placed in the pharynx to record changes associated with acid escape into the pharynx (39). This latter technique has helped discriminate between healthy volunteers, GERD patients, and those with GE-reflux-related posterior laryngitis. The use of the three-site pH system enables the physi-

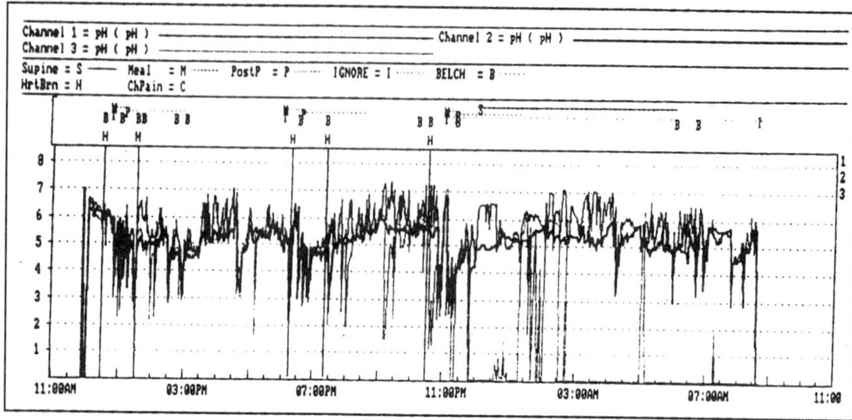

Figure 4 Three-site pH recording (two probes in esophagus; one probe in hypopharynx) of GERD events over a 24-h period in patient TD. Explanations for letters are noted at the top. A total of 10 pharyngeal acid events were recorded during this period.

cian to determine whether the pH changes recorded proximally are temporally associated with distal acid reflux events. Some concern about recording pH in the hypopharynx has been raised because of the existence of upper-airway mucus and possible entrapment of the pH probe and the relatively capacious region of the oropharynx that could conceivably influence pH recording (40). However, when a decrease in hypopharyngeal pH is considered abnormal only when it correlates with a simultaneous acid reflux event in the distal esophagus below, these concerns about pH recording artifact are minimized.

Although a recent study has shown reproducibility of reflux parameters in the distal esophagus of a small group of GERD patients (9 of 11; 82%), variability in the proximal esophagus was pointed out (41). Only six of 11 patients (55%) had pH values reproduced in the proximal zone of the esophagus. However, another recent report utilizing multiple esophageal pH probes demonstrated a linear decrease in the number of reflux events with increasing distance above the LES zone (42). Based upon the information from this study and an extensive literature review, it is estimated that the normal range of total acid exposure when the pH probe is positioned beneath the UES is approximately 0–1% over 24 h (40). However, a significantly higher percentage of distal reflux episodes reached the proximal esophagus in a group of laryngitis patients compared to control groups and the number of pharyngeal reflux episodes and time of acid exposure were also significantly higher in the pharyngitis group (39). The extent and duration of hypopharyngeal acid reflux events during a 24-h ambulatory pH recording is shown in Figure 4.

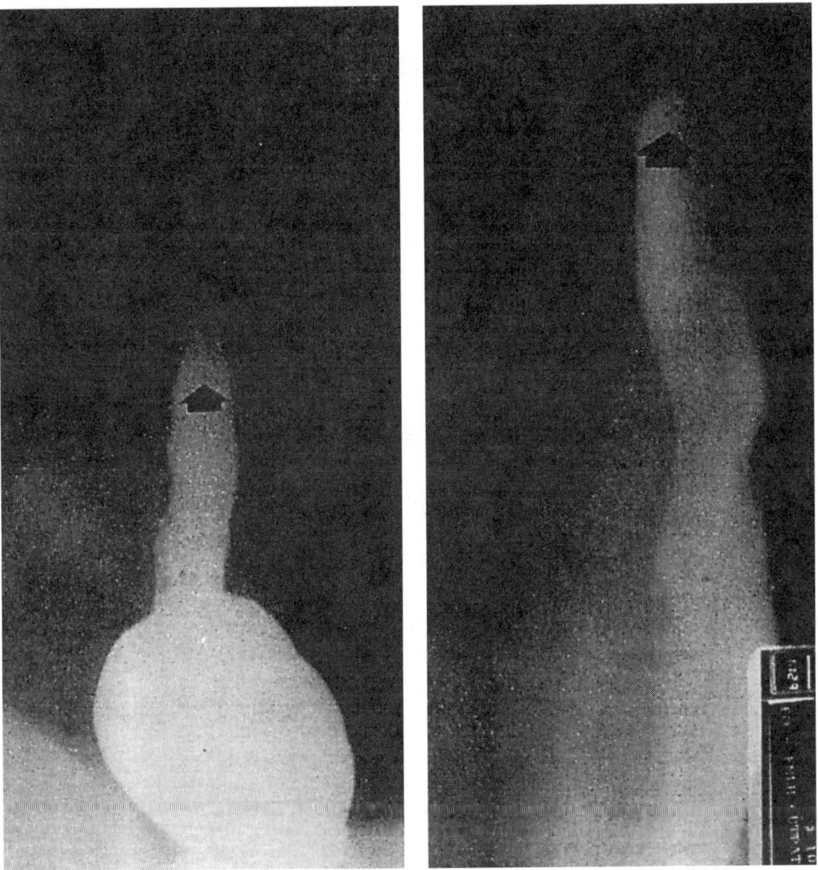

Figure 5 Spontaneous barium reflux to the level of the aortic arch is demonstrated in this esophagogram on patient SG. The patient exhibited this finding on several occasions during the study.

Acid reflux values for the distal esophageal pH probe vary from laboratory to laboratory. The most meaningful computed values are those indicating the total time of esophageal exposure (pH less than 4.0) and a differentiation of total acid exposure in the upright versus the supine position. In a study performed in our laboratory (43) in a group of patients and control subjects who underwent four separate pH studies during a 24-h monitoring period, several interesting findings were determined. The quantitative pH values provided suboptimal discrimination between the two groups! The majority of reflux events and total acid exposure occur when subjects are upright rather than supine. Finally, a "standard-

Table 2 24-Hour Ambulatory pH Monitoring: Controls Versus Patients, Acid Reflux Values for Distal Probe (Mean ± SD) (Comparison of Two Diets)

Group	Subject (*n*)	Standard diet (% pH < 4.0)			Ad-lib diet (% pH < 4.0)		
		24 h	Upright	Supine	24 h	Upright	Supine
Controls	14	6 ± 5	7 ± 6	5 ± 7	7 ± 8	8 ± 8	7 ± 12
Patients	12	13 ± 5	16 ± 7	9 ± 11	14 ± 6	16 ± 8	9 ± 9

Source: Ref. 43.

ized diet'' does not increase test discrimination or reproducibility (43). These values for 24-h pH monitoring for our laboratory are shown in Table 2.

Gastroesophageal reflux has been estimated to occur in 75% of asthmatics (5). In the more recent study using dual-electrode ambulatory pH monitoring, distal acid exposure was prevalent in patients with chronic cough (50%), asthma (44%), and unexplained chest pain (54%). In addition, prevalence of abnormal proximal esophageal acid exposure was significantly higher in chest pain patients without pulmonary complaints (44%) than in patients with either asthma (24%) or chronic cough (11%) (44).

In patients with unexplained chronic cough, devoid of other symptoms, the initial study of choice to assess the possibility of acid reflux is the 24-h ambulatory pH study (45). In one report, the ambulatory intraluminal esophageal pH was the only method used to diagnose GERD in approximately 32% of patients with chronic unexplained cough (46). In another report, esophageal pH monitoring had a positive predictive value of 89–100% and a negative predictive value of 100% in diagnosing GERD as a cause of chronic cough (47). The necessity for the use of ambulatory pH studies in patients with chronic unexplained cough is reinforced by the fact that between 50 and 75% of patients with this problem have no discernible reflux symptoms whatsoever (48).

Despite the many glowing reports concerning the use of the 24-h ambulatory pH test, in patients with suspected gastroesophageal reflux complications, it is an exaggeration to call this procedure the ''gold standard.'' Although the 24-h esophageal pH test is the best current diagnostic tool available to implicate GERD and its possible role in supraesophageal disorders, the sensitivity and specificity of this test is open to challenge (43).

Upper Gastrointestinal Endoscopic Examination

Demonstrating signs of esophageal inflammation at endoscopic examination does not per se incriminate GERD as the possible etiology in a supraesophageal disorder. However, it does help build a possible scenario for the role of acid reflux and alerts the clinician to a possible explanation for the patient's problems. Unfortunately, the presence of esophagitis detected at endoscopic examination is not a constant finding in patients with suspected supraesophageal complications of GERD. In one report based on a comprehensive literature review, there was only a 40% incidence of esophageal mucosal damage from acid reflux in asthmatic patients (18). In another report by the same group, in a consecutive series of asthmatics, esophageal erosions or ulcerations were found at endoscopy in only 39% of asthmatics while 13% had Barrett's esophagus (49). Noteworthy was the fact that the authors eliminated from this study any patients who were referred for workup because of gastrointestinal symptoms or who were not part of a consecutive asthmatic protocol. A recent study of U.S. military veterans evaluated the significance of esophagitis associated with various pulmonary and laryngeal problems (6). The highest odds ratio of GERD with pulmonary disorders was bronchial asthma (OR 1.51) and pulmonary fibrosis (OR 1.36). The association between esophagitis and laryngitis was also significant (OR 2.10) as was the association with laryngeal stenosis (OR 2.02). Although the absence of physical damage to the esophagus in the majority of patients with suspected supraesophageal complications of GERD appears at first glance to be an apparent paradox, nonetheless, most investigators in this field have come to accept this fact. It is worthwhile to point out one other compounding feature; often patients with suspected supraesophageal complications of GERD have been treated with antacids at doses acceptable for healing esophagitis but inadequate for treating the suspected supraesophageal complications. In these situations, a macroscopic inflammation of the esophageal lining may have disappeared completely. The presence of subtle distal esophageal scars and pitting above the GE junction are hallmarks of gastroesophageal reflux. Obviously, the presence of Barrett's columnar lining with or without associated esophageal inflammation indicates the presence of acid reflux disease.

Radiological Examination of the Esophagus

A demonstration of a structural abnormality on a barium contrast esophagram may supply useful clues to the presence of GERD, e.g., the presence of hiatal hernia or distal esophageal lumen compromise. The former finding may be a clue; the latter is evidence of damage secondary to GERD. Although reflux of gastric barium into the esophagus during fluoroscopy is not specific for diagnosing a "reflux" condition, spontaneous, frequent barium reflux to the aortic arch correlates well in our experience with patients who have massive "acid reflux." We believe that this is a valuable clue for the association of GERD with supraesophageal complications (Fig. 5).

In one report of 28 patients with severe asthma (50), 64% of the patients had a hiatal hernia while 46% had reflux of barium demonstrated during fluoroscopy. In another report, 11 of 15 asthmatic patients had an abnormal barium X-ray suggesting a prevalence rate of 73% in this patient group (51). Contrary to our experience, neither the frequency or height of the refluxed barium column (noted at fluoroscopy) nor the presence of a hiatal hernia is correlated with clinically significant gastroesophageal reflux disease in this report.

Scintiscan Study

The use of radiolabeled gastric contents (scintiscan) has found little clinical use in adults; it has been used primarily in infants and children to detect aspiration and delayed gastric emptying (52). A group of 32 patients with chronic bronchial disease ranging from recurring unexplained cough to pulmonary infection were studied using a scintigraphic technique. Lung contamination by gastric radiolabeled content was reported in 75% of this patient group (53). Despite theoretical advantages of overnight gastroesophageal scintigraphy, there are a number of compounding issues associated with this test that have prevented its use as a standard diagnostic modality to detect pulmonary microaspiration of gastric contents.

MANAGEMENT OF SUSPECTED SUPRAESOPHAGEAL REFLUX COMPLICATIONS

Medical Management

GERD-related supraesophageal complications are most effectively treated with a proton pump inhibitor (PPI). PPIs are the most effective drugs in treating gastroesophageal reflux disease involving the esophagus proper. Acid reflux events are decreased by >80% and healing of esophagitis is reported in 80–90% of patients. The response to medical therapy in patients with suspected supraesophageal complications of GERD is not as efficacious as that noted in GERD disease of the gullet, however (54). Although use of PPIs appears to be effective in asthmatics, higher doses and longer duration of therapy are necessary compared to those required for esophageal GERD disease. In one study using increasing omeprazole doses from 20 to 60 mg daily, esophageal pH monitoring was performed until reflux was controlled in 30 patients with heartburn symptoms (55). The treatment was continued for 3 months during which time 73% of patients had alleviation of their symptoms as monitored by both the GERD symptoms score and peak expiratory flow rates. In this study it was pointed out that at least one-third of the patients required an omeprazole dose ≥ 40 mg daily and a prolonged duration of therapy ≥ 3 months before maximal improvement in asthma was demonstrated. Similar recommendations for the treatment of suspected supraesophageal complications of GERD with PPI therapy were recommended by the Working Party at the First Multi-Disciplinary International Symposium on Supraesophageal Complications of Gastroesophageal Reflux Disease (56). At that meeting it was recommended that a double standard dose of PPI therapy was initially indicated in patients with suspected supraesophageal complications of GERD and that treatment be continued for at least 3 and possibly 6 months. At the completion of this initial trial, assessment of the patient's symptomatology and the responsiveness to that therapy would be critically evaluated. A similar approach has been recommended for the role of impaired therapy in treatment of idiopathic chronic cough. In choosing a medical therapy, consideration was recommended for initially giving maximal rather than submaximal therapy (57). Maximal medical therapy for this disorder was felt to take 2 or 3 months before beginning to show efficacy and on an average, 5–6 months was required before optimal results were noted. If coughing has not improved by 3 months, 24-h esophageal pH monitoring was recommended while the patient was on therapy to determine whether GERD was still a likely cause of cough or possibly that the patient had failed maximal medical therapy.

Before medical therapy can be considered a ''failure'' adequate esophageal and gastric acid suppression should be documented. In one study, 70% of patients on omeprazole or lansoprazole twice daily had nocturnal gastric acid recovery (pH below 4) (58). Recently, a study reported the results of PPI therapy in 16 patients with persistent posterior laryngitis who had failed H_2-receptor therapy. Omeprazole treatment ranged from 6 to 24 weeks with a dosage of 40 mg of omeprazole at nighttime. (This was increased to 40 mg twice daily for 6 weeks in four patients with continuing symptoms.) At the conclusion of the study, both the laryngoscopy scores and the esophageal symptom indices improved significantly. Symptoms recurred, however, after the discontinuation of acid suppressant therapy suggesting that acid reflux was indeed the underlying etiology (59).

In the treatment of chronic laryngitis, the importance of long-term treatment is stressed because the injury to the epithelium is a chemical burn and takes weeks to months to resolve. For most patients, an 8-week course of antisecretory treatment is required therapy. Recurrence of symptoms is common in patients who require PPI therapy for initial treatment (60).

At present there are major problems with the interpretation of therapeutic trials using PPIs for treatment of patients with suspected supraesophageal complications. Studies contain small groups of patients, treatment durations are very short, and no control groups have been used. Future studies using PPIs in patients with suspected supraesophageal GERD require properly designed control protocols to fully evaluate treatment efficacy.

H_2-receptor antagonists and prokinetic medications have not for the most part found an effective role in treating patients with suspected supraesophageal GERD complications. Because the efficacy of diagnostic testing is relatively poor in substantiating the role of GERD supraesophageal disorders, currently a therapeutic trial is a physician's only recourse. In this situation, attempts at maximal acid suppression are critical and require potent PPI therapy.

Operative Therapy

The only randomized therapeutic trial to date was a surgical trial involving 31 patients comparing operative therapy to H_2-receptor antagonist or placebo (61). The mean symptom score and medicine score significantly improved in the surgical group and the cimetidine group compared to the placebo group at 6-month follow-up. At 5 years, only the surgical group had maintained its symptom-free status; the cimetidine and placebo groups were unchanged. A second randomized study, which has only been reported in abstract form, involved 73 patients with both GERD and asthma randomized to antacids, cimetidine 150 mg three times daily, or antireflux surgery (62). The efficacy of surgical correction of reflux was demonstrated at 5 years. There was a decreased need for medication and elimination of symptoms with improvement of pulmonary function in the surgical group.

The apparent advantage of operative therapy is that it corrects the antireflux barrier at the LES, it repairs the hiatal herniation of the stomach, and it prevents the reflux of most stomach contents. Additionally, the coughing episodes or asthmatic attacks significantly increase intra-abdominal pressure. If the LES is incompetent, gastroesophageal reflux will occur and this has been demonstrated in patients during coughing (63). Another recent publication demonstrated the alleviation of supraesophageal complications following surgical control of gastroesophageal reflux (64). Following 6 months on medication, 21 patients with severe pulmonary symptoms and demonstrable gastroesophageal reflux underwent antireflux surgery. Respiratory symptoms were improved in 86% of the patients after the operation.

Several large series demonstrate the positive effects of laparoscopic operative treatment of gastroesophageal reflux (65,66).

The candidates for antireflux surgery are often patients who require continuous or increasing doses of medication to maintain their symptoms of reflux. The case has been made for the young patient, the noncompliant patient, the patient who chooses to have this type of therapy. Often, financial concerns of the patient have been a reason for a fundoplication operation. Although the long-term efficacy of laparoscopic fundoplication is not available, 80–90% of patients are reported to be asymptomatic or have minimal symptoms following conventional fundoscopic operation; in a 10-year follow-up after open-fundoplication surgery, 91% of patients continued to have control of their symptoms (67). Short-term outcome results following laparoscopic fundoplication detail the control of symptoms in 85–90% of patients with acceptably low morbidity rates (68).

The recent introduction of ''minimally invasive'' laparoscopic surgery has replaced conventional open-fundoplication operation. Subsequently, an increasing number of patients are undergoing laparoscopic fundoplication encouraged by this new technology to greater acceptance on the part of their treating physician because many surgeons with little experience in esophageal physiology or traditional fundoplication operation have begun to perform this procedure. Not unexpectedly, the number and severity of complications resulting from laparoscopic fundoplication have increased (69). For that reason, this operation should not be ''first-line'' therapy for simple GERD patients or patients with ''suspected'' supraesophageal complications of GERD. Only in dramatic situations such as obvious regurgitation and aspirating or laryngospasm should surgery be the first-line therapy. In fact, demonstration of the effectiveness of acid suppression therapy should be the major criterion for predicting successful outcome of fundoplication operation. The morbidity associated with fundoplication operations varies but may be significant. The frequency of postoperative dysphagia ranges from 0 (70) to 17% (71) in large reported series.

Finally, fundoplication surgery is championed as the treatment of choice particularly for the young patient with significant GERD who faces a ''lifetime'' of medical treatment with potentially negative impact on life-style. Although this scenario seems reasonable, few have questioned the long-term integrity of the fundoplication wrap structure. Reports vary concerning the long-standing durability of the fundoplication wrap, but at least one long-term study showed a significant ''breakdown'' of the fundoplication wrap 20 years after the open fundoplication operation (72).

The strongest evidence to date that GERD is either the cause or contributing factor to asthma has resulted from surgical correction of gastroesophageal reflux. The dramatic improvement provided by surgery suggests that eliminating all gastric reflux rather than just reducing acid reflux may be the treatment of choice. Currently, studies are now under way to determine whether gastric acid suppression or PPIs are as effective as total gastric content suppression by laparoscopic fundoplication in the treatment of patients with suspected supraesophageal complications of GERD.

SUMMARY

Supraesophageal complications of GERD are becoming more frequently recognized or suspected by clinicians. Unfortunately, positive proof of the association between the two is often difficult or impossible to substantiate and the majority of these patients lack the characteristic symptoms of heartburn or objective findings of esophageal inflammation. Acid reflux has been demonstrated in the majority of patients with asthma and perhaps a quarter of patients with otolaryngological problems. Because GERD is the most common disorder in the population, it is quite possible that suspected supraesophageal complications of GERD may actually be independent disorders occurring in the same patient.

The suspected mechanism of GERD-associated asthma appears to be directed through vagal reflexes and hypersensitivity of the tracheobronchial tree. GERD-related otolaryngological manifestations are more apt to be caused by microaspiration with resulting damage by surface contact. The best diagnostic modality available to the clinician to help identify this association between GERD and supraesophageal complications is the ambulatory two-site/three-site pH probe recording technique. Although this test can be quite helpful, its overall sensitivity and specificity for recording acid reflux events particularly in the proximal esophagus has been seriously questioned.

Although sophisticated clinical studies have aided in identifying the role for gastroesophageal reflux and suspected supraesophageal complications of GERD, only one prospective controlled study has shown positive effects of preventing reflux of gastric contents in a group of asthmatic patients.

In many patients with suspected supraesophageal complications of GERD, ''intent to treat'' is both the primary therapy and diagnostic tool available to the physician. High-dose PPI therapy for prolonged periods is the recognized mode of conservative therapy. Operative therapy, i.e., a fundoplication operation, is the procedure of choice in situations where overt regurgitation is clinically manifested. In situations where significant GERD is demonstrated in patients with suspected supraesophageal complications of GERD, an operative treatment is a viable option but only after intense medical treatment has been demonstrated to effectively alter or influence the supraesophageal complication.

Future controlled clinical trials are necessary and more sophisticated techniques are required before we can definitely determine which markers predict the definite cause and effect between acid reflux above and beyond the esophagus with these supraesophageal complications. Until this time, the general medical community needs to be aware of the possibility of the association between GERD and supraesophageal complications to possibly define and effectively treat the patient's GERD-related complications.

REFERENCES

1. A Gallup Organizational National Survey. Heartburn Across America. Princeton, NJ: Gallup Organization, 1988.
2. Graham DY, Smith JL, Patterson DJ. Why do apparently healthy people use antacid tablets? Am J Gastroenterol 1983; 78:257–260.
3. Thompson WJ, Heaton KW. Heartburn and globus in apparently healthy people. Can Med Assoc J 1982; 126:46–48.

4. Locke GR III, Talley NJ, Fett SL, Zinsmeister AR, Milton LJ III. Prevalence and clinical spectrum of gastroesophageal reflux: a population-based study in Olinstead County, Minnesota. Gastroenterology 1997; 112:1448–1456.
5. Sontag S, O'Connell S, Khandelwal S, Miller T, Nemchausky B, Serlovsky R. Most asthmatics have gastroesophageal reflux with or without bronchodilator therapy. Gastroenterology 1990; 99:613–620.
6. El-Serag HB, Sonnenberg A. Comorbid occurrence of laryngeal or pulmonary disease with esophagitis in United States military veterans. Gastroenterology 1997; 113: 755–760.
7. Gaynor EB. Otolaryngolic manifestations of gastroesophageal reflux. Am J Gastroenterol 1991; 86:801–805.
8. Kaufman JH. The otolaryngolic manifestations of gastroesophageal reflux (GERD): a clinical investigation of 225 patients using ambulatory 24 hour pH study. Laryngoscope 1991; 101:1–78.
9. Mansfield LE, Stein MR. Gastroesophageal reflux and asthma: a possible reflex mechanism. Ann Allergy 1978; 41:224–226.
10. Belsey R. The pulmonary complications of oesophageal disease. Br J Dis Chest 1960; 54:1342–1348.
11. Gastol OL, Castell JA, Castell DO. Frequency and site of gastroesophageal reflux in patients with reflux symptoms. Chest 1994; 106:1793–1796.
12. Ing AJ, Ngu MC, Breslin AB. Chronic persistent cough and clearance of esophageal acid. Chest 1992; 102:1668–1671.
13. Harding SM, Schan CA, Guzzo MR, Alexander RW, Bradley LA, Richter JE. Gastroesophageal reflux induced bronchoconstriction: is microaspiration a factor? Chest 1995; 108:1220–1227.
14. Wesseling G, Brummer RJ, Wouters FF, TenVeldi GP. Gastric asthma? No change in respiratory impedance during intraesophageal acidification in adult asthmatics. Chest 1993; 104:1733–1736.
15. Gudmundsson K, Kristleifsson G, Theodors A, Holbrook WP. Tooth erosion, gastroesophageal reflux and salivary buffer capacity. Oral Surg Oral Med Oral Pathol Oral Radiol Endodont 1995; 79:185–189.
16. Neurman JH, Toskala J, Nuutmen P, Klemetti F. Oral and dental manifestations in gastroesophageal reflux disease. Oral Surg Oral Med Oral Pathol Oral Radiol Endont 1994; 78:583–589.
17. Schroeder PL, Filler SJ, Ramirz B, Lozarchik DA, Vaezi MF, Richter JE. Dental erosions and acid reflux disease. Ann ENT Med 1995; 122:809–815.
18. Sontag S. Why do the published data fail to clarify the relationship between GER and asthma? Proceedings from the Second Multi-Disciplinary International Symposium on Supraesophageal Complications of Reflux Disease, 1998. Am J Med 2000; 108(4A):159–169.
19. Jack CL, Calvery PM, Donnelly RJ, Tran J, Russel G, Hind CR, Evans CC. Simultaneous tracheal and esophageal pH measurements in asthmatic patients with gastroesophageal reflux. Thorax 1995; 50:201–204.
20. Shaker R, Dodds WJ, Helm J, Kern MK, Hogan WJ. Regional esophageal distribution and clearance of refluxed acid. Gastroenterology 1991; 101:355–359.

21. Medda BK, Lang IM, Layman R, Hogan WJ, Dodds WJ, Shaker R. Characterization and quantification of a pharyngo-UES contractile reflex in cats. Am J Physiol 1994; 267:G972–G983.
22. Sengupta JN, Saha JK, Goyal RK. Stimulus-response function studies of esophageal mechanosensitive nociceptors in sympathetic afferents of opossum. J Neurophysiol 1990; 64:796–812.
23. Wallin L, Boesby S, Madsen T. The effect of HCl infusion in the lower part of the esophagus on the pharyngoesophageal sphincter pressure in normal subjects. Scand J Gastroenterol 1978; 13:821–826.
24. Vakil NB, Kahrilas PJ, Dodds WJ, Vanagunas A. Absence of an upper esophageal sphincter response to acid reflux. Am J Gastroenterol 1989; 84:606–610.
25. Wilson JA, Pryde A, Macintrye CCA, Heading RC. Effect of esophageal acid exposure on upper esophageal sphincter pressure. J Gastrointest Motil 1990; 2:117–120.
26. Shaker R, Dodds WJ, Ren J, Hogan WJ, Arndorfer RC. Esophagoglottal closure reflex: a mechanism of airway protection. Gastroenterology 1992; 102:857–861.
27. Shaker R, Ren J, Medda B, Lang I, Cowles V, Jaradeh S. Identification and characterization of the esophagoglottal closure reflex in the feline model. Am J Physiol 1994; 266:G147–G153.
28. Shaker R, Ren J, Hogan WJ, Lui J, Podvrsan B, Sui Z. Glottal function during postprandial gastroesophageal reflux. Gastroenterology 1993; 104:A58.
29. Ren J, Shaker R, Medda B, Bonnevier J, Kern M, Durn B. Effect of acute esophagitis on the esophagoglottal closure reflex in a feline model. Gastroenterology 1995; 108: A677.
30. Nishino T. Swallowing as a protective reflex for the upper respiratory tract. Anesthesiology 1993; 79:588–601.
31. Shaker R, Ren J, Zamir Z, Sarna S, Lui J, Sui Z. Effect of aging, position and temperature on the threshold volume triggoring pharyngeal swallows. Gastroenterology 1994; 107:396–402.
32. Patterson WG. Neuromuscular mechanisms of esophageal responses at and proximal to a distending balloon. Am J Physiol 1991; 260:6148–6155.
33. Ren J, Shaker R, Dua K, Trifan A, Podvran B, Sui Z. Glottal adduction response to pharyngeal water stimulation: evidence for pharyngoglottal closure reflex. Gastroenterology 1994; 106:A558.
34. Shaker R, Ren J, Kern M, Dodds WJ, Hogan WJ, Li Q. Mechanisms of airway protection and UES opening during belching. Am J Physiol 1992; 262:G621–G628.
35. Ing AJ, Ngu MC, Breslin AB. Chronic persistent cough and clearance of esophageal acid. Chest 1992; 102(6):1668–1671.
36. Jindal JR, Milbrath MM, Hogan WJ, Shaker R, Toohill RJ. Gastroesophageal reflux disease as a likely cause of ‘‘idiopathic’’ subglottic stenosis. Ann Otol Rhinol Laryngol 1994; 103:186–191.
37. Lazarchik DH, Filler SJ. Effects of gastroesophageal reflux on the oral cavity. Am J Med 103(5A):107S–113S.
38. Dobhan R, Castell DO. Normal and abnormal proximal esophageal acid exposure: results of ambulatory dual-probe pH monitoring. Am J Gastroenterol 1993; 88:25–29.

39. Shaker R, Milbrath M, Ren J, Toohill R, Hogan WJ, Qun L, Hofmann C. Esophagopharyngeal distribution of refluxed gastric acid in patients with reflux laryngitis. Gastroenterology 1995; 109:1575–1582.
40. Richter JE. Ambulatory esophageal pH monitoring. Am J Med 1997; 103(5A):1305–1345.
41. Valzi MF, Schroeder PL, Richter JE. Reproducibility of proximal probe pH parameters in 24-hour ambulatory esophageal pH monitoring. Am J Gastroenterol 1997; 92:825–829.
42. Weusten BL, Akkermans LM, vonBerge-Henegouwen GP, Smout AJ. Spatiotemporal characteristics of physiological gastroesophageal reflux. Am J Physiol 1994; 226: G357–G362.
43. Shaker R, Helm JF, Dodds WJ, Hogan WJ. Revelations about ambulatory esophageal pH monitoring. Gastroenterology 1988; 94(5):A421.
44. Gastul OL, Castell JA, Castell DU. Frequency and site of gastroesophageal reflux in patients with chest symptoms. Chest 1994; 106:1793–1796.
45. Ing AJ. Cough and gastroesophageal reflux. Am J Med 1997; 103:915–965.
46. Irwin RS, Curley FJ, French CL. Chronic cough: The spectrum and frequency of causes, key components of the diagnostic evaluation and outcome of specific therapy. Am Rev Respir Dis 1990; 141:640–647.
47. Smyrnios NA, Irwin RS, Curley FJ. Chronic cough with a history of excessive sputum production. Chest 1995; 108:991–997.
48. Ing AJ, Ngu MC, Breslin ABX. Pathogenesis of chronic persistent cough associated with gastroesophageal reflux. Am J Respir Crit Care Med 1994; 149:160–161.
49. Sontag SJ, Schnell TG, Miller TQ, Khandelwal S, O'Connell S, Chyfec G, Greenlec H, Seidel UJ, Brand L. Prevalence of esophagitis in asthmatics. Gut 1992; 33:872–876.
50. Mays EE. Intrinsic asthma in adults: association with gastroesophageal reflux. JAMA 1976; 236:2626–2628.
51. Rodriguez-Villarrel H, et al. Refluxo gastroesofagio associado a asthma bronquial. Bol Md Hosp Infant Mex 1988; 45:442.
52. Ruth M, Carlsson S, Mansson I, Bengtsson W, Sundberg N. Scintigraphic detection of gastro-pulmonary aspiration in patients with respiratory disorders. Clin Physiol 1993; 13:19–33.
53. Crannaz FM, Faver G. Aspiration of solid food particles into lungs of patients with gastroesophageal reflux and chronic bronchial disease. Chest 1988; 93:376–378.
54. Katzka DA, Paoletti V, Leite L, Castell DO. Prolonged ambulatory pH monitoring in patients with persistent gastroesophageal reflux disease symptoms: testing while on therapy identifies the need for more aggressive anti-reflux therapy. Am J Gastroenterol 1996; 10:2110–2113.
55. Harding SM, Richter JK, Guzzo MR, et al. Asthma and gastroesophageal reflux: acid suppressive therapy improves asthma outcome. Am J Med 1996; 100:395–405.
56. Hogan WJ, Hinder R, Dent JD, de Caestecker J, Filler S, Pope C, Sontag S. First Multi-Disciplinary International Symposium on Supraesophageal Complications of Gastroesophageal Reflux Disease. Am J Med 1997; 103(5A):149–150.
57. Irwin RS. Anatomical diagnostic protocol in evaluating chronic cough with specific reference to GERD. Proceedings from the Second Multi-Disciplinary International

Symposium on Supraesophageal Complications of Reflux Disease, 1998 (Seattle, WA). Am J Med 2000; 108(4):126–130.

58. Peghini P, Katz P, Beldassy A, Bracy N, Gideon M, Paoletti V, Castell J, Castell DO. Nocturnal acid breakthrough during twice daily (bid) administration of proton pump inhibitor (PPI). Gastroenterology 1997; 112:A255.
59. Kamel PL, Hanson D, Kahrilas PJ. Omeprazole for the treatment of posterior laryngitis. Am J Med 1994; 96:321–326.
60. Hanson DG. Diagnosis and management of chronic irritative laryngitis. Proceedings from Second Multi-Disciplinary International Symposium on Supraesophageal Complications of Reflux Disease, 1998 (Seattle, WA). Am J Med 2000; 108(4): 112–119.
61. Larrain A, Carrasco E, Galleguillos F, Sepulveda R, Pope C. Medical and surgical treatment of non-allergic asthma associated with gastroesophageal reflux. Chest 1991; 99:1330–1336.
62. Sontag SJ, O'Connell S, Khandewal S, Greenlee H, Chejfec G, Nemchausky B, Schnell T, Miller T, Brand CL. Anti-reflux surgery in asthmatics with reflux improves pulmonary symptoms and function. Gastroenterology 1990; 98(2):A128.
63. Pellegrini CA, DeMeester TR, Johnson LF, Skinner DB. Gastroesophageal reflux and pulmonary aspiration, incidental functional abnormality and results of surgical therapy. Surgery 1979; 86:110–119.
64. Wetscher GI, Glaser K, Hinder RA, et al. Respiratory symptoms in patients with gastroesophageal reflux disease following medical therapy and following anti-reflux surgery. Am J Surg 1997; 174:639–643.
65. Hinder RA, Filipi CJ, Wetscher GJ, et al. Laparoscopic Nissen fundoplication is an effective treatment for gastroesophageal reflux disease. Ann Surg 1994; 220:471–488.
66. Perkikis G, Hinder RA, Wetscher GJ. Nissen fundoplication for gastroesophageal reflux disease: laparoscopic Nissen fundoplication—technique and results. Dis Esoph 1996; 9:272–277.
67. DeMeester TR, Bonavina L, Albertucci M. Nissen fundoplication for gastroesophageal reflux disease. Evaluation of primary repair in 100 consecutive patients. Ann Surg 1986; 204:9–20.
68. Peters JH, Heimbucher J, Incarbone R, et al. Clinical and physiologic comparison of laparoscopic and open fundoplication. J Am Coll Surg 1995; 180:385–393.
69. Kozarek RA, Low DE, Raltz SL. Complications associated with laparoscopic antireflux surgery: one multi-specialty clinic's experience. Gastrointest Endosc 1997; 46:527–531.
70. Cadiere GB, Houben JJ, Bruyns J, Himpens J, Panzer FM, Gelin M. Laparoscopic Nissen fundoplication: technique and preliminary results. Br J Surg 1994; 81:400–403.
71. Jamieson CG, Watson DI, Brittin-Jones R, Mitchell PC, Anvaro M. Laparoscopic Nissen fundoplication. Ann Surg 1994; 220:137–145.
72. Luostarinen M, Isolaurs J, Laitinen J, Koskinen M, Keyrilaine O, Markkula H, Lehtinen E, Uusitole A. Fate of Nissen fundoplication after 20 years: a clinical, endoscopical and functional analysis. Gut 1993; 34:1015–1020.

10
Medical Therapy of Gastroesophageal Reflux Disease

Guido N. J. Tytgat
Academic Medical Center, Amsterdam, The Netherlands

INTRODUCTION: THE MANY FACES OF GERD

Before discussing in depth the medical therapy of gastroesophageal reflux disease (GERD), it is important to draw attention to four conditions that have major bearing on understanding the possibilities and limitations of current medical therapy.

First, it is essential to realize that the spectrum of GERD is enormously wide, varying from very mild or very intermittent symptoms to virtually daily continuous heartburn and acid regurgitation.

Also the symptom pattern is highly complex, varying from characteristic symptoms of heartburn and acid regurgitation to massive nocturnal regurgitation and occasionally aspiration to very nonspecific symptoms corresponding either to dysmotility-like or gastroparesis-like dyspepsia or other atypical symptoms such as hoarseness, retrosternal pain, nausea, and vomiting.

Moreover, there is tremendous confusion in the endoscopic grading of mucosal damage, particularly for grade I. Some grading systems define grade I when the so-called minor or equivocal changes are present (erythema, blurring of the squamocolumnar mucosal junction, etc.), whereas other systems define grade I as the presence of solitary, usually linear mucosal erosive defects without confluence.

Finally, the conclusions drawn from trials with inherent selection bias may be of limited relevance to the mainstream GERD patients encountered by physicians in primary care. Often the focus of evaluation is directed to short-term clinical efficacy and not to long-term clinical effectiveness. All cost estimations are based on calculations and assumptions made in the artificial environment generated in clinical trials.

These four factors are responsible for substantial confusion. Clinicians should realize that virtually no pharmacological study takes these four factors into account. We know, for example, very little of the efficacy of life-style modifications, when symptoms are nonspecific. Neither do we know how to compare pharmacological efficacy in the various types of "grade I esophagitis."

This overview of medical therapy in GERD will summarize our current state of knowledge focusing especially on the latest achievements. The reader is referred to some of the excellent overviews for more detailed information (1–5).

AIMS OF MEDICAL THERAPY

As symptoms are the driving force, symptom reduction is the dominant aim of medical therapy. In addition, regression of endoscopic mucosal damage and thereby prevention of complications is a secondary aim. In contrast with the prevailing surgical views, for physicians full histological normalization is not a primary aim of medical therapy. However, prevention of further worsening of mucosal abnormalities to a more unfavorable stage such as columnar metaplasia should also be aimed for. Patients seek medical care for symptoms and in devising the optimal therapy one should therefore focus on symptom severity. Ranked from least to most potent, medical therapies for GERD can be stratified as follows: life-style modifications, antacids/alginates, H_2-receptor antagonists (H_2RAs) and prokinetics of promotility agents (PMAs) (cisapride), and proton pump inhibitors (PPIs). Given that the dominant aim of therapy is symptom relief, there is great appeal to the concept of a therapeutic trial with one of the above therapeutic principles.

SELF-MEDICATION

Antacid therapy is common and popular. Antacids are considered effective in providing symptom relief because of their ability to neutralize refluxed acid. Neutralization of acid results in a rapid increase in pH, which, in turn, inactivates pepsin. The studies to prove symptom relief and mucosal healing are controversial. Antacids provide rapid relief of postprandial heartburn and epigastric pain by neutralizing gastric acid in the stomach and esophagus. However, the effectiveness of antacids in providing more sustained relief of heartburn has not been demonstrated adequately. Despite this, antacids are used extensively either as prescribed medication or, more usually, as an over-the-counter (OTC) product taken as required (6).

Also alginate/antacids are often used successfully as self-medication by nonconsulting refluxers. Alginic acid, combined with sodium bicarbonate or other antacids, reacts with saliva to form a viscous solution that is thought to float on the surface of the gastric fluid pool, acting as a mechanical barrier to reflux. The combination of antacids with alginate seems more effective than antacids alone (7,8).

Also H_2RAs are useful in patients with mild disease and can also be administered on demand. As OTC medication they may eventually replace antacids as a first-line symptomatic therapy (9). Even with low doses of H_2RAs (ranitidine 25, 75, 125 mg; famotidine 10 mg), there is a dose-related decrease in intragastric acidity, lasting up to 9 h after dosing (10,11). Moreover they have a sustained effect on postprandial nocturnal intragastric acidity (12,13). Famotidine 10 mg taken before an evening meal has been shown to prevent postprandial and nocturnal heartburn (11). A special wafer formulation of famotidine allowing very rapid dissolution of the tablet in the oral cavity facilitates ingestion. Low-dose H_2RAs are available in many countries without a prescription for the short-term self-medication of heartburn (cimetidine 200 mg, ranitidine 75 mg, famotidine 10 mg).

H_2RAs have also been produced in effervescent formulation for rapid and sustained rise of pH. Effervescent formulations provide more rapid absorption and almost immediate clinical benefit. Combining antacids with low-dose H_2RA is particularly appropriate for such use. Because of the immediate (antacid) and the longer-lasting (H_2RA) effect, effervescent formulations of H_2RAs are particularly well suited for on-demand treatment (14).

EMPIRICAL THERAPY

There are several factors in support of an initial empirical approach in the management of GERD. The prevalence of heartburn and acid regurgitation, the most typical symptoms of GERD, is high in the community. The prevalence of esophagitis is far lower. Less than half the patients with GERD symptoms have endoscopic abnormalities, and most of the latter have only mild-to-moderate abnormalities. Therefore, endoscopy has, at best, only a relatively low diagnostic yield in everyday practice.

The natural history of GERD varies substantially. For specialists GERD usually presents as a chronic relapsing condition, often in need of maintenance drug therapy. The severity of endoscopic abnormalities at initial endoscopy is to some extent predictive of the therapeutic response and the risk of recurrence after cessation of therapy. In contrast, for primary-care physicians, GERD is usually a less severe disease, often only presenting with intermittent symptoms. Most patients are "endoscopy-negative" or have at the most mild esophagitis

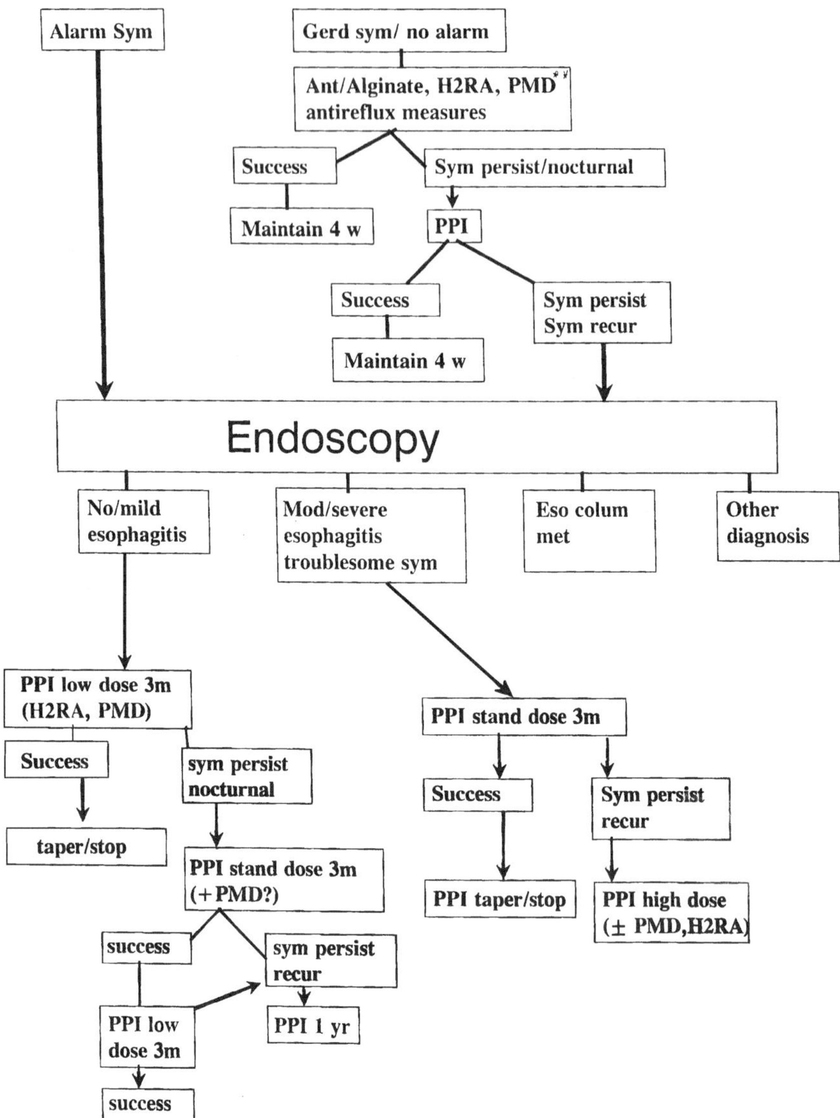

Figure 1 GERD: Management algorithm.

with little risk of worsening in time. In most patients lesions never develop or, if present, wax and wane without further worsening. Early endoscopic assessment is therefore not advisable or necessary for all patients with GERD symptoms.

In clinical practice, the diagnosis can be made reliably when typical symptoms of heartburn and regurgitation are present and dominant. A firm diagnosis can also be made in endoscopy-negative patients provided dominant typical symptoms are present and in those patients where a significant relationship between symptoms and acid reflux event can be demonstrated at ambulatory pH monitoring.

Symptom relief is now largely accepted as the primary goal of medical treatment. Symptom relief even on prolonged observation is highly predictive of endoscopic healing (15,16). Therefore, no endoscopic monitoring is required if a patient becomes and remains symptom-free.

Because of the above reasons, an empirical approach in GERD is acceptable provided the symptoms are typical, and provided alarming or sinister symptoms are absent (17) particularly for the younger patient population (Fig. 1). A 4–8-week empirical treatment intended to relieve heartburn and regurgitation can be performed with excellent efficacy and safety (17). One of the major issues concerning empirical treatment is the choice of drug therapy. The classical ''step-up'' strategy calls for the use at first of less effective drugs in responders (H_2RAs, PMAs) reserving PPIs for nonresponders. The ''top-down'' strategy goes directly to PPI either at low-dose or standard dose. Both strategies have theoretical advantages and disadvantages and inconveniences. Controversial results have been published concerning the most cost-effective strategy (18,19).

LIFE-STYLE CHANGES

Any approach to a patient with reflux disease begins with explanation of the disorder, inquiry about potentially correctable abnormalities, and advice for life-style modification whenever appropriate (Table 1). Of those measures, early-evening meal, low fat content of the diet, avoidance of chocolate, and raising the head of the bed are obviously the most important. How many patients with moderate/severe reflux disease do follow those measures in real life is unknown. Compliance with life-style changes is often poor. Moreover, because the majority of patients are daytime refluxers, the efficacy of raising the head of the bed at night may be questioned. Bed elevation turns out to be a difficult measure because of induction of back pain and various other logistic problems. Some physicians question the necessity of many of the above measures in view of the effectiveness of current pharmacological possibilities, but life-style modifications are the likely

Table 1 GERD Therapy: Lifestyle Modification

Elevation of head of bed; avoid waterbed; use foam rubber wedge on top of mattress
Dietary modifications
early-evening meal; no food prior to sleeping
low-calorie, low-fat evening meal
avoid specific irritants [citrus juices, tomato products, coffee, alcoholic beverages (e.g., white wine), chocolate]
weight loss, if overweight in presence of hiatal hernia
Avoid potentially harmful medications
sedatives/tranquilizers; theophylline, prostaglandins, calcium channel blockers, progesterone anticholinergics (?)
Avoid lying down after meals; avoid bending and stooping
Do not wear tight clothing
Avoid excessive repetitive straining at stool
Avoid smoking

means for getting patients off medication and this is obviously to be preferred over lifelong medication.

PHARMACOTHERAPY: HEALING THERAPY, MAINTENANCE THERAPY

Many patients experiencing reflux symptoms have self-medicated with OTC antacids, antacid/alginates, or OTC H_2RAs (7,8). A large proportion of the GERD spectrum can be treated adequately with such therapy. Only when the symptoms become more bothersome, or are insufficiently controlled by OTC medication, is medical advice sought.

In essence two main avenues are available for the practicing physician: attempts at improving the underlying motor disorder or reducing the noxious effects of the refluxate through inhibition of acid secretion. Mucosal protectants such as sucralfate have been used in the past, but are now superseded by acid suppressants and promotility drugs because of their limited clinical efficacy.

It is customary to distinguish a healing phase and a maintenance phase in medical therapy. The latter is necessary because for many patients GERD is a chronic relapsing disease. Stopping therapy after healing rapidly leads to reappearance of symptoms and mucosal damage. This is to be expected because the underlying motor disorder is hardly improved during healing therapy.

THERAPY WITH PROKINETICS OR PROMOTILITY AGENTS (PMAs)

The most important prokinetic agents at present are 5HT4 agonists, exemplified by cisapride. In the past bethanecol, a cholinergic agent, and domperidone, a dopamine antagonist, have been used in the therapy of GERD, but today these therapies are more or less considered obsolete. These therapies will therefore no longer be discussed.

Cisapride (5-, 10-, 20-mg tablets) activates 5HT4 receptors and thereby releases acetylcholine at the neuromuscular junction of cholinergic motor neurons. Through activation of nicotinic receptors, smooth-muscle contractility is enhanced. The overall effect of prokinetics in GERD encompasses the following areas: improvement of esophageal body motility and esophageal clearance capability (20); elevation of basal lower-esophageal sphincter (LES) pressure, especially late postprandially and during periods of fasting; acceleration of gastric emptying, especially when delayed; and improvement of gastroduodenal coordination and enhancement of salivary flow (21).

First-pass metabolism reduces bioavailability to 40–50%. Also hypochlorhydria reduces bioavailability. Intake 15 min prior to meals improves bioavailability.

Several studies have shown that cisapride effectively decreases esophageal acid exposure and improves esophageal clearing capacity (22,23). The overall efficacy of cisapride in symptom relief and mucosal healing is roughly comparable to what can be obtained with H_2RAs (24) (as summarized in Table 2). Symptom improvement and mucosal healing are mainly seen in the milder forms of reflux disease. Quadruple 10-mg daily dosing is equivalent to 20 mg twice daily (25). When cisapride is combined with H_2RAs, synergistic efficacy can be shown. Head-to-head comparison between cisapride and PPIs has not been carried out.

It is often stated that GERD patients with concomitant dysmotility-like dyspepsia should be particularly eligible for cisapride therapy in view of the well-documented efficacy of cisapride in patients with dysmotility-like dyspepsia. Such symptoms that favor prokinetic therapy include nocturnal predominance of symptoms and concurrent gastroparesis-like symptoms such as bloating, fullness, regurgitation, early satiety, and nausea. According to Schütze et al. (25), associated dyspeptic symptoms improve remarkably with cisapride, but whether such patients indeed do have a superior response to cisapride compared to acid suppression remains unknown.

Large-scale trials have been carried out to study the maintenance efficacy of cisapride, as summarized in Table 2. It is obvious that cisapride can maintain remission especially when healing was induced either with cisapride itself or with

Table 2 Prokinetics: Healing and Maintenance Therapy

	n	Duration	PLA	CIS	Alg	H_2RA	PPI	CIS+H_2RA	CIS+PPI
Healing (% Healed)									
Martin-Abreu (53)	174	6 wk	G66	S83					
Silveira (54)	145	8 wk		68		72			
Maleev (55)	129	8–12 wk		63		56			
Geldof (56)	155	6 wk				81		83	
McKenna (57)	344	12 wk				71		82[a]	
Schütze (25)	407	8–12 wk		73					
Poynard (8)	353	4 wk		S76	S89[a]				
Castell (52)	398	4 wk	S43[b]	S67					
Maintenance (% Remission)									
Silveira (54)	83	12 mo		67		66			
Tytgat (58)	298	6 mo	43	53					
Blum (59)	443	12 mo	49	67					
Vigneri (60)	175	12 mo	49	54		49	80	66	89
Hatlebakk (26)	535	6 mo	33	39					

Only selection of studies with at least 100 patients enrolled.
[a] Stat. sign.
[b] S, symptomatic relief.

H_2RAs but not with PPIs. Two studies failed to find efficacy for cisapride after prior healing with PPIs (26,27). This lack of efficacy is worrisome and difficult to explain. Selection of more recalcitrant patients, responding only to PPIs, is unlikely to be the entire explanation. However, which other mechanisms are involved is currently unexplored: Acid rebound? Aggravation of corpus/cardia inflammation enhancing the reflux tendency?

Therapy with cisapride is usually well tolerated. A minority of patients will complain of diarrhea. Cisapride is extensively metabolized mainly via the CYP-3A4 enzymes. Coadministration of ketoconazole, macrolides, and other CYP-3A4 enzyme inhibitors may result in increased electrocardiographic QTc intervals and torsades de pointe. Concomitant use of the above drugs is strictly contraindicated. Care should also be taken when prescribing cisapride in patients with cardiac arrhythmias or QT prolongation or with uncorrected electrolyte disturbances (hypokalemia, hypomagnesemia). EKG monitoring prior to drug administration is indicated.

The development of prokinetic drugs was obviously an important step forward. Yet clinicians should be aware of the limitations of that therapy. It is still not clear what their most important mode of action is: improving the clearing capacity or acceleration of gastric emptying; it is unfortunate that cisapride has little effect on postprandial LES tone or on transient LES relaxations (28). To what extent cisapride can diminish duodenogastroesophageal or biliary reflux is insufficiently documented but may well be of substantial importance. Why cisapride is less efficacious after prior healing with PPIs is unclear. Whether the GERD patients with concomitant dysmotility-like dyspeptic symptoms or with dominant regurgitation especially at night should be particularly eligible for cisapride therapy awaits further documentation. Despite these shortcomings several new 5HT4 agonists, 5HT3 antagonists, drugs with combined action such as mosapride (29) and motilides, variants of the erythromycin macrolide molecule without antimicrobial efficacy, are being developed. Some of those new compounds are substantially more powerful in their motor actions than cisapride. However, as yet no clinical efficacy data have been published in GERD patients.

ACID SUPPRESSANTS

Acid suppression is now established as first-line therapy. Indeed Bell et al. (30) demonstrated a significant correlation between the degree of gastric acid suppression and the reduction in esophageal acid exposure in patients with GERD. The primary determinants of esophageal healing are the duration of treatment and the proportion of the 24-h period during which intragastric pH is maintained above 4.0. The longer the treatment maintains intraesophageal pH > 4, the higher the healing rate. The time above pH 4 is significantly longer with PPIs than with

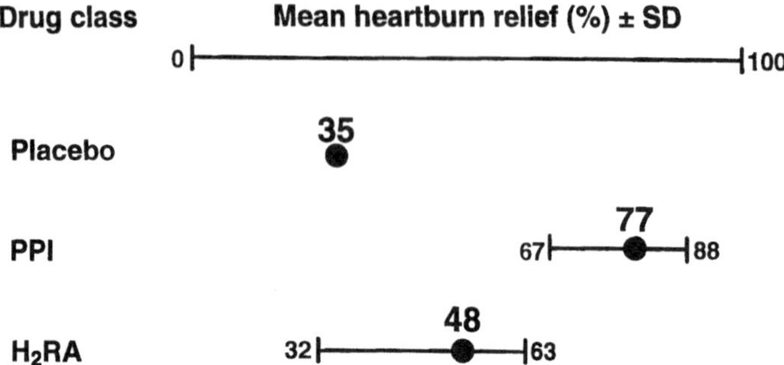

Figure 2 Heartburn relief in Grade II–IV esophagitis: A meta-analysis by drug class.

H_2RAs (30–32). The healing time curves for GERD (grades II–IV) are shifted to the left by the PPIs, which heal a significantly greater proportion of patients earlier than do H_2RAs. Chiba et al. (33) carried out a meta-analysis to compare the speed of healing and symptoms relief, as summarized in Figures 2 and 3.

ACID SUPPRESSANTS—H_2-RECEPTOR ANTAGONISTS (H_2RAs)

H_2RAs interfere mainly with the histamine receptor, particularly at the level of the parietal and ECL cells. Histamine is an important mediator in the activation cascade of parietal cells. Many studies have been carried out comparing H_2RAs to placebo and comparing H_2RAs to PPIs, as summarized in Tables 3–5. Those studies can be summarized as follows: H_2RAs are efficacious in symptom relief and healing mucosal abnormalities, but the efficacy is particularly obvious for

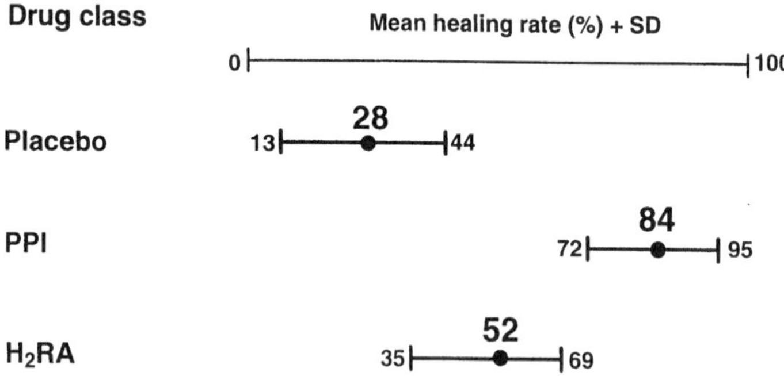

Figure 3 Healing in Grade II–IV GERD: A meta-analysis by drug class.

Table 3 Acid Suppressants: Healing Therapy

		Symptom relief/end H/4 wk									Symptom relief/end H/8 wk								
Author	n	PLA	RAN 150.2	OME 20	>20	LAN15	LAN 30	>30	PAN 40	>40	PLA	RAN 300.2	OME 20	>20	LAN15	LAN 30	>30	Pan 40	>40
Havelund (61)	162		39	77								60	91						
Damman (62)	178		51	61															
Zeitoun (63)	156		45	81								66	95						
Sandmark (64)	150		31	67								50	85						
Bate (65)	283		30	57								38	69						
Benhaim (66)	177		40			55	80					53			82	91			
Hatlebakk (67)	229			65			63						87			85			
Corallo (68)	145			84			86						88			88			
Eriksson (69)	935	33	41	S65[a]/65[a]								50	77[a]						
Bardhan (70)	229		39				84	72				53				92	91		
Robinson (71)	242		52				82					70				92[a]			
Mössner (72)	286			S86/78					S83/74				94					90	
Koop (73)	249		57						69			67						82[a]	
Corinaldesi (74)	208			79					79				91					94	
Dammann (75)	723		Ran 54						75[a]			66							87[a]
	734		Pan 48						69[a]			62							83[a]
Jansen (76)	133		42				79					66				91			
Mulder (77)	211				81		88							93		96			
Castell (78)	1284	33		82		75	83				40		91		79	90			
Hotz (79)	521			75					77				92					81	
Van Rensburg (80)	192								78	72								95	94
Mee (81)	604			57			62						71			75			
Gallo (82)	315		58						78			74						94	
Van Zyl (83)	201	58	55						S88/84			78						96	
Vicari (84)	243			83					87			90						93	
Ramirez-Barba (85)	271		74						90			88						96	
Dupas (86)	H227						78		79										
	P234						83		83										
Green (87)	196		33	72															
Lundell (88)[b]	98		R600 47		63							38			86[a]				
McTavish (89)[b]												38			80[a]				
Bianchi Porro (90)[b]	60		21		50							35			79[a]				
Sontag (91)[b]	159		22				75					22				82			
Feldman (92)[b]	95		33				80					38				89			

[a] Stat. sign.
[b] H_2RA-resistant patients.

Table 4 Acid Suppressants: Maintenance (% Remission)

Author	n	PLA	RAN 300/600	OME 10	20	LAN 15	30	PAN 20	40
Dent (93)	159		25	58	89				
Hallerback (94)	392		45	62	72				
Bate (95)	193	14		50	74				
Sontag (96)	146	17				62	61		
Gough (97)	266		32			69	80		
Robinson (98)	173	24				80	91		
Baldi (99)	986				87	73	86		
Van Rensburg (100)	157								87
Carlsson (101)	919	11	52	72	82				
Poynard (102)	206					87	90		
Hatlebakk (103)	103					73	85		
Escourrou (104)	396							72	89
Plein (105)	433							75	72
Bate (106)	166								
Jansen (107)	206					76	78		

Table 5 Symptom Relief with Low-Dose PPI

Author	n	Duration	PLA	Ome 10	Ome 20	Lan 15	Cis	ant/alg 10 ml QID	Ran
Hungin (108) primary care	424	4 wk			59				27
Goves (109) primary care	674	4 wk		64				30	
Mason[a] (110) primary care	725	4 wk		62				36	
Bate (111)		4 wk	19		57				
Venables GP (112)	994	4 wk		49	61				40
Galmiche (113)	426	4 wk		42	55		29		
Bardhan (114)	448	2 wk		40	55				26
Jones (115)	609	4 wk		49		60			
Lind (116)	509	4 wk	14	32	48				
Carlsson (101)	261	4 wk	19	35	41				
Lauritsen (117)	1959	4 wk	24	53	60		46		46
Blom (118)	195			58	80				45
Maintenance—relapse free			*Symptomatic remission*						
Venables GP (119)	495	6 mo	48	73					
Lundell (120)	424	6 mo	56	69	83				

[a] Step up to omeprazole 20 or 40 mg or, respectively, ranitidine 150 mg twice a day or four times a day when required.

the milder end of the spectrum of reflux disease. The majority of patients report symptomatic relief during the first few days of treatment with H_2RAs at prescription doses. The efficacy in healing more severe mucosal abnormalities is rather limited. Overall the efficacy of H_2RAs in GERD is substantially less spectacular than what has been seen in peptic ulcer disease.

Studies have also been performed to find out whether high-dose H_2RAs could improve the symptomatic and healing results. Higher and more frequent doses of H_2RAs do appear to be more effective in achieving satisfactory endoscopic healing, but only in a limited way. Euler et al. (34) and Roufail et al. (35) reported healing in 79% and 83%, respectively, of patients with grade II–IV esophagitis treated with ranitidine 150 mg four times daily for 12 weeks. Unfortunately increasing the dose further, for example, ranitidine 300 mg four times daily, did not improve the healing rates further in patients with more advanced disease. This is in all probability due to some loss of efficacy due to tachyphylaxis.

The limited efficacy of H_2RAs is mainly explained by the fact that these drugs insufficiently antagonize diurnal meal-stimulated acid secretion. Usually twice-daily dosing is necessary and there is undeniable tachyphylaxis. In contrast, H_2RAs are highly efficacious in decreasing nocturnal acid secretion. For the rare patient with almost intractable disease, PPIs may be combined with H_2RAs administered before retiring (36). Overall the safety profile of H_2RAs is excellent. There are very few, if any, clinically relevant side effects.

ACID SUPPRESSANTS—PROTON PUMP INHIBITORS (PPIs)

PPIs, substituted benzimidazoles, are prodrugs that, once trapped and activated in the acid milieu of the parietal cells, potently suppress gastric secretion of acid and, secondarily, raise pH also of pepsin activity. PPIs have a slow onset of action, which makes them unsuited for on-demand therapy. PPIs are irreversible blockers of the activated $H+/K+$-ATPase or proton pump. Timing of medication intake may be important. Plasma levels of PPIs are substantially higher following morning compared to evening administration.

Numerous studies have proven the symptom relief and mucosal healing capabilities of PPIs. The latter are markedly superior to standard-dose H_2RAs or prokinetics. PPIs are also efficacious in H_2RA-resistant GERD (37) (Tables 3 and 4). They are also superior to H_2RAs in patients with reflux-induced stricturing upon dilation therapy. Occasionally dosing PPIs once a day is insufficient and twice-daily dosing is required for full healing.

PPIs are also markedly superior to H_2RAs in maintaining remission. Several studies have now shown that most patients presenting with GERD symptoms can be maintained in symptomatic remission with low-dose PPI once symptom relief has been achieved, irrespective of their initial degree of esophagitis. Moreover, if the presence of esophagitis is not known, which is often the case in general practice, the physician can be confident that once the patient's symptoms have resolved, low-dose PPI will afford significant protection against the likelihood of relapse. At least 80% of patients remain healed over the course of 1 year, regardless of the initial degree of endoscopic mucosal damage. Occasionally the maintenance dose needs to be increased gradually for reasons poorly understood. Relapse rates at 1 year on omeprazole 20 mg daily in H_2RA-refractory esophagitis vary from 28% to 69%, being on average 36% (pooled from 298 patients) (38). Koop and Arnold (39) observed a 40% relapse at 3 years and Klinkenberg-Knol et al. (40) reported a 47% relapse in 86 patients treated for a mean of 4 years (range 36–64 months). According to Brunner et al. (41), none of 53 patients maintained at 40 mg omeprazole daily relapsed during treatment for 1–6.5 years.

Several recent studies looked at the symptom-relieving potential of low-dose PPI particularly in patients with so-called endoscopy-negative GERD. The results of those trials are summarized in Table 5 and do indicate that low-dose PPI is superior to any other pharmacological modality in acute and long-term symptom relief.

Whether there is any clinically relevant difference between the various PPIs currently available (omeprazole, lansoprazole, pantoprazole, rabeprazole) remains a vexing question. Several studies have shown that the acid-suppressing effect of lansoprazole appears to be greater than that of omeprazole in the first few days of therapy, perhaps related to lansoprazole's increased bioavailability. Pantoprazole has reportedly a tighter pharmacokinetic profile with reduced inter-individual variability, not altered by concomitant food or antacid administration.

Despite their obvious clinical superiority PPIs do have shortcomings. Not uncommonly in the more severe end of the spectrum dose escalation is necessary and even then some patients do fail to heal or to become symptom-free. Although omeprazole 20 mg or lansoprazole 30 mg or pantoprazole 40 mg/once a day is usually sufficient to control the symptoms, in more severe reflux disease, standard dose of PPI given once daily may occasionally be insufficient (42). Not uncommonly, nocturnal intragastric acidity remains high in those circumstances. A split regime of BID dosing provides superior acid suppression compared with single-dosing regimens with increased PPI dose qAM or qPM (43). But even with BID PPI dosing, some reflux patients continue to have high intragastric acidity (44). Peghini et al. (45) defined nocturnal acid breakthrough as intragastric pH < 4 over 1 h, which occurred in 75% of patients with GERD. This decrease in intragastric pH occurs between 1 and 2 AM, corresponding to approximately 7.5 h after intake of the evening dose of PPI. According to those authors, esophageal acid exposure occurs in roughly 70% of chronic GERD patients during this period of acid breakthrough and may be especially injurious because of delayed clearance at night (46). Intragastric nocturnal acidity is mainly histamine driven, which explains the high and superior efficacy of H_2RA blockade before retiring compared to PPI dosing hs. PPIs only inhibit actively secreting proton pumps in the secretory canaliculi, sparing those at rest in the tubulovesicles (47). PPIs have a relatively short half-life of approximately 50 min. Therefore, the fraction of active and hence PPI-susceptible pumps during the period of therapeutic plasma levels theoretically determines the efficacy of a dose of PPI. Food-related stimuli increase acid secretion (hence active pumps) up to 10 times (48). Bedtime dose of a PPI not accompanied by a meal mostly encounters resting pumps. In contrast, the action of an H_2RA does not depend on food intake. A dose of 150 mg ranitidine has peak plasma concentrations within 1–3 h and a duration of action up to 12 h (49).

In GERD patients infected with *Helicobacter pylori*, long-term PPI therapy leads to worsening of the inflammation, especially in the proximal part of the stomach. Although still controversial, most studies would indicate that even the development of atrophic changes is accelerated in those individuals. Many clinicians would therefore advise healing the mucosa first through *H. pylori* eradication before embarking on long-term PPI acid suppressive therapy. The downside of curing the infection is that the overall efficacy of PPIs in acid reduction diminishes. The effect of *H. pylori* status on sensitivity to antisecretory drugs has significant implications for the management of GERD. In the absence of infection current dosing with PPIs may result in insufficient acid control for optimal treatment of GERD. The corollary of this is that in some patients the dose needs to be increased again to raise the pH sufficiently to render the patient symptom-free and to keep the mucosal lesions healed.

Finally, evidence for acid rebound upon stopping therapy or tachyphylaxis is insufficiently studied, but well probable. High recurrence rates of symptoms and reflux esophagitis have been reported when treatment with robust acid suppressants is discontinued. Rebound acid hypersecretion has been suggested as an explanation. However, any rebound is usually rather short-lived and therefore unlikely to be responsible. A more plausible explanation is the lack of improvement of the underlying motor abnormalities, allowing damaging reflux to occur as soon as the acid suppression is stopped. In contrast, patients who are free of heartburn during maintenance therapy, be it with prokinetics or with acid suppression, are most unlikely to develop a relapse of esophagitis. The high predictive value of absence of heartburn for maintenance of healing supports a simple follow-up approach of symptom evaluation rather than reliance on endoscopy and of adjusting ''step-down'' dosing to the lowest effective level.

Omeprazole undergoes hydroxylation of the pyridinyl methyl group, mediated mainly by the polymorphic CYP2C19. Poor metabolizers due to allelic mutation may have higher gastric pH levels. Decreased metabolic clearance of omeprazole with increasing age may result in greater bioavailability; a low dose of 10 mg daily may be an appropriate initial maintenance dose in patients over 65 years of age. Lansoprazole is 5-hydroxylated at the benzimidazole ring, mediated mainly by CYP3A4. Pantoprazole's low affinity for specific cyp enzymes explains its low potential for drug interaction. The bioavailability of lansoprazole (86–91%) is higher and more constant compared to the bioavailability of omeprazole, rising from 35% to 63% after multiple dosing (50).

"STEP-UP" OR "TOP-DOWN" THERAPY?

A hotly debated controversy relates to the overall approach in clinical practice. Some would advocate a ''step-up'' approach starting with the least efficacious therapy and gradually intensifying the therapy depending upon the response of the patient (19) (Fig. 4). The ''step-up'' approach follows the principle of applying the minimum pharmacological force necessary to achieve a stated therapeutic objective. This approach targets more powerful and costly therapy selec-

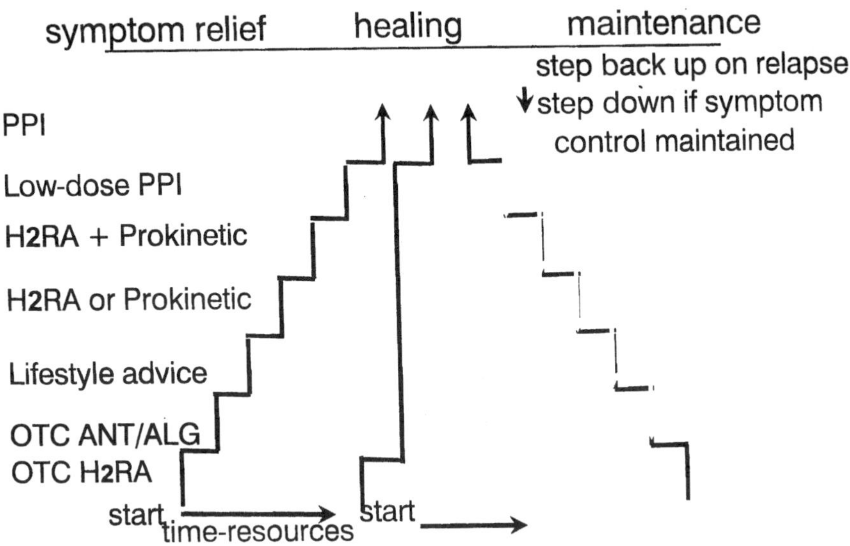

Figure 4 GERD: Step up or top down treatment.

tively toward patients with proven therapeutic need for such intensive treatment. Others would advise starting immediately with the most powerful therapy to bring the patient quickly into symptomatic and mucosal remission and then to gradually step down while monitoring symptoms. The principal characteristic in this "top-down" approach is the universal application of powerful costly therapy in patients in whom less intensive interventions may have been adequate. The "top-down" approach has been acclaimed as being the most cost-effective treatment option (51). It is the decision of the physician to choose the approach that he feels to be optimal for this patient. Respective advantages and disadvantages, summarized in Table 6, may be useful as a guide. Beyond doubt, the overall clinical applicability of the PPIs is constantly increasing.

HOW TO CHOOSE?

Symptom relief is beyond doubt the most important aim of medical therapy. The majority of patients using antacid/alginate alone are most likely to simply self-medicate. Ideally, those in need of more powerful antireflux therapy should explore which drug or drug combinations are most effective in controlling symptoms and inducing patient satisfaction. To let the patient sort it out in practice, comparing prokinetics, H_2RAs, and PPIs on an individual basis, is not realistic. Physicians

Table 6 GERD: Step Up or Top Down

Advantages step up	Advantages top down
emphasizes lifestyle modifications	faster and better symptom relief
less consumption of PPIs	faster and better lesion healing
step down less problematic	
less potential for long-term complications	
reduced drug cost (?)	
Disadvantages step up	Disadvantages top down
slow and partial symptom relief	higher drug cost (?)
slow and partial healing	greatest alteration of normal physiology
	limits on chronic use in some countries
	occasional dose escalation

need to guide the patient in his/her pharmacological exploration. In view of the superiority of PPIs, it comes as no surprise that the latter application keeps expanding especially in those countries where no restriction is provided by the regulatory authorities. Routine medical practice is, however, not always scientifically sound. There would be little scientific support for the common combination therapy of PPIs and prokinetics as often seen in the United States, where combination therapy is more common than prokinetic monotherapy. Exception to this statement concerns the patient with dominant (dysmotility-like) dyspeptic symptoms.

Sridhar et al. (18) critically reviewed the published economic studies of the cost-effectiveness of treatments for GERD. These authors conclude that PPIs are considered the best choice for the management of grades II–IV esophagitis and are more cost-effective than H_2RAs because of their fast healing of esophagitis, early relief of symptoms, and prevention of recurrent esophagitis and complications.

CONCLUDING REMARKS

The currently available pharmaceutical armamentarium allows successful medical therapy of virtually every patient with GERD with respect to the characteristic reflux symptoms and to mucosal healing. Deciding whether a step-up or step-down approach is most appropriate should be based on a case-by-case evaluation. Many different algorithms have been presented throughout the years. The one shown in Figure 1 reflects a personal preference.

In patients with severe, highly symptomatic GERD, certainly when refractory to conventional treatment, PPIs should be considered because they are the most potent healing agents and have proven to keep patients, even with aggressive GERD, in remission. In patients with recurrent GERD presenting with dysmotility-like dyspeptic symptoms, promotility agents should be considered to improve gastric emptying, to relieve postprandial symptoms, and to speed up intestinal transit in the constipated individual. For patients with mild-to-moderate reflux symptoms the choice remains between prokinesis, H_2RAs, low- or standard-dose PPI, and should be decided on a case-by-case basis.

Patients with esophageal columnar metaplasia (Barrett's esophagus) should be treated in a similar fashion as non-Barrett patients, the symptom severity and the endoscopic severity being the driving parameters. When it is necessary to differentiate reactive changes from genuine dysplastic changes, maximally intense PPI therapy, dosed twice daily, is mandatory. Full-dose PPI therapy is also indicated whenever ablative therapy is carried out for removal of dysplastic or nondysplastic Barrett's mucosa. Truly asymptomatic individuals should not be treated medically even when a segment of columnar metaplasia is present.

Patients who develop a ''peptic'' stricture should in principle be treated lifelong with full-dose PPI therapy to prevent recurrent stricturing after adequate dilation therapy. Also patients with extraintestinal manifestations of GERD (e.g., asthma, chronic laryngitis, etc.) usually require prolonged, powerful acid-suppressant therapy. This usually requires PPI therapy, especially when those patients are *H. pylori*–negative.

It should be realized that GERD is a constantly evolving field that necessitates regular adaptation. Currently there is a gradual expansion of PPI-induced acid suppression, which largely reflects their pharmacological and clinical superiority. Different dosing possibility further facilitates their applicability and in fact fits with the concept of a step-up approach. Unsolved problems relate to the proper indication of H_2RAs for mild/intermittent reflux symptomatology and particularly for suppression of nocturnal acidity and the response to acid suppression of dysmotility-like dyspeptic symptoms. The latter do seem to respond to prokinetic drugs but to what extent they also regress upon acid suppression is largely unknown. Unsolved also is the proper indication of promotility drugs in mild to moderate GERD despite some recent interesting data obtained by the American Cisapride Investigator Group (52). Only carefully conducted studies with meticulous symptom monitoring will clarify when and how combination of acid suppression and prokinesis is justified.

REFERENCES

1. Tytgat GNJ, Bianchi Porro G, Feussner H, Pace F, Richter JE, Siewert JR. Long term strategy for the treatment of gastro-oesophageal reflux disease. Gastroenterol Int 1991; 4:21–32.

2. De Boer WA, Tytgat GNJ. Drug therapy for reflux oesophagitis. Aliment Pharmacol Ther 1994; 8:147–157.
3. Hatlebakk JG, Berstad A. Pharmacokinetic optimisation in the treatment of gastro-oesophageal reflux disease. Clin Pharmacokinet 1996; 31:386–406.
4. Dent J. Management strategies for gastro-oesophageal reflux disease. Aliment Pharmacol Ther 1997; 11(suppl 2):99–105.
5. De Vault KR, Castell DO, for the Practice Parameters Committee of the American College of Gastroenterology. Guidelines for the diagnosis and treatment of gastroesophageal reflux disease. Arch Intern Med 1995; 155:2165–2173.
6. Penston JG, Pounder RE. A survey of dyspepsia in Great Britain. Aliment Pharmacol Ther 1996; 10:83–89.
7. Poynard T and a French Co-operative Study Group. Relapse rate of patients after healing of oesophagitis—a prospective study of alginate as self-care treatment for 6 months. Aliment Pharmacol Ther 1993; 7:385–392.
8. Poynard T, Vernisse B, Agostini H. Randomized, multicentre comparison of sodium alginate and cisapride in the symptomatic treatment of uncomplicated gastro-oesophageal reflux. Aliment Pharmacol Ther 1998; 12:159–165.
9. Simon TJ, Berlin RG, Gardner AH, Stauffer LA, Gould AL, Getson AJ. Self-directed treatment of intermittent heartburn: a randomized, multicenter, double-blind, placebo-controlled evaluation of antacid and low doses of an H_2-receptor antagonist (famotidine). Am J Ther 1995; 2:304–313.
10. Wyeth JW, Pounder RE, Sercombe JC, Snell CCL. The effects of low doses of ranitidine on intragastric acidity in healthy men. Aliment Pharmacol Ther 1998; 12:255–261.
11. Mann SG, Cottrell J, Murakami A, Stauffer L, Rao AN. Prevention of heartburn relapse by low-dose famotidine: a test meal model for duration of symptom control. Aliment Pharmacol Ther 1997; 11:121–127.
12. Grimley CE, West JM, Loft DE, Cottrell J, Mann SG, Stauffer L, Nwokolo CU. Early and late effects of low-dose famotidine, ranitidine or placebo on pentagastrin-stimulated gastric acid secretion in man. Aliment Pharmacol Ther 1996; 10:743–747.
13. Grimley CE, Cottrell J, Mann SG, Stauffer L, Nwokolo CU. Nocturnal intragastric acidity after over-the-counter doses of famotidine, ranitidine or placebo. Aliment Pharmacol Ther 1997; 11:881–885.
14. Engzelius JM, Solhaug JH, Knapstad LJ, Kjaersgaard P. Ranitidine effervescent and famotidine wafer in the relief of episodic symptoms of gastro-oesophageal reflux disease. Scand J Gastroenterol 1997; 32:513–518.
15. Tytgat GNJ, Blum AL, Verlinden M. Prognostic factors for relapse and maintenance treatment with cisapride in gastro-oesophageal reflux disease. Aliment Pharmacol Ther 1995; 9:271–280.
16. Carlsson R, Galmiche J-P, Dent J, Lundell L, Frison L. Prognostic factors influencing relapse of oesophagitis during maintenance therapy with antisecretory drugs: a meta-analysis of long-term omeprazole trials. Aliment Pharmacol Ther 1997; 11: 473–482.
17. Talley NJ, Silverstein MD, Agréus L, Nyren O, Sonnenberg A, Holtmann G. Amer-

ican Gastroenterological Association. AGA technical review: evaluation of dyspepsia. Gastroenterology 1998; 114:582–595.
18. Sridhar S, Huang J, O'Brien BJ, Hunt RH. Clinical economics review: cost-effectiveness of treatment alternatives for gastro-oesophageal reflux disease. Aliment Pharmacol Ther 1996; 10:865–873.
19. Eggleston A, Wigerinck A, Huijghebaert S, Dubois D, Haycox A. Cost effectiveness of treatment for gastro-oesophageal reflux disease in clinical practice: a clinical database analysis. Gut 1998; 42:13–16.
20. Paterson WG, Wang H, Beck IT. The effect of cisapride in patients with reflux esophagitis: an ambulatory esophageal manometry/pH-metry study. Am J Gastroenterol 1997; 92:226–230.
21. Verlinden M. Review article: a role for gastrointestinal prokinetic agents in the treatment of reflux oesophagitis. Aliment Pharmacol Ther 1989; 3:113–131.
22. Tytgat GNJ, Janssens J, Reynolds JC, Wienbeck M. Update on the pathophysiology and management of gastro-oesophageal reflux disease: the role of prokinetic therapy. Eur J Gastroenterol Hepatol 1996; 8:603–611.
23. Heading RC, Baldi F, Holloway RH, Janssens J, Jian R, McCallum RW, Richter JE, Scarpignato C, Sontag SJ, Wienbeck M. Prokinetics in the treatment of gastro-oesophageal reflux disease. Eur J Gastroenterol Hepatol 1998; 10:87–93.
24. Iskedjian M, Einarson TR: Meta-analyses of cisapride, omeprazole and ranitidine in the treatment of GERD. Implications for treating patient subgroups. Clin Drug Invest 1998; 16:9–18.
25. Schütze K, Bigard MA, Van Waes L, Hinojosa J, Bedogni G, Hentschel E. Comparison of two dosing regimens of cisapride in the treatment of reflux oesophagitis. Aliment Pharmacol Ther 1997; 11:497–503.
26. Hatlebakk JG, Johnsson F, Vilien M, Carling L, Wetterhus S, Thøgersen T. The effect of cisapride in maintaining symptomatic remission in patients with gastro-oesophageal reflux disease. Scand J Gastroenterol 1997; 32:1100–1106.
27. McDougall NI, Watson RGP, Collins JSA, McFarland RJ, Love AHG. Maintenance therapy with cisapride after healing of erosive oesophagitis: a double-blind placebo-controlled trial. Aliment Pharmacol Ther 1997; 11:487–495.
28. Holloway RH, Downton J, Mitchell B, Dent J. Effect of cisapride on postprandial gastro-oesophageal reflux. Gut 1989; 30:1187–1193.
29. Ruth M, Hamelin B, Röhss K, Lundell L. The effect of mosapride, a novel prokinetic, on acid reflux variables in patients with gastro-oesophageal reflux disease. Aliment Pharmacol Ther 1998; 12:35–40.
30. Bell NJV, Burget D, Howden CW, Wilkinson J, Hunt RH. Appropriate acid suppression for the management of gastro-oesophageal reflux disease. Digestion 1992; 51(suppl 1):59–67.
31. Hunt RH. The relationship between the control of pH and healing and symptom relief in gastro-oesophageal reflux disease. Aliment Pharmacol Ther 1995; 9(suppl 1):3–7.
32. Howden CW, Freston JW. Setting the "gold standards" in the management of gastroesophageal reflux disease. Gastroenterol Today 1996; 6:13–16.
33. Chiba N, De Gara CJ, Wilkinson JM, Hunt RH. Speed of healing and symptom

relief in grade II to IV gastroesophageal reflux disease: a meta-analysis. Gastroenterology 1997; 112:1798–1810.

34. Euler AR, Murdock RH, Wilson TH, Silver MT, Parker SE, Powers L. Ranitidine is effective therapy for erosive esophagitis. Am J Gastroenterol 1993; 88:520–524.
35. Roufail W, Belsito A, Robinson M, Barish C, Rubin A, and the Glaxo Erosive Esophagitis Study Group. Ranitidine for erosive esophagitis: a double-blind placebo-controlled study. Aliment Pharmacol Ther 1992; 6:597–608.
36. Castell DO, Katz PO. The acid suppression test for unexplained chest pain. Gastroenterology 1998; 115:222–224.
37. Sontag SJ, Kogut DG, Fleischmann R, Campbell DR, Richter J, Robinson M, McFarland M, Sabesin S, Lehman GA, Castell D. Lansoprazole heals erosive reflux esophagitis resistant to histamine H2-receptor antagonist therapy. Am J Gastroenterol 1997; 92:429–437.
38. Bardhan KD. Is there any acid peptic disease that is refractory to proton pump inhibitors? Aliment Pharmacol Ther 1993; 7(suppl 1):13–24.
39. Koop H, Arnold R. Long-term maintenance treatment of reflux esophagitis with omeprazole. Prospective study in patients with H_2-blocker-resistant esophagitis. Dig Dis Sci 1991; 36:552–557.
40. Klinkenberg-Knol EC, Festen HPM, Jansen JBM, et al. Long-term treatment with omeprazole for refractory reflux esophagitis: efficacy and safety. Ann Intern Med 1994; 121:161–167.
41. Brunner GHG, Lamberts R, Creutzfeldt W. Efficacy and safety of omeprazole in the long term treatment of peptic ulcer and reflux oesophagitis resistant to ranitidine. Digestion 1990; 47(suppl 1):64–68.
42. Hendel J, Hendel L, Hage E, Hendel J, Aggestrup S, Nielsen OH. Monitoring of omeprazole treatment in gastro-oesophageal reflux disease. Eur J Gastroenterol Hepatol 1996; 8:417–420.
43. Kuo B, Castell DO. Optimal dosing of omeprazole 40 mg daily: effects on gastric and esophageal pH and serum gastrin in healthy controls. Am J Gastroenterol 1996; 91:1532–1538.
44. Katzka DA, Paoletti V, Leite L, Castell DO. Prolonged ambulatory pH monitoring in patients with persistent gastroesophageal reflux disease symptoms-testing while on therapy identifies the need for more aggressive antireflux therapy. Am J Gastroenterol 1996; 91:2110–2113.
45. Peghini PL, Katz PO, Bracey NA, Castell DO. Nocturnal recovery of gastric acid secretion on thrice-daily proton pump inhibitors. Am J Gastroenterol 1998; 93:763–767.
46. Anderson C, Katz PO, Khoury R, Castell DO. Distal esophageal reflux accompanies nocturnal gastric acid breakthrough in patients with gastroesophageal reflux disease (GERD) on proton pump inhibitor (PPI) BID. Gastroenterology 1998; 114:A56.
47. Cederberg C, Andersson T, Skanberg I. Omeprazole: pharmacokinetics and metabolism in man. Scand J Gastroenterol 1989; 24(suppl 166):33–40.
48. Blair JA, Feldman M, Barnett C, Walsh JH, Richardson CT. Detailed comparison of basal and food-stimulated gastric acid secretion rates and serum gastric concentrations in duodenal ulcer patients and normal subjects. J Clin Invest 1987; 79:582.

49. Fields JB, Friedman LS, Isselbacher KJ. Ranitidine: a new H_2-receptor antagonist. N Engl J Med 1983; 309:1368–1373.
50. Dammann HG, Von Kleist DH. Efficacy and tolerability of pantoprazole versus ranitidine and famotidine in patients with gastro-oesophageal reflux disease: multicentre, open, randomised, controlled studies. In: International Clinical Practice Series. German Phase IV Pantoprazole Programme. Kent, England: Wells Medical, 1997.
51. Freston JW, Malagelada JR, Petersen H, McCloy RF. Critical issues in the management of gastroesophageal reflux disease. Eur J Gastroenterol Hepatol 1995; 7:577–586.
52. Castell DO, Sigmund C, Patterson D, Lambert R, Hasner D, Clyde C, Zeldis JB, and the CIS-USA-52 Investigator Group. Cisapride 20 mg b.i.d. provides symptomatic relief of heartburn and related symptoms of chronic mild to moderate gastroesophageal reflux disease. Am J Gastroenterol 1998; 93:547–552.
53. Martin-Abreu L. Cisapride controls chronic gastro-oesophageal reflux symptoms in patients with oesophagitis. Today's Ther Trends 1988; 6:1–11.
54. Silveira JCB, Barbosa J, Barramos J, Balja B, Ferreira SA, Fremas J, Gautier A, Leal FC, Marcaing M, Mendes V, Noronha R, Pinho C, Rodrigues J, Santos JM, Soares C, Trancoso V, Vigeant Gomes M. Cisapride versus ranitidine in the treatment and prevention of recurrent oesophagitis. Hellen J Gastroenterol 1992; 5(suppl):324.
55. Maleev A, Mendizova A, Popov P, et al. Cisapride and cimetidine in the treatment of erosive esophagitis. Hepato-Gastroenterology 1990; 37:403–407.
56. Geldof H, Hazelhoff B, Otten MH. Two different dose regimens of *cisapride* in the treatment of reflux oesophagitis: a double-blind comparison with ranitidine. Aliment Pharmacol Ther 1993; 7:409–415.
57. McKenna CJ, Mills JG, Goodwin C, Wood JR. Combination of ranitidine and cisapride in the treatment of reflux oesophagitis. Eur J Gastroenterol Hepatol 1995, 7. 817–822.
58. Tytgat GNJ, Anker Hansen OJ, Carling L, De Groot GH, Geldof H, Glise H, Efskind P, Elsborg L, Karvonen AL, Ohlin B, Solhaug OH, Vermeersch B & other Scanedcis trialists. Effect of cisapride on relapse of reflux oesophagitis, healed with an antisecretory drug. Scand J Gastroenterol 1992; 27:175–183.
59. Blum AL, Adami B, Bouzo MH, Brandstätter G, Fumagalli I, Galmiche JP, Hebbeln H, Hentschel E, Hüttemann W, Schütz E, Verlinden M, and the Italian Eurocis Trialists. Effect of cisapride on relapse of esophagitis. A multinational, placebo-controlled trial in patients healed with an antisecretory drug. Dig Dis Sci 1993; 38: 551–560.
60. Vigneri S, Termini R, Leandro G, Badalamenti S, Pantalena M, Savarino V, Di Mario F, Battaglia G, Mela GS, Pilotto A, Plebani M, Davi G. A comparison of five maintenance therapies for reflux esophagitis. N Engl J Med 1995; 333:1106–1110.
61. Havelund T, Laursen LS, Skoubo-Kristensen E, et al. Omeprazole and ranitidine in treatment of reflux esophagitis: double blind comparative trial. Br Med J 1988; 296:89–92.
62. Dammann HG, Blum AL, Lux G, et al. Different healing tendencies of reflux esoph-

agitis following omeprazole and ranitidine. Results of a German-Austrian-Swiss multicentre study. Dtsch Med Wochenschr 1986; 111:123–128.

63. Zeitoun P, Rampal R, Barbier P, et al. Omeprazole (20 mg om) vs. ranitidine (150 mg bid) in reflux esophagitis. Results of a double-blind randomised trial. Gastroenterol Clin Biol 1989; 13:457–462.
64. Sandmark S, Carlsson R, Fausa O, Lundell L. Omeprazole or ranitidine in the treatment of reflux esophagitis. Scand J Gastroenterol 1988; 23:625–632.
65. Bate CM, Crowe J, Dickinson RJ. Reflux esophagitis resolves more rapidly with omeprazole 20 mg once daily than with ranitidine 150 mg twice daily. Omeprazole 40 mg once daily produces further benefit in unresponsive patients. Br J Clin Res 1991; 2:133–148.
66. Benhaim MC, Evreux M, Salducci J, et al. Lansoprazole and ranitidine in treatment of reflux oesophagitis: double-blind comparative trial. Gastroenterology 1990; 98: A20.
67. Hatlebakk JG, Berstad A, Carling L, et al. Lansoprazole versus omeprazole in short term treatment of reflux oesophagitis. Scand J Gastroenterol 1993; 28:224–228.
68. Corallo J, Vicari F, Forestier S, et al. Lansoprazole in acute treatment of reflux esophagitis. Gastroenterology 1993; 104:A58.
69. Eriksson S, Langstrom G, Rikner L, Carlsson R, Naesdel J. Omeprazole and H_2-receptor antagonists in the acute treatment of duodenal ulcer, gastric ulcer and reflux oesophagitis: a meta-analysis. Eur J Gastroenterol Hepatol 1995; 7:467–475.
70. Bardhan KD, Hawkey CJ, Long RG, et al. Lansoprazole versus ranitidine for the treatment of reflux oesophagitis. Aliment Pharmacol Ther 1995; 9:145–151.
71. Robinson M, Sahba B, Avner D, et al. A comparison of lansoprazole and ranitidine in the treatment of erosive oesophagitis. Aliment Pharmacol Ther 1995; 9:25–31.
72. Mössner J, Hölscher AH, Herz R, Schneider A. A double-blind study of pantoprazole and omeprazole in the treatment of reflux oesophagitis: a multicentre trial. Aliment Pharmacol Ther 1995; 9:321–326.
73. Koop H, Schepp W, Dammann HG, et al. Comparative trial of pantoprazole and ranitidine in the treatment of reflux esophagitis: results of a German multicenter study. J Clin Gastroenterol 1995; 20:192–195.
74. Corinaldesi R, Valentini M, Belaïche J, et al. Pantoprazole and omeprazole in the treatment of reflux oesophagitis: a European multicentre study. Aliment Pharmacol Ther 1995; 9:667–671.
75. Dammann HG, Von Kleist DH. Efficacy and tolerability of pantoprazole versus ranitidine and famotidine in patients with gastro-oesophageal reflux disease: multicentre, open, randomised, controlled studies. Int Clin Pract Ser 1997; 15:9–12.
76. Jansen JBJM, Hazenberg BP, Tan TG, Meijer WW. Lansoprazole (30 mg) is more effective than high-dose ranitidine (2×300 mg) in achieving endoscopic healing and relief of symptoms in moderate to severe reflux oesophagitis (grades II and III). A Dutch multicenter trial. Data on file, Hoechst Marion Roussel.
77. Mulder CJ, Dekker W, Gerretsen M, on behalf of the Dutch Study Group. Lansoprazole 30 mg versus omeprazole 40 mg in the treatment of reflux oesophagitis grade II, III and IVa (a Dutch multicentre trial). Eur J Gastroenterol Hepatol 1966; 8: 1101–1106.

78. Castell DO, Richter JE, Robinson M, et al. Efficacy and safety of lansoprazole in the treatment of erosive reflux esophagitis. Am J Gastroenterol 1996; 91:1749–1757.
79. Hotz J, Gangl A, Heinzerling H. Pantoprazole vs. omeprazole in acute reflux esophagitis. Gastroenterology 1996; 110(suppl):A136.
80. Van Rensburg CJ, Honiball PJ, Grundling H de K, et al. Efficacy and tolerability of pantoprazole 40 mg versus 80 mg in patients with reflux oesophagitis. Aliment Pharmacol Ther 1996; 10:397–401.
81. Mee AS, Rowley JL, and the Lansoprazole Clinical Research Group. Rapid symptom relief in reflux oesophagitis: a comparison of lansoprazole and omeprazole. Aliment Pharmacol Ther 1996; 10:757–763.
82. Gallo S, Dibildox M, Moguel A, Di Silvio M, Rodriguez F, Almaguer I, Garcia C, and the Mexican Group of Pantoprazole Study in GERD. Clinical superiority of 40 mg pantoprazole (PANTO) compared to 2 × 150 mg ranitidine (RANI) in the healing of reflux esophagitis (GERD II/III). Gastroenterology 1997; 112(suppl): A123.
83. Van Zyl JH, Grundling H de K, Van Rensburg CJ, Retief FJ, O'Keefe SJD, Theron I, Bethke T. Efficacy and tolerability of 20 mg pantoprazole versus 300 mg ranitidine in patients with GERD, stage 1. Gastroenterology 1997; 112(suppl):A322.
84. Vicari F, Belin J, Marek L. CREGG. Pantoprazole 40 mg versus omeprazole 20 mg in the treatment of reflux oesophagitis: results of a French multicentric double-blind comparative trial. Gastroenterology 1998; 114(suppl):A324.
85. Ramirez-Barba EJ, Di Silvio M, Dibildox M, Moguel A, Rodriguez F, Almaguer I, Andrade P, Fischer R, Klein M, Wurst W, and the Mexican Pantoprazole Study Group in GERD. Superiority of 20 mg fantoprazole vs. 150 mg ranitidine in healing and symptom relief of patients with mild reflux esophagitis. Gastroenterology 1998; 114(suppl):A264.
86. Dupas J-L, Houcke PH, Giret-d'Orsay G, Samoyeau R. First comparison pantoprazole versus lansoprazole in hospital and private practice patients with reflux esophagitis. Gastroenterology 1998; 114(suppl):A110.
87. Green JRB, Tildesley G, Theodossi A, Bate CM, Copeman MB, Taylor MD, et al. Omeprazole 20 mg to 40 mg once daily is more effective than ranitidine 300 mg to 600 mg daily in providing complete symptom relief and endoscopic healing in patients with reflux oesophagitis. Br J Clin Res 1995; 6:63–76.
88. Lundell L, Backman L, Ekström P, et al. Omeprazole or high dose ranitidine in the treatment of patients with reflux esophagitis not responding to "standard doses" of H_2 receptor antagonists. Aliment Pharmacol Ther 1990; 4:145–155.
89. McTavish D, Buckley MMT, Heel RC. Omeprazole. An updated review of its pharmacology and therapeutic use in acid related disorders. Drugs 1991; 42:138–170.
90. Bianchi Porro G, Pace F, Peracchia A, Bonavina L, Vigneri S, Scialabba A, Franceschi M. Short-term treatment of refractory reflux esophagitis with different doses of omeprazole or ranitidine. J Clin Gastroenterol 1992; 15:192–198.
91. Sontag S, Kurucar C, Murray S, Greski-Rose P, Jennings D, and the Lansoprazole Study Group. Lansoprazole heals erosive reflux esophagitis resistant to histamine H_2-receptor antagonist therapy. Gastroenterology 1992; 102:A167.
92. Feldman M, Harford WV, Fischer RS, et al. Treatment of reflux esophagitis resis-

tant to H_2-receptor antagonists with lansoprazole, a new H+/K+-ATPase inhibitor: a controlled, double-blind study. Am J Gastroenterol 1993; 88:1212–1217.
93. Dent J, Yeomans ND, Mackinnon M, et al. Omeprazole v ranitidine for prevention of relapse in reflux oesophagitis. A controlled double blind trial of their efficacy and safety. Gut 1994; 35:590–598.
94. Hallerback B, Unge P, Carling L, et al. Omeprazole or ranitidine in long-term treatment of reflux esophagitis. Gastroenterology 1994; 107:1305–1311.
95. Bate CM, Booth SN, Mountford RA, et al. Omeprazole 10mg or 20mg once daily in the prevention of recurrence of reflux oesophagitis. Gut 1995; 36:492–498.
96. Sontag SJ, Kogut DG, Fleischmann R, et al. Lansoprazole prevents recurrence of erosive reflux esophagitis previously resistant to H_2-RA therapy. Am J Gastroenterol 1996; 91:1758–1765.
97. Gough AL, Long RG, Cooper BT, et al. Lansoprazole versus ranitidine in the maintenance treatment of reflux oesophagitis. Aliment Pharmacol Ther 1996; 10:529–539.
98. Robinson M, Lanza F, Avner D, et al. Effective maintenance treatment of reflux esophagitis with low-dose lansoprazole. Ann Intern Med 1996; 124:859–867.
99. Baldi F, Bardhan KD, Borman BC, et al. Lansoprazole maintains healing in patients with reflux esophagitis. Gastroenterology 1996; 110:A55.
100. Van Rensburg CJ, Honiball PJ, de K. Grundling H, Van Zyl JH, Spies SK, Eloff FP, Simjee AE, Marks IN, Theron I, Bethke T. Prophylactic efficacy and safety of 40 mg pantoprazole against relapse in patients with healed reflux oesophagitis—a one year study. Gut 1996; 39(suppl):A603.
101. Carlsson R, Dent J, Watts R, Riley S, Sheikh R, Hatlebakk J, Haug K, de Groot G, van Oudvorst A, Dalväg ZA, Junghard O, Wiklund I, and the International GORD Study Group. Gastro-oesophageal reflux disease in primary care: an international study of different treatment strategies with omeprazole. Eur J Gastroenterol Hepatol 1998; 10:119–124.
102. Poynard T, Staub JL, Lemerez M, Deltenre M, Rekacevicz C, Sallerin V, and multicentric group. Efficacy and safety of lansoprazole 15 mg QAD or 30 mg QAD as one year maintenance treatment for erosive reflux esophagitis. A randomized trial. Gastroenterology 1995; 108(suppl):A195.
103. Hatlebakk JG, Berstad A. Lansoprazole 15 and 30 mg daily in maintaining healing and symptom relief in patients with reflux oesophagitis. Aliment Pharmacol Ther 1997; 11:365–372.
104. Escourrou J, Fiasse R, Saggioro A, Vaira D, Geldof H, Fischer R, Maier C. Pantoprazole 40 mg and 20 mg are equivalent in prevention of relapse of reflux esophagitis. Gastroenterology 1998; 114:A115.
105. Plein K, Hotz J, Wurzer H, Fumagalli I, Tenor H, Schneider A. Pantoprazole 20 mg is as effective as pantoprazole 40 mg in prevention of relapse of reflux esophagitis. Gastroenterology 1998; 114:A259.
106. Bate CM, Green JRB, Axon ATR, Tildesley G, Murray FE, Owen SM, Emmas C, Taylor MD. Omeprazole is more effective than cimetidine in the prevention of recurrence of GERD-associated heartburn and the occurrence of underlying oesophagitis. Aliment Pharmacol Ther 1998; 12:41–47.
107. Jansen JBMJ, Haeck PWE, Snel P, Tan TG, Hazenberg BP, Wetzels AMH, Harlaar

C (on behalf of the Dutch investigators group). What is the preferred dose of lansoprazole in the maintenance therapy of reflux oesophagitis? The results of a Dutch multi-center comparative trial. Gastroenterology 1998; 114:A160.

108. Hungin AP, Gunn SD, Bate CM, Turbitt ML, Wilcock C, Richardson PDI. A comparison of the efficacy of omeprazole 20 mg once daily with ranitidine 150 mg bd in the relief of symptomatic gastro-oesophageal reflux disease in general practice. Br J Clin Res 1993; 4:73–88.
109. Goves J, Oldring JK, Kerr D, Dallara RG, Roffe EJ, Powell JA, Taylor MD. First line treatment with omeprazole provides an effective and superior alternative strategy in the management of dyspepsia compared to antacid/alginate liquid: a multicentre study in general practice. Aliment Pharmacol Ther 1998; 12:147–157.
110. Mason I, Millar LJ, Sheikh RR, Evans WMI, Todd PL, Turbitt ML, Taylor MD, on behalf of the complete research group. The management of acid-related dyspepsia in general practice: a comparison of an omeprazole versus an antacid-alginate/ranitidine management strategy. Aliment Pharmacol Ther 1998; 12:263–271.
111. Bate CM, Griffin SM, Keeling PWN, et al. Reflux symptom relief with omeprazole in patients without unequivocal oesophagitis. Aliment Pharmacol Ther 1996; 10: 547–555.
112. Venables TL, Newland RD, Patel AC, Hole J, Wilcock C, Turbitt ML. Omeprazole 10 mg once daily, omeprazole 20 mg once daily, or ranitidine 150 mg twice daily, evaluated as initial therapy for the relief of symptoms of gastro-oesophageal reflux disease in general practice. Scand J Gastroenterol 1997; 32:965–973.
113. Galmiche J-P, Barthelemy P, Hamelin B. Treating the symptoms of gastro-oesophageal reflux disease: a double-blind comparison of omeprazole and cisapride. Aliment Pharmacol Ther 1997; 11:765–773.
114. Bardhan KD. Management issues and economic implications in erosive oesophagitis—a case-illustrated discussion. Eur J Clin Res 1997; 9:85–89.
115. Jones RH, Crouch SL, and the Lansoprazole Study Group. Low dose lansoprazole provides greater relief of heartburn and epigastric pain than low dose omeprazole in patients with a CID-related dyspepsia. Gastroenterology 1997; 112:A162.
116. Lind T, Havelund T, Carlsson R, et al. Heartburn without oesophagitis: efficacy of omeprazole therapy and features determining therapeutic response. Scand J Gastroenterol 1997; 32:974–979.
117. Lauritsen K. Management of endoscopy-negative reflux disease: progress with short-term treatment. Aliment Pharmacol Ther 1997; 11(suppl 2):87–92.
118. Blom H, for the multicenter study group. Omeprazole vs ranitidine in the management of patients with heartburn. Gastroenterology 1997; 112:A73.
119. Venables TL, Newland RD, Patel AC, Hole J, Copeman MB, Turbitt ML. Maintenance treatment for gastro-oesophageal reflux disease: a placebo-controlled evaluation of 10 mg omeprazole once daily in general practice. Scand J Gastroenterol 1997; 32:627–632.
120. Lundell L. New information relevant to long-term management of endoscopy-negative reflux disease. Aliment Pharmacol Ther 1997; 11(suppl 2):93–98.

11
Surgical Treatment of Gastroesophageal Reflux Disease

Lars R. Lundell
Sahlgren's University Hospital, Gothenburg, Sweden

BACKGROUND

For many patients gastroesophageal reflux disease (GERD) is a chronic relapsing problem. This becomes readily apparent when confronted with the very rapid and almost universal symptomatic and/or endoscopic relapse after prior healing of reflux-induced esophageal damage with acid inhibitory drugs (1). One explanation for the chronic nature of GERD is the failure of medical therapy to correct the underlying motor abnormalities responsible for GERD. As no medical therapy is capable of providing permanent correction of the motor disorders, it is to be expected that reflux will recur as soon as therapy is stopped (2,3). However, with modern medical therapy, in the form of proton pump inhibitors (PPIs), patients can be kept in clinical remission for years (4,5).

There are, however, shortcomings and drawbacks with pharmacological maintenance therapy. H_2-receptor antagonists insufficiently interfere with food-stimulated acid production and the striking tachyphylaxis and subsequent acid rebound is frequently seen (6,7). For more severe reflux disease twice-daily doses of PPIs are often necessary and occasionally acid rebound is also demonstrable after cessation of PPI therapy (3,8,9). Furthermore, there is sometimes an insufficient control of volume reflux, nocturnal symptoms, and the retrosternal pain. With time clinical data have suggested that dose escalation is necessary and particularly divided doses of acid inhibitory drugs are required (4). Acid breakthrough during the night has recently been recognized and a novel medical management strategy has subsequently been designed with the use of nighttime H_2-receptor antagonist therapy. Another aspect causing some concern is, of course, the worsening of the inflammation of the gastric mucosa, especially within the corpus area in *Helicobacter pylori*–infected patients. This topic has been quite vigorously debated recently (10–12). The ongoing controversy relating to nonacid reflux (bile and pancreatic juice reflux) and its potential effect on the occurrence of columnar metaplasia, and therefore also the increasing problem with adenocarcinoma of the esophagus, must always be borne in mind (12–15). The rising incidence of adenocarcinoma of the esophagus and gastric cardia has recently been shown to be strongly associated with chronic reflux particularly in obese patients (16). These many concerns will in the future have important impact on the attitudes toward complete control of reflux and the reconstruction of the physiology of the gastroesophageal junction by an antireflux operation.

INDICATIONS FOR ANTIREFLUX SURGERY

Surgical treatment of gastroesophageal reflux disease has previously been limited to patients with chronic complicated reflux or those with very long-standing severe symptoms (17,18). There is now an increasing tendency in many countries to utilize surgery in the early stage of reflux. This is due to changes in the surgical technique (the introduction of laparoscopic surgery), and also perhaps paradoxically because of improvement in medical therapy. Patients with reflux can be divided into two groups: those who have complicated reflux and those with straightforward disease without complications.

Peptic Stricture

The treatment of peptic strictures has been greatly improved by the introduction of proton pump inhibitors (13,19). In the past surgery was the only effective treatment for strictures and when the stricture was tight and fibrotic, this often required a resection of the esophagus. Resection is still indicated in extremely dense and undilatable fibrotic strictures with shortening of the esophagus. However, dilatable strictures in young, healthy patients are still an indication for fundoplication and dilatation.

Respiratory Complications

Gastroesophageal regurgitation with aspiration of gastric juice into the respiratory tree causes respiratory illness, including recurrent pneumonia, bronchitis, asthma, and also laryngitis (20–24). This is a firmly established indication for antireflux surgery although we must admit that the scientific evidence for the true benefit of antireflux surgery is still to be gained. Related to that, we consequently also have difficulties in precisely selecting patients with concomitant reflux and respiratory symptoms in whom a beneficial effect of antireflux surgery easily could be predicted. Again it is probably a wise strategy to consistently evaluate the effect of profound and maintained acid inhibition therapy, over a defined period, to select those with concomitant respiratory symptoms who might benefit from antireflux surgery (25).

Columnar Metaplasia of the Esophagus (CLE)

There is no consensus on whether Barrett's esophagus (CLE) remains an absolute indication for antireflux surgery. Evidence, however, suggests that continued reflux may be deleterious for the process of neoplastic changes in the esophageal mucosa, and in fact the results of a randomized trial, presented some years ago, suggested that antireflux surgery had advantages over medical therapy (26–28). The modern, updated use of PPIs, however, has to be compared to antireflux surgery to reach a more comprehensive view of the potential merits of respective therapies. Another important aspect is, of course, the data suggesting that dysplastic lesions do not occur after successful antireflux surgery as compared to the situation in those who experienced relapse after the surgical procedure (27). Recent circumstantial information would also indicate that antireflux surgery has the potential to reverse the metaplastic lesions in the cardiac region, but continued follow-up and more extensive clinical research are required to allow a firm view on these delicate issues (26).

At present it seems, however, justified to conclude that antireflux surgery should aim at controlling reflux symptoms in patients with Barrett's esophagus rather than to prevent progression or induce regression of the columnar-lined mucosa per se. However, as most clinicians regard columnar-lined esophagus as being at the severe end of the reflux spectrum it seems advisable, until proven otherwise, to regard it as a strong indicator for consideration of antireflux surgery (27).

Uncomplicated Reflux

Antireflux surgery used to be indicated in cases where medical treatment could not prevent the disorder from having a significant impact on patients' quality of life. This indication still remains valid but modern medical therapies are so effective that only a small minority of patients do not get substantial or complete relief of their symptoms. However, if patients cease their use of PPIs, reflux symptoms recur rapidly and sometimes even with greater severity than before treatment. This may relate to acid rebound and the parietal cell hyperplasia, which seems to occur in *Helicobacter pylori*–negative patients (3,8,9). Also, many patients with reflux do not want to be reliant on a form of medication that is yet to establish its record of safety over many years (>10 years) of continuous use. Historically, failure to respond to medical treatment has been the main determinant for those referred for antireflux surgery. With the availability of modern antisecretory drugs most patients with chronic GERD can control their symptoms adequately by these means (4). Although some may require adjustment of the dose to adequately control the symptoms, one relevant question today is whether patients who do not respond adequately to PPI are suitable candidates for antireflux surgery? Some data from a recent study may have a bearing on this important clinical question (29). Depending on the design of the trial, 34 patients out of 310 enrolled into a randomized clinical trial comparing open antireflux surgery with omeprazole therapy did not initially have their symptoms properly controlled by omeprazole 40 mg daily but were eventually therefore offered antireflux surgery according to the protocol. The remaining symptoms in these patients were predominantly regurgitations, although not of acid nature. The outcome in these 34 patients, however, compared well with that of the main group of patients who initially had adequate control of reflux symptoms before randomization. The important message is therefore that continuing symptoms of reflux and only a partial response to PPIs should not be regarded as indicators of an unfavorable postoperative course after antireflux surgery.

HOW DO ANTIREFLUX OPERATIONS WORK?

Fundoplication, or some variation of it, is the most frequently performed major antireflux operation. It is likely that total fundoplication, such as Nissen (Fig. 1A), and partial fundoplication (Fig. 1B and C), whether anterior or posterior, work in similar fashions. This may be through both a mechanical and a physiological process, as these procedures are effective not only when placed in the chest in vivo but also when tested in animal viscera ex vivo (30,31). The principles of fundoplication are to mobilize the lower esophagus and to wrap the fundus of the stomach either partially or totally around the esophagus (Fig. 1). When the esophageal hiatus is enlarged, it is narrowed by sutures to prevent paraesophageal herniation postoperatively and also to prevent the wrap from being pulled up into the chest. In case of reflux complications, such as fibrotic stricturing with shortened esophagus, an esophageal-lengthening procedure is sometimes undertaken to allow the esophagus to reach the abdomen (18). The laparoscopic fundoplication was first reported in 1991 and it has rapidly established itself as the procedure of choice for reflux due to the typical laparoscopic advantages of lower wound morbidity, shorter hospital stay, and shorter time of work (32,33).

The antireflux barrier can conceptually be divided into three main components: (1) the esophagus acting as a conduit and peristaltic pump to clear itself of reflux material, (2) the lower esophageal sphincter as a selective barrier between the esophagus and the stomach, and (3) the stomach as a reservoir for

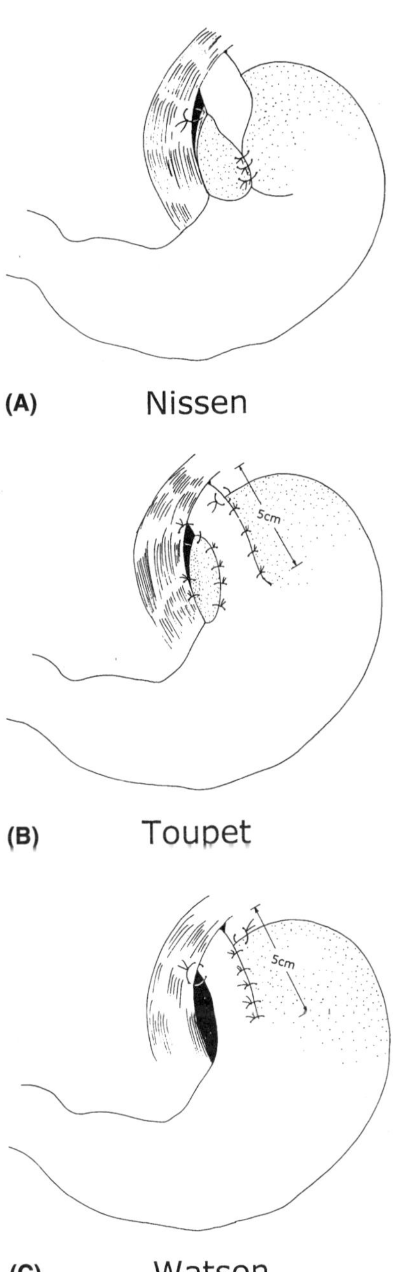

(A) Nissen

(B) Toupet

(C) Watson

Figure 1 Fundoplication operations are either total 360° wraps as in the (A) Nissen or partial wraps as in the (B) 180–200° Toupet or (C) 90–100° Watson procedures. Partial wraps may be performed either anterior or posterior.

swallowed food bolus and a trigger zone for the transient lower esophageal sphincter relaxations (34–39). Most common is a defect in the function of the lower esophageal sphincter, and accumulated data also suggest that the increased acid pepsin bile exposure into the esophagus including reduced propulsive force of the esophagus and sometimes the poor salivary function and gastric emptying disorders might contribute. Antireflux maneuvers focus on three main objectives: The first is the anatomical repositioning of the lower esophageal sphincter into the abdominal positive pressure environment. The operation reduces the hiatal hernia by the dissection and the mobilization of the esophagus and positioning of the crural sutures. This anatomical restoration per se might also have the potential to prevent reflux by reducing the hiatal hernia and by improving esophageal clearance and crural function. Second is the increased resting pressure of the lower esophageal sphincter (LES) and the lengthening of the intra-abdominal portion of the sphincter. By using different measuring techniques numerous studies have shown an increase in LES tone after a variety of fundoplication procedures (40–42). In a continuous assessment of LES tone over a longer time period, by use of a sleeve sensor, it was revealed that the LES pressure was considerably higher after a total fundoplication than after a partial posterior fundoplication. In the latter group the pressure levels reported in the LES were very close to what is seen in normal healthy controls (43). In this context it must be borne in mind that a total fundoplication might even overcorrect the mechanical deficiencies in the gastroesophageal junction, eliciting a supercompetent cardia. Irrespective of which type of fundoplication is carried out, basal LES tone assessment has shown that pressure never reaches a level at which free reflux is considered to occur. Third, the number of transient lower-esophageal-sphincter relaxations and also the proportion of those associated with reflux are substantially reduced (43,44). A low frequency of transient LES relaxations has been found after both a total and a partial fundoplication, both in the recumbent and in the upright body position. After similar operations, gas insufflation into the stomach seldom elicited transient LES relaxations. This contrasts to the situation in GERD patients when this stimulus triggers repeated relaxations of the LES accompanied by acid reflux. There are, however, important differences between a total and a partial fundoplication in that there is a tendency toward more transient LES relaxations after gas insufflation into the stomach in patients having a partial fundoplication with a similar trend toward lower nadir pressure during these relaxations (43). Furthermore, venting of air from the stomach occurs significantly more often after a partial fundoplication than in patients having a total fundic wrap as indicated by the occurrence of common cavities during manometry. It has been suggested that transient LES relaxations, triggered from the stomach, react to inhibitory neural impulses via long vagovagal reflexes (45,56). However, incomplete LES relaxation after fundoplication operations might also be induced by other neural mechanisms since mobilization of the fundus of the stomach divides connection between the gastric mechanoreceptors in that area and the esophageal sphincter region.

HOW TO INVESTIGATE AND SELECT PATIENTS FOR ANTIREFLUX SURGERY?

Fundoplication operations are designed to correct anatomical deficiencies and reconstruct the defects in the physiology of the gastroesophageal junction with permanent control of GERD with minimal levels of postfundoplication complaints. Therefore, the precision by which the diagnosis of chronic GERD is established is vital for the subsequent success rate of therapy. The primary approach by which the diagnosis of GERD is reached is by a comprehensive symptom analysis. With a frequent use of a structured questionnaire, using descriptive terms, the sensitivity of symptom analysis in the diagnosis of the disease is high but the specificity has to be assessed (47). Second, the response to therapy is important, which, in the years to come, will occupy an even more significant clinical role (25). Endoscopy is the most readily available diagnostic tool for GERD but its strength and limitation should be appreciated (48). The advantages of endoscopy include the ability to directly assess esophageal mucosal damage, complications, and structure abnormalities resulting from or associated with GERD. In this context it is important to emphasize that there is no relationship between the postoperative success rate after antireflux surgery and the preoperative grading of esophagitis (49).

Biopsies should be taken for histological examination in case of columnar-lined esophagus and strictures. There is still no consensus of the place of endoscopy in the management of GERD, but a majority consider a ''once in a lifetime'' endoscopy mandatory to recognize, for instance, Barrett's esophagus. There is a consensus among surgeons that endoscopy should be done before resorting to antireflux surgery. However, endoscopy is not a perfect diagnostic tool since at least 40% of patients with chronic typical reflux symptoms do not have, and most likely will not develop, endoscopically apparent esophagitis (48).

MANOMETRY AND 24-h pH MONITORING

Twenty-four-hour pH monitoring has been considered important to further document the diagnosis of GERD particularly in patients with either normal or equivocal endoscopic findings (50). If the study is done to confirm excessive acid exposure, it should be carried out after withholding the antisecretory drug for 1 week or more and a symptom reflux correlation should be aimed for in the analysis. Twenty-four-hour pH monitoring is particularly helpful in patients who have reflux symptoms or supposed reflux symptoms that are relieved insufficiently by acid suppression therapy. This test is also important in endoscopy-negative reflux disease and in patients with atypical symptoms such as noncardiac chest pain and in patients with supposed respiratory complications of GERD.

MANOMETRY

With the task to define the risk profile of those who subsequently might fail after fundoplication procedures the role of manometry has received a special attention in the preoperative evaluation of GERD patients. Is it even possible that antireflux operations in fact are done in patients in whom the diagnosis is not properly established? One aspect of this important issue can be understood from an analysis of the literature covering reoperations for failed antireflux procedures. The figures vary from series to series, but in about 10% of patients referred for reoperation, the index operation has in fact been done on a patient with a primary motor disorder of the esophagus and/or gastroesophageal junction and not with GERD (51–53).

It is generally recognized that the pathogenesis of GERD is multifactorial. Motility defects in the esophageal body have been described that per se cause impaired esophageal clearance of reflux material (39,54,55). Although the figures vary between different series, as many as 40% of patients with severe GERD might have delayed gastric emptying, which per se may also facilitate reflux of noxious material into the esophagus. Recent data have demonstrated an association between impaired motor function recorded in the esophagus and delayed emptying of food components from the stomach in these patients (56). An important question is therefore whether patients with severe motor disturbances in the esophagus and/or stomach may benefit from antireflux surgery, and if not, is it possible to define the profile of those who potentially may fail?

Esophageal manometry has been recommended to be carried out in all patients prior to antireflux surgery (57–59). Although an important objective for the manometry is to adequately localize the lower esophageal sphincter to position the pH probe for ambulatory pH monitoring, additional information of clinical importance can be gained. Contraction amplitudes below the 25th percentile of the normal, at any level of the esophagus, are considered failed contractions. Contraction velocity between two contraction peaks of 20 cm/s or more renders the peristaltic wave simultaneous rather than peristaltic. Using these definitions, failure of esophageal body motor function can be identified by the presence of a contraction amplitude below 20 mmHg in one or more of the three lowest 5-cm esophageal segments, or a prevalence of more than 20% simultaneous waves in these segments. Furthermore, impaired bolus clearance follows a peristaltic amplitude $\leq$30 mmHg in the distal third of the esophagus. A selection of surgical approaches has been based on assessment of esophageal contractility and sphincter length. For example, a transabdominal approach has been advocated in patients with normal esophageal contractility and sphincter length, and in those with poor contractility, a transthoracic approach was selected with construction of a partial fundoplication to prevent bolus obstruction by the fundic wrap. In a review of 104 patients selected on a similar basis, 66% were operated on by use of a transabdominal Nissen fundoplication of whom ≥90% were ''cured,'' whereas less favorable results were achieved in the transthoracic partial fundoplication group. Another approach to the problem was taken by Mughal and coworkers (60), who in a prospective, cross-sectional study evaluated esophageal manometry and studied 126 consecutive patients who had a floppy Nissen transabdominal fundoplication, irrespective of the manometric findings regarding both the body of the esophagus and the LES area. Poor results were largely due to recurrent reflux, technical failure, or irritable bowel syndrome. An unsatisfactory result was not more likely in those with upright reflux, esophageal motility disorder, or an incompetent cardia as defined by manometry. Baigrie and co-workers (61) studied 31 patients who had disordered peristalsis preoperatively and reported postoperatively very similar clinical results in these patients compared to a larger group of patients with normal motor function of the esophagus, which suggested to the authors that these manometric abnormalities are not a contraindication to a Nissen fundoplication.

We recently (62) reported a randomized, clinical study where 106 patients had a long-term follow-up after either a Nissen Rossetti total fundic wrap (n = 53) or a Toupet posterior partial fundoplication (n = 53). These patients were allocated to respective fundoplication procedure irrespective of the preoperative manometric findings. Consequently, the manometric observations were blinded for the operating surgeon as well as for the clinical observer making the postoperative assessment of the patients. No relationship at all was found between the clinical outcome and the preoperative manometric findings with similar favorable results in the two fundoplication groups. When selecting patients into groups of more severe motor disturbances (peristaltic amplitude $<$ 30 mmHg, failed primary peristalsis, and $>$ 20% simultaneous contractions) we recruited 33 and 34 patients in each study group, respectively. Again we observed no difference between the two fundoplication groups. Therefore, the present state of knowledge suggests that the principle of tailored fundoplication strategy, based on the preoperative motor function of the esophagus in chronic GERD patients, lacks firm scientific support. Similarly the alleged preference of a transthoracic approach in obese patients found no support by results from a similar study (62). We were unable to demonstrate any impact of the level of obesity on the long-term outcome of antireflux surgery when performed through the abdominal route. Therefore, the most obvious objectives for the manometric investigation, in the preoperative setting, should be to exclude other than non-GERD causes of symptoms and to establish a physiological reference point to which the positioning of the pH electrode for 24-h pH monitoring can be related.

GASTRIC EMPTYING

Although a proportion of patients with chronic GERD seems to have delayed gastric emptying of both solid and liquid diet components, it is still a matter of debate which pathophysiological role these disturbances might play. For routine clinical practice, assessment of gastric emptying cannot be recommended in the preoperative evaluation of patients being referred for antireflux surgery depending on the following facts: Even in patients with delayed gastric emptying a significant improvement in gastric motor function will ensue after fundoplication procedures. Second, until now no clear-cut picture has emerged relating the preoperative motor characteristic of the stomach to the subsequent long-term course after antireflux surgery (63–65). These data suggest that meaningful prognostic information cannot be gained from similar preoperative investigations.

OTHER INVESTIGATIONS

Testing for bilirubin reflux by use of modern technology (Bilitec) is a useful scientific tool for assessing nonacid reflux components. For clinical practical purposes there seems to be no role for these technologies at present. A barium swallow is usually considered indicated to properly assess stricture cases. Scintigraphic investigations are used only for investigational, scientific purposes.

CONTROL TRIALS IN SURGERY FOR GERD

Surgical attention was originally focused on the anatomical defects in the hiatus in the form of the hernia rather than the problem of physiological defect of incompetence in the reflux-preventing mechanisms. Nissen discovered that the fundic wrap prevented reflux when he studied a patient many years after a partial esophagectomy (66). Fundoplications have subsequently become the most widely used from of antireflux surgery, and the efficacy, side effects, and reoperation rates have been established by clinical and endoscopic follow-up and also by esophageal 24-h pH monitoring, irrespective of whether it is performed by an open, conventional technique or by use of modern laparoscopic technology (Fig. 2 and Table 1).

Over the past years, a number of modifications of the original fundoplication operations have been launched, but not every surgeon using the actual tech-

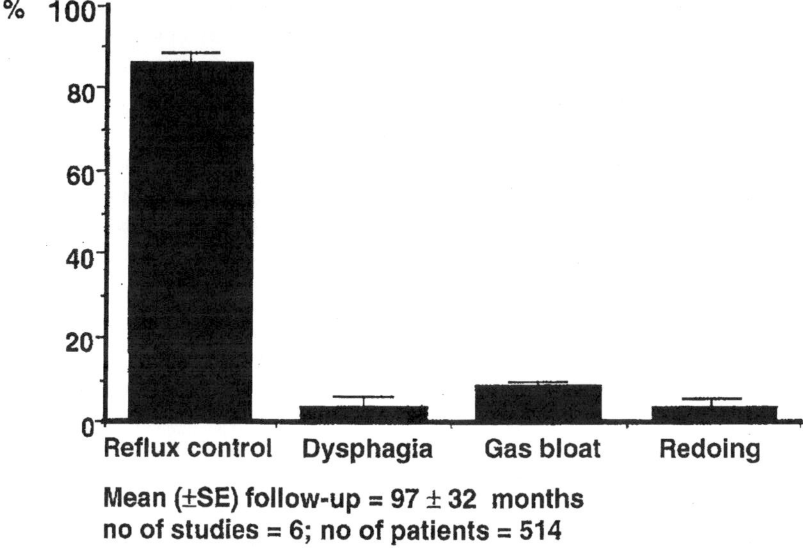

Figure 2 Long-term efficacy, complications, and frequency of reoperation as assessed in controlled, randomized clinical trails published during the last 5 years. Means and standard error are given.

Table 1 Clinical Efficacy, Technical Characteristics, and Operative Approaches Relating to Different Fundoplication Procedures Frequently Used in Clinical Practice

Type of operation	Efficacy	Esophageal wrapping (degrees)	Operative approach
Belsey Mark IV	?	270	Thoracotomy, thoracoscopy
Nissen, Nissen-Rossetti	+++	360	Laparotomy, laparoscopy
Lind (posterior, partial)	+	270	Laparotomy, laparoscopy
Toupet (posterior, partial)	+	180–200	Laparotomy, laparoscopy
Watson (anterior, partial)	+	90–100	Laparotomy, laparoscopy
Thal (anterior, partial)	?	90	Laparotomy, laparoscopy
Hill (posterior, gastropexy)	+	?	Laparotomy, laparoscopy

The efficacy refers to objective assessment (endoscopy ± 24 h pH-metry) extending ≥12 months postoperatively. The number of + indicates the amount of scientific support.

nique is as satisfied with the clinical outcome as the originator. When compiling data from controlled clinical trials it can be concluded that obvious clinical differences in the efficacy between different antireflux procedures seem not to prevail when the outcome is judged with regard to the cumulative GERD relapse rate (67–79). Excellent control of gastroesophageal reflux symptom can be obtained with the total fundic wrap, a 270° fundoplication, and a 180° fundoplication provided each operation involves the reduction of hiatal hernia coupled with the reconstruction of the reflux-preventing mechanisms to reestablish gastroesophageal competence. The problem is, however, that published results usually represent the best results in the field of antireflux surgery and the local expertise can vary considerably (80–82). Accordingly, it is reasonable to propose that antireflux surgery should be performed only in centers where the expertise has been assembled in the management of GERD as well as in the essential diagnostic facilities.

The most comprehensive and scientifically valid way of establishing an eventual advantage of one therapeutic strategy over another is to carry out comparative, randomized, and clinical trials. There are a number of obstacles that make the design and logistics of similar trials in the surgical field complicated. Since the introduction of the Nissen total fundoplication there has been some concern about the incidence of troublesome mechanical complications, which has necessitated several modifications reducing the overall incidence of these complications to about 15%. Increasing knowledge of the pathophysiology of the total fundic wrap has revealed that these complications are associated with a supracompetent high-pressure zone in the LES area that relaxes incompletely on swallowing accompanied by abolition of gas reflux (inability to belch) and reflux of noxious fluid material (83,84). Partial fundoplication procedures, which augment various constituents of the valvuloplastic component of competence and utilize a lesser degree of fundoplication, seem to be associated with a lower incidence of mechanical complications, but the argument has been made that reflux control may be suboptimal and less durable than after a Nissen fundoplication. However, several good objective, comparative studies and prospective, randomized trials have conformed that well-conducted partial fundoplication procedures are as effective and durable in reflux control as a total fundoplication (73,75, 79,84). However, the former are associated with a lower incidence of mechanical complications. This debate has been even more intensified with the advent of laparoscopic technique for fundoplications, and several reports have highlighted the increased incidence of mechanical complications following a laparoscopic total fundic wrap when compared to the conventional open-laparotomy approach. A higher incidence of impaired lower-esophageal sphincter relaxations have been reported after laparoscopic operations also associated with obstructive complaints and these consequences are believed to be associated with altered geometry, lack of tactile feedback, and other factors inherent in the laparoscopic technique (85). Several prospective studies are in progress comparing laparoscopic partial and total fundoplication and the continuance of these studies as well as those underway that compare different partial fundoplication procedures is important to form a firm basis for the choice of the most appropriate antireflux operation.

POSTFUNDOPLICATION COMPLAINTS

Although antireflux surgery is generally very effective in controlling gastroesophageal reflux, some failures are proven unavoidable (63,86,87). Persistent postprandial adverse symptoms, in the form of dysphagia, inability to belch and vomit, postprandial fullness, bloating, pain, and socially embarrassing rectal flatus, can mar an otherwise excellent result in a small but significant group of patients after similar procedures (Table 2). The frequency with which these postfundoplication symptoms have been reported varies considerably between series. Dysphagia is frequently reported during the early postoperative period but seems to diminish with the passage of time as do some other postfundoplication symptoms as well. As we lack effective treatment of established severe postfundoplication symptoms, prevention is a primary concern. A number of technical considerations have been focused on and alleged to relieve some of these problems. There is a widespread consensus among experienced surgeons that if a complete 360° wrap is done, it has to be both floppy and short. However, a large randomized clinical trial (75) has reported that a posterior partial fundoplication according to Toupet was associated with less troublesome complaints of gas bloat/rectal

Table 2 Postfundoplication Complaints After Open and Laparoscopic Nissen Fundoplications (Literature Review)

No of Patients	Dysphagia (%)	Flatulence (%)	Bloating (%)	Inability to belch (%)	Postprandial fullness (%)
		Open technique			
1922	35 (0–71)	41 (30–67)	26.5 (5.7–38)	20 (2.6–60)	30.5 (7–50)
		Laparoscopy			
308	11 (0–31)	Incomplete data	17 (1–33)	Incomplete data	Incomplete data

Median and ranges are given.

flatus. Furthermore, a laparoscopic anterior fundoplication seems to have a similar advantage (79).

IN CASE OF FAILURE?

Failure of the fundoplication to control reflux symptoms occurs in 4–9% of the patients. There are reports with a considerably higher failure rate (Table 3) and it is important to emphasize that essentially all failures occurs early in the postoperative period, indicating the importance of adhering to technical details. There are no data available to suggest that the failure rate is higher after laparoscopic fundoplication than traditionally seen after the open operations. The only tendency is toward a more frequent occurrence of paraesophageal herniations with its inborn threat of severe complications (88,89). In case of suggested failure, endoscopy and barium swallow investigations are mandatory to fully explore the anatomical deficiencies occurring in the postsurgical situation. Furthermore, the presence of reflux relapse should be also documented by use of 24-h pH monitoring and the role of manometry could in similar situations be more obvious. Issues such as a tight fundoplication or slipped fundoplication have to be addressed by use of similar functional tests. The use of a sleeve sensor (90) adapted to the manometric assembly is of particular value in these situations. Scintigraphic investigations of esophageal function primarily directed toward gastric motor function may sometimes be indicated.

The success rate after reoperation for failed primary operations is generally lower than after the index operations. This should be taken into consideration together with the fact that the postoperative morbidity and mortality are many times higher. These facts should form a strong plea for referring these patients to specialized centers for assessment and careful investigations but also to ensure adequate surgical expertise to minimize the risk and to optimize the functional outcome.

Table 3 Technical Failures and Reoperation Rates After Antireflux Surgery (Literature Review)

Disruption of the wrap (%)	Slipping of the wrap (%)	Herniation of the wrap (%)	Reoperation (%)
7.2 (0–14.3)	2.5 (0–25)	4.8 (0–7.7)	3.5 (0–25)

Median and ranges are given.

FUTURE DEVELOPMENTS

Cost-effectiveness analyses have shown that the laparoscopic reflux operations are associated with obvious advantages over the conventional open approach in the form of less morbidity and pain, shorter hospital stay, and a smoother postoperative recovery (91–94). Despite some investigators' problem in coping with the complexity of minimal invasive surgical technology, data have accumulated to show that the long-term results after minimal invasive operations are very similar to what has been documented previously after open surgical procedures. Therefore, this technology will be the main avenue for surgical therapy for GERD in the years to come. Cost-effectiveness analyses have also shown that the laparoscopic approach carries a cost that after 3 years equals that of modern medical therapy (94,95). There are reasons to believe that laparoscopic antireflux surgery seems to be the most cost-effective long-term alternative in the long-term management of chronic GERD. With the development of modern anesthesiology and also further improvement of minimally invasive surgical technology, day care antireflux surgery will be further developed and offered to an increasing proportion of GERD patients.

With the further development of clinical research programs for the refinement of antireflux procedures, reconstruction of the physiology of the gastroesophageal junction will be optimized enabling patients to adequately vent air from the stomach to prevent important postfundoplication complaints. In addition, we will see further innovations in the field of technology allowing endoscopic procedures to be done, either transgastrically or via the endoluminal route to reconstruct the physiology of the reflux-preventing mechanisms. Prototype devices have already been developed for either suturing or application of staples.

REFERENCES

1. Spechler SJ. Epidemiology and natural history of gastro-oesophageal reflux disease. Digestion 1992; 51:24–29.
2. Fennerty MB, Lieberman D. H2-receptor antagonists in the treatment of complicated gastroesophageal reflux disease: ''for whom the bell tolls.'' Gastroenterology 1994; 107:1545–1548.
3. Lundell L. Acid suppression in the long term treatment of peptic strictures in Barrett's oesophagus. Digestion 1992; 51(suppl 1):49–58.
4. Klinkenberg-Knol E, Festen H, Jansen J, Lamers C, Nelis F, Snel P. Long-term treatment with omeprazole for refractory reflux esophagitis: efficacy and safety. Ann Intern Med 1994; 121:161–233.
5. Bardhan KD. The role of the proton pump inhibitors in the treatment of gastroesophageal reflux disease. Aliment Pharmacol Ther 1995; 9(suppl 1):15–25.

6. El-Omar E, Benerjee S, Wirz A, Penman I, Ardill JE, McColl KE. Marked rebound acid hypersecretion after treatment with ranitidine. Am J Gastroenterol 1996; 91: 355–359.
7. Scarpignato C, Galmice JP. The role of H_2 receptor antagonist in the area of proton pump inhibitors. In: Lundell L, ed. Guidelines for Management of Symptomatic Gastroesophageal Reflux Disease. London: Science Press, 1998:55–66.
8. Leite LP, Johnston BT, Just RJ, Castell DO. Persistent acid secretion during omeprazole therapy: a study of gastric acid profiles in patients demonstrating failure of omeprazole therapy. Am J Gastroenterol 1996; 91:1527–1531.
9. Gillen D, Wirz AA, Ardill JE, McColl KEL. Rebound hypersecretion after omeprazole and its relation to on-treatment acid suppression and Helicobacter pylori status. Gastroenterology 1999; 116:239–247.
10. Kuipers EJ, Lundell L, Klinkenberg-Knol E, Havu N, Festen HP, Liedman B, Lamers CB, Jansen JB, Dalenbäck J, Snel P, Nelis GF, Meuwissen SG. Atrophic gastritis in *Helicobacter pylori* infection in patients with reflux esophagitis treated with Omeprazole or fundoplication. N Engl J Med 1996; 334:1018–1022.
11. Lundell L, Mietinen P, Myrvold HE, Pedersen SA, Thor K, Andersson A, Hattlebakk J, Havu N, Janatuinen E, Levander K, Liedman B, Nyström P. Lack of effect of acid suppression therapy and gastric atrophy. Results from a randomized clinical study. Gastroenterology 1999; 117(2):319–326.
12. Correa P. Human gastric carcinogenesis: a multistep and multifactorial process—1st Am Cancer Society Ward Lecture on the Cancer Epidemiology and Prevention Cancer Res 1992; 52:6735–6740.
13. Pera AM, Cameron AJ, Trastec VF. Increasing incidence in adenocarcinoma of the esophagus and esophagogastric junction. Gastroenterology 1993; 104:510–513.
14. Peters JH, Clarke GXNW, DeMeester TR. Do all adenocarcinomas of the esophagus arise in Barrett's mucosa? In: Giuli RR, Tytgat GNJ, DeMeester TR, Calmiech E, eds. The Esophageal Mucosa. Amsterdam: Elsevier, 1994:1109–1115.
15. Attwood SE, Smyrk TC, DeMeester TR. Duodenoesophageal reflux and the development of adenocarcinoma in rats. Surgery 1992; 111:503–510.
16. Lagergren J, Bergström R, Lindgren A, Nyrén O. Symptomatic gastroesophageal reflux as a risk factor for esophageal adenocarcinoma. N Engl J Med 1999; 340(11): 825–831.
17. Rossetti M, Hell K. Fundoplication for the treatment of gastroesophageal reflux in hiatal hernia. World J Surg 1977; 1:439–443.
18. Jamieson GG, Durancĕau AC, Deschamps C. Surgical treatment of gastroesophageal reflux disease. In: Jamieson GG, Duranceau AC, eds. Gastroesophageal Reflux. Philadelphia: WB Saunders, 1988:10–35.
19. Smith PM, Kerr CD, Cockel R, Ross BA, Bate CM, Brown P, Dronfield MW, Green JR, Hislop WS, Theodossi A. A comparison of omeprazole and ranitidine in the prevention of recurrence of benign oesophageal stricture. Gastroenterology 1994; 107:1312–1318.
20. Allen CJ, Newhouse MT. Gastroesophageal reflux and chronic respiratory disease. Am Rev Respir Dis 1984; 129:645–647.
21. Sonntag SJ, O'Connell S, Khandelwall S, Miller T, Nemchausky B, Schnell G, Ser-

lovsky R. Most asthmatics have gastroesophageal reflux with or without broncho dilator therapy. Gastroenerol 1990; 99:613–620.
22. DeMeester TR, Bonavina L, Iascone C, Courtney JV, Skinner DB. Chronic respiratory symptoms and occult gastroesophageal reflux: a prospective clinical trial and results of surgical therapy. Ann Surg 1990; 211:337–345.
23. Ford GA, Oliver PS, Prior JS, Butland RJ, Wilkinson SP. Omeprazole in the treatment of asthmatics with nocturnal symptoms and gastroesophageal reflux: a placebo controlled cross over study. Post Grad Med J 1994; 70:350–354.
24. Ruth M, Bake B, Sandberg N, Olbe L, Lundell L. Pulmonary function in gastroesophageal reflux disease. Effects of reflux controlled by fundoplication disease of the esophagus. Dis Esophagus 1994; 7:268–275.
25. Muller C, Lissner S. The role of therapeutic trial in the assessment of patients with reflux-like symptoms. In: Lundell L, ed. Guidelines for Management of Symptomatic Gastroesophageal Reflux Disease. London: Science Press, 1998:39–44.
26. Öberg S, Peters JH, DeMeester TR, Chandrasoma P, Hagen JA, Ireland AP, Ritter MP, Mason RJ, Crookes P, Bremner CG. Inflammation and specialized intestinal metaplasia of cardiac mucosa is a manifestation of gastroesopahgeal reflux disease. Ann Surg 1997; 226:522–532.
27. Csendes A, Braghetto I, Burdiles P, Punte G, Korn O, Diaz JC, Maluenda F. Long-term results of classic antireflux surgery in 152 patients with Barrett's esophagus: clinical radiologic, endoscopic, manometric and acid reflux test analyses before and late after operation. Surgery 1998; 123:645–657.
28. Ortiz A, Martinez de Haro LF, Parrilla P, Morales G, Molina J, Bermejo J, Liron R, Aguilar J. Conservative treatment vs antireflux surgery in Barrett's oesophagus: long-term results of a prospective study. Br J Surg 1996; 83(2):274–278.
29. Lundell L, Dalenbäck J, Hattlebakk J, Janatuinen E, Levander K, Miettinen P, Myrvold HE, Pedersen SA, Thor K, Junghard O, Andersson A. Nordic GORD-study Group. Outcome of open antireflux surgery as assessed in a Nordic multicentre, prospective clinical trial. Eur J Surg 1998; 164:751–757.
30. Little AG. Mechanism of action of antireflux surgery: theory and facts. World J Surg 1992; 16:320–325.
31. Watson DI, Mathew G, Pike GK, Jamieson GG. Comparison of anterior, posterior and total fundoplication using a viscera model. Dis Esophagus 1997; 10:110–114.
32. Dallemagne B, Weerts JM, Jehaes C, Markiewicz S, Lombard R. Laparoscopic Nissen fundoplication: preliminary report. Surg Laparosc Endosc 1991; 1:138–143.
33. Perdikis G, Hinder RA, Lund RJ, Raiser F, Katada N. Laparoscopic Nissen fundoplication: where do we stand? Surg Laparosc Endosc 1997; 7:17–21.
34. Schoeman MN, Tippett MD, Akkermans LM, Dent J, Holloway RH. Mechanisms of gastroesophageal reflux in ambulant healthy human subjects. Gastroenterology 1995; 108:83–91.
35. Mittal RK, Holloway RH, Penagini R, Blackshow LA, Dent J. Transient lower esophageal sphincter relaxation. Gastroenterology 1995; 109:601–610.
36. Holloway RH, Kocyan P, Dent J. Provocation of transient lower esophageal sphincter relaxations by meals in patients with symptomatic gastroesophageal reflux. Dig Dis Sci 1991; 36:1034–1039.

37. Dodds WJ, Dent J, Hogan WJ, Helm JF, Hauser R, Patel GK, Egide MS. Mechanisms of gastroesophageal reflux in patients with reflux esophagitis. N Engl J Med 1982; 307:1547–1552.
38. Dodds M, Dentj, Hogan, Helm F, Hauser R, Patel GK, et al. Mechanisms of gastroesophageal reflux in patients with reflux esophagitis. N Engl J Med 1982; 307:1547–1552.
39. Kahrila PJ, Dodds WJ, Hogan WJ. Effect of peristaltic dysfunction on esophageal volume clearance. Gastroenterology 1988; 94:73–80.
40. Bancewicz J, Mughai M, Marples M. The lower esophageal sphincter after floppy Nissen fundoplication. Br J Surg 1987; 74:162.
41. Bjerkeset T, Nordgard K, Schjonsby H. Effect of Nissen fundoplication operation on the lower esophageal sphincter. Scand J Gastroenterol 1980; 15:213.
42. DeMeester TR, Wernly JA, Brian GH, et al. Clinical and in vitro analysis of determinants of gastroesophageal competence: a study of the principles of antireflux surgery. Am J Surg 1979; 137:39.
43. Rydberg L, Ruth M, Lundell L. Mechanism of action of antireflux procedures. Br J Surg 1999; 86:405–410.
44. Johnsson F, Holloway RH, Ireland AC, Jamieson GG, Dent J. Effect of fundoplication on transient lower oesophageal sphincter relaxation and gas reflux. Br J Surg 1997; 84:686–689.
45. Martin CJ, Patrikios J, Dent J. Abolition of gas reflux and transient lower esophageal sphincter relaxation by vagal blockade in the dog. Gastroenterology 1986; 91:890–896.
46. Martin CJ, Franzi SJ, Dent J, Cox MR. The effect of sham fundoplication on transient lower esophageal sphincter relaxations (TLESRs in the dog), (abstr). Gastroenterology 1988; 94:A285.
47. Carlsson R, Dent J, Bolling-Sternevald E, et al. The usefulness of a structured questionnaire in the assessment of symptomatic gastroesophageal reflux disease. Scand J Gastroenterol 1998; 33:1023–1029.
48. De Caestecker JS, Bennett JR. The role of endoscopy in gastroesophageal reflux disease. In: Lundell L, ed. Guidelines for Management of Symptomatic Gastroesophageal Reflux Disease. London: Science Press, 1998:15–24.
49. Watson DI, Foreman D, Devitt PG, Jamieson GG. Preoperative endoscopic grading of oesophagitis vs. outcome after laparoscopic Nissen fundoplication. Am J Gastroenterol 1997; 92:222–225.
50. Armstrong D, Emde C, Inauen W, Blum AL. Diagnostic assessment of gastrooesophageal reflux disease: what is possible vs. what is practical? Hepatogastroenterology 1992; 39:3–13.
51. Skinner DB. Surgical management after failed antireflux operations. World J Surg 1992; 16:359–363.
52. Stein HJ, Feussner H, Siewert JR. Failure of antireflux surgery: causes and management strategies. Am J Surg 1996; 171:36–39.
53. Jacob P, Kahrilas PJ, Vanagunas A. Peristaltic dysfunction associated with nonobstructive dysphagia in reflux disease. Dig Dis Sci 1990; 35:939–942.
54. Maddern GJ, Jamieson GG. Oesophageal emptying in patients with gastroesophageal reflux. Br J Surg 1986; 73:615–617.

55. Olsen AM, Schlegel JF. Motility disturbances caused by oesophagitis. J Thorac Cardiovasc Surg 1965; 150:706–712.
56. Lundell L, Myers JC, Jamieson GG. Is motility impaired in the entire upper intestinal tract in patients with gastroesophageal reflux disease? Scand J Gastroenterol 1996; 31:131–135.
57. Waring JP, Hunter JG, Oddsdottir M, Wo J, Katz E. The preoperative evaluation of patients considered for laparoscopic antireflux surgery. Am J Gastroenterol 1995; 90:35–38.
58. Fuchs KH, Heimbucher J, Freys SN, Thide A. Management of gastrooesophageal reflux disease 1995. Tailored concept of antireflux operations. Dis Esophagus 1994; 7:250–254.
59. Kauer WK, Peters JH, DeMeester TR, Heimbucher J, Ireland AP, Bremner CG. A tailored approach to antireflux surgery. J Thorac Cardiovasc Surg 1995; 110(1):141–146.
60. Mughal MM, Bancewics J, Marpies M. Oesophageal manometry and pH recording does not predict the bad results of Nissen fundoplication. Br J Surg 1990; 77:543–561.
61. Baigrie RJ, Watson DI, Myers JC, Jamieson GG. Outcome of laparoscopic Nissen fundoplication in patients with disordered preoperative peristalsis. Gut 1997; 40: 381–385.
62. Rydberg L, Ruth M, Abrahamsson H, Lundell L. Tailoring of antireflux surgery. A concept subjective to a randomize clinical trial. World J Surg 1999; 23(6):612–618.
63. DeMeester TR, Stein HJ. Minimizing the side effects of antireflux surgery. World J Surg 1992; 16:335–336.
64. DeMeester TR. Surgical management of gastro-oesophageal reflux disease. In: Castell DO WC, Ott DJ, eds. Gastro-oesophageal Reflux Disease. Pathogenesis, Diagnosis, Therapy. New York: Futura, 1985: 243–280.
65. Lundell LR, Myers JC, Jamieson GG. Delayed gastric emptying and its relation to symptoms of "gasbloat" after antireflux surgery. Eur J Surg 1994; 1106:161–166.
66. Nissen R. Eine einfache Operation zur Be-einflussung der Refluxösophagitis. Scheweitz Med Wochenschr 1956; 86:590–592.
67. Lundell L, Abrahamsson H, Ruth M, Sandberg N, Olbe L. Lower esophageal sphincter characteristics and esophageal acid exposure following partial or 360° fundoplication: results of a prospective, randomized, clinical study. World J Surg 1991; 15: 115.
68. DeMeester TR, Johnson LF, Kent AH. Evaluation of current operations for the prevention of gastroesophageal reflux. Ann Surg 1974; 180:511.
69. Gear MWL, Gillison EW, Dowling BL. Randomised prospective trial of the Angelchik antireflux prosthesis. Br J Surg 1984; 71:681.
70. Kimiot WA, Kirby RM, Akinola D, Temple G. Prospective randomised trial of Nissen fundoplication and Angelchik prosthesis in the surgical treatment of medically refractory gastroesophageal reflux disease. Br J Surg 1991; 78:1181.
71. Stuart RD, Dawson K, Keeling P, Byrne PJ, Hennessy TPJ. A prospective randomized trial of Angelchik prosthesis versus Nissen fundoplication. Br J Surg 1989; 76: 86.

72. Thor KBA, Silander T. A long-term randomized prospective trial of the Nissen procedure versus a modified Toupet technique. Ann Surg 1989; 210:719.
73. Walker SJ, Holt S, Sanderson CJ, Stoddard CJ. Comparison of Nissen total and Lind partial transabdominal fundoplication in the treatment of gastroesophageal reflux. Br J Surg 1992; 79:410.
74. Washer BF, Gear MWL, Dowling BL, Gillison EW, Royston CMS, Spencer J. Randomised prospective trial of Roux-en-Y duodenal diversion vs. fundoplication for severe reflux esophagitis. Br J Surg 1984; 71:181.
75. Lundell L, Abrahamsson H, Ruth M, Rydberg L, Lönroth H, Olbe L. Long-term results of a prospective randomized comparison of total fundic wrap (Nissen-Rossetti) or semifundoplication (Toupet) for gastro-oesophageal reflux. Br J Surg 1996; 83:830–835.
76. Johansson J, Johnson F, Joelsson BE, Florén CH, Walther B. Outcome from 5 year after 360° fundoplication for gastroesophageal reflux disease. Br J Surg 1993; 80: 46.
77. Watson DI, Pike GK, Bagrie RJ, Mathew G, Devitt PG, Britten-Jones R, Jamieson GG. Prospective double-blind randomised trial of laparoscopic Nissen fundoplication with division and without division of short gastric vessels. Ann Surg 1997; 226(5):642–652.
78. Watson A, Jenldnson LR, Ball CS, Barlow AP, Norris TL. A more physiological alternative to total fundoplication for the surgical correction of resistans gastrooesophageal reflux. Br J Surg 1991; 78:1088–1094.
79. Watson DI, Jamieson GG, Pike GK, Davies N, Richardson M, Game PH, Devitt PG. Laparoscopic anterior partial fundoplication versus laparoscopic Nissen fundoplication—a prospective randomised double blind trial. Br J Surg 1999; 86(1): 123–130.
80. Viljakka M, Luostarinen M, Isolauri J. Incidence of antireflux surgery in Finland 1988–1993. The influence of proton pump inhibitors and laparoscopic technique. Scand J Gastroenterol 1997; 2:415–418.
81. Watson DI, Baigrie RJ, Jamieson GG. A learning curve for laparoscopic fundoplication. Definable, avoidable, or a waste of time? Ann Surg 1996; 224:198–203.
82. Loustarinen MES, Isolauri JO. Surgical experience improves the long-term results of Nissen fundoplication. Scand J Gastroenterol 1999; 34:117–120.
83. Watson A. Surgical management of gastro-oesophageal reflux disease. Br J Surg 1996; 83:1313–1315.
84. Watson A. Update: total versus partial laparoscopic fundoplication. Dig Surg 1998; 15:172–180.
85. Bais JE, van Lanschot JJB, Bonjer HJ, Klinkenberg EC, Smout AJPM, Go PNY, Nadrop JHSM, Cuesta MA, Gooszen HG. A randomized study comparing laparoscopic and conventional Nissen fundoplication. Patient inclusion ended after interim analysis. Gastroenterology 1999; 116:A117.
86. Garstin WI, Hohnston GW, Kennedy TL, Spencer ES. Nissen fundoplication: the unhappy 15%. J Roy Coll Surg Edinb 1986; 31:207.
87. Negre JB. Post-fundoplication symptoms. Do they restrict the success of Nissen fundoplication? Ann Surg 1983; 198:698.
88. Seeling MH, Hinder RA, Klinger PJ, Floch NR, Branton SA, Smith SL. Paraesopha-

geal herniation as a complication following laparoscopic antireflux surgery. J Gastrointest Surg 1999; 3:95–99.
89. Edye MB, Canin-Endres J, Gattorno F, Salky BA. Durability of laparoscopic repair of paraesophageal hernia. Ann Surg 1998; 228(4):528–535.
90. Dent J. A new technique for continuous sphincter pressure measurement. Gastroenterology 1976; 71:263–267.
91. Van den Boom G, Go PMMYH, Hameeteman W, Dallemagne B. Cost effectiveness of medical versus surgical treatment in patients with severe or refractory gastroesophageal reflux disease in the Netherlands. Scand J Gastroenterol 1996; 31:1–9.
92. Heudebert G, Marks R, Wilcox C, Centor R. Choice of long-term strategy in the managements of patients with severe esophagitis: a cost-utility analysis. Gastroenterology 1996; 112:1078–1086.
93. Blomqvist A, Dalenbäck J, Lönroth H, Ruth M, Wiklund I, Lundell L. Quality of life assessment after laparoscopic and open fundoplications. Results of prospective clinical studies. Scand J Gastroenterol 1996; 31:1052–1058.
94. Blomqvist AMK, Lönroth H, Dalenbäck J, Lundell L. Laparoscopic or open fundoplication? A complete cost analysis. Surg Endosc 1998; 12(10):1209–1212.
95. Myrvold HE, Lundell L, Liedman B, Hattlebakk J, Miettinen P, Janatuinen E, Pedersen SA, Thor K, Lewander K, Nyström P, Stålhammar NO, and the Nordic GERD Study Group. The cost of omeprazole versus open anti-reflux surgery in the long-term management of reflux esophagitis. Gastroenterology 1998; 114:A238.

12
Gastroesophageal Reflux Disease in Infants and Children

Susan R. Orenstein
University of Pittsburgh School of Medicine and Children's Hospital of Pittsburgh, Pittsburgh, Pennsylvania

Gastroesophageal reflux disease (GERD) in children has much in common with that in older individuals. However, there are important differences between these age groups that impact the natural history, presenting symptoms, diagnosis, differential diagnosis, and therapy in crucial ways (1). Thus a clinician must be aware not only of the differences in drug doses in pediatric patients, but also of the differences in the array of differential diagnostic considerations, the pathophysiology, and the natural history. Furthermore, much has been learned in the past decade or so, making even recently utilized diagnostic and therapeutic modalities obsolete and sometimes actively harmful; a number of poorly understood areas remain, challenging us to rationalize diagnosis and therapy further in the next decade. This chapter will review current understanding of pediatric GERD in light of this rapid growth of knowledge, focusing on areas in which children and adults differ.

INCIDENCE, PREVALENCE, NATURAL HISTORY

Infant vs. Older Child vs. Adult

Infants, i.e., children in the first year of life, differ more from older children than older children differ from adults, with regard to many aspects of GERD. This was initially recognized by the most evident infantile symptom of GERD, regurgitation, which rarely occurs in adults, and only occasionally occurs in older children (i.e., between 1 year and 18 years). Even the less common symptoms of GERD in infants, such as apnea, are essentially isolated to this age group, while presentations such as asthma exacerbations are more common in older children and adults than in infants. The second notable difference is the natural history of the disorder, which resolves in the majority of infants by 1, or occasionally 2, years of age, whereas reflux disease in older children tends to recur, as it does in adults (2,3). As will be discussed, pathophysiology and therapy are also considerably different in infants. Because of these differences, this chapter will focus on GERD in infants, discussing older children particularly when they differ from adults.

Natural History

The true natural history of GERD in infancy is difficult to define. Initial studies, which could have identified the natural history in untreated patients because effective treatment was unavailable, were limited in their identification of children with GERD. Nonregurgitant reflux was rarely appreciated, and respiratory manifestations of GERD were unheard of. In fact, the earliest studies of natural history equated reflux (or ''chalasia'' as it was sometimes termed) with hiatal hernia (''partial thoracic stomach''), which is currently identified uncommonly in infants and children with GERD. Furthermore, it is likely that children with disorders other than GERD, such as those with vomiting due to food allergy, were included. Through a combination of retrospective and prospective evaluation, Carre calculated that about 60% of these babies with reflux would resolve by 2 years of age, 30% would have vomiting and/or dysphagia (but without stricture) persisting until at least 4 years of age, 5% would develop a stricture, and nearly 5% more would die of malnutrition (4). A later study indicated that one-third of these hiatal hernias ''resolved'' spontaneously (5).

These early studies did, however, identify the same phenomenon we still recognize in infants: spontaneous resolution of GERD in the majority of infants. Though there are few untreated infants with GERD today, most children treated during infancy will no longer require treatment by 1 year of age, and very few persist symptomatic after 18 months of age. Those occasional children who remain in need of therapy beyond that time are unlikely to outgrow their infantile GERD.

Another way to envision the developmental history of reflux (rather than GERD) during childhood is to review the data obtained from pH probe and radiographic studies in children without GERD. Although the pH probe values for esophageal acid reflux show remarkably similar values throughout life (likely due to the infant's consumption of buffering milk formula every few hours), the post-(barium-)meal data from fluoroscopic studies show decreasing amounts of reflux as children age (Figs. 1 and 2) (6).

Still unanswered today, however, is the question of whether infantile reflux that seems to resolve merely ''goes underground,'' and, by no longer manifesting with regurgitation, escapes attention until it resurfaces in older adults with Bar-

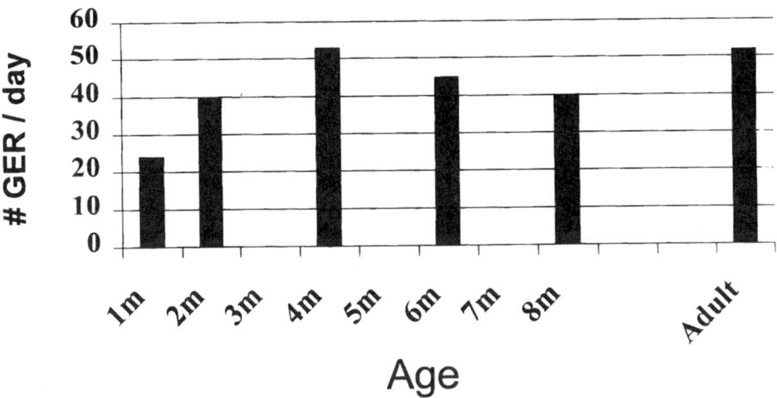

Figure 1 Epidemiology: normal range of pH-probe-documented acid reflux during development. Graphic representation of normal ranges (mean + 2 SD) for acid reflux in children of various ages (n = 285) and in adults (n = 15). (Data derived from Vandenplas Y, Sacre-Smits L. Continuous 24-hour esophageal pH monitoring in 285 asymptomatic infants 0–15 months old. 1987; 6:220–224, and from Johnson LF, DeMeester TR. Twenty-four-hour pH monitoring of the distal esophagus: a quantitative measure of gastroesophageal reflux. Am J Gastroenterol 1974; 62:325–332.)

rett's esophagus (7). This is a critical area for future research, because it would greatly change how we manage infantile reflux, and whether we can continue to regard resolution of symptoms as equivalent to resolution of disease.

Incidence, Prevalence

Recent work has indicated that the prevalence of GERD may be similar at all ages, with respect to varying degrees of disease. Thus, nearly half of all adults have mild symptoms suggesting reflux, but not necessarily GERD, and the same is true of babies during the first year of life; only the type of symptom is different. Likewise, the prevalence of more severe disease, prompting physician consultation and treatment, or even subspecialist referral and invasive testing, is similar in adults and infants. This has prompted adaptation of the GERD "iceberg," described by Castell, to infants (Fig. 3). Differentiation between reflux and reflux disease often challenges the clinician (8).

Infantile GERD generally becomes symptomatic enough to prompt investigation by 1–2 months of age, peaks by 4 or 5 months of age, and begins to wane by about 8 months, when increased torso tone allows the baby to sit upright unsupported, rather than slumping semisupine. Complete resolution, by 10–12 months, usually occurs when the infant gains enough tone and strength to assume

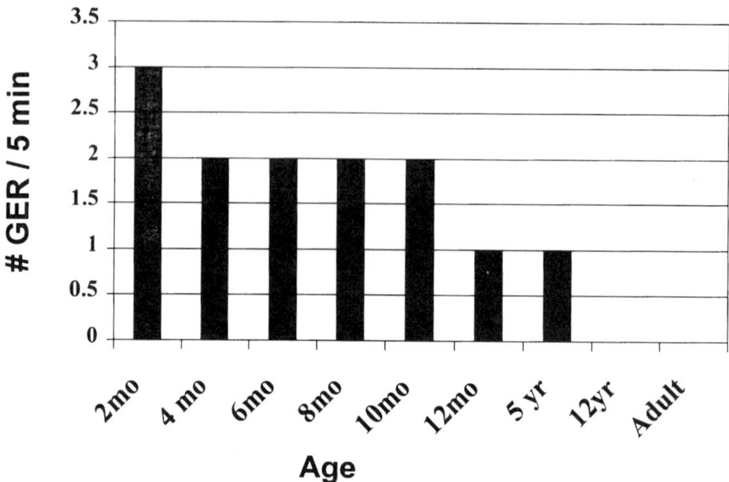

Figure 2 Epidemiology: normal range of fluoroscopically documented volume reflux during development. Histogram depicting the upper range of normal subjects for the number of reflux episodes observed fluoroscopically during 5 min following a barium meal (# GER/5 min). Reflux episodes occur more frequently (and also reach a higher level in the esophagus, not shown here) at younger ages. (Data from Cleveland RH, Kushner DC, Schwartz AN. Gastroesophageal reflux in children: results of a standardized fluoroscopic approach. Am J Roentgenol 141:53–56, 1983.)

sitting and standing positions independently. The prevalence of symptoms of regurgitation during various portions of the first year of life in normal infants is parallel to this progression in infants with GERD (Fig. 4) (9).

Older children more frequently present with esophagitis than with vomiting, and their course tends to be recurrent in half (10). This relapsing and remitting course makes the concept of ''incidence'' more complicated than it is in diseases with a discrete onset and resolution. In addition, because the disease symptoms are less ''visible,'' the incidence and prevalence are less clear than in infants. The annual incidence may be a bit less than in adulthood, because of the shorter lifetime duration of acid exposure and the more limited provocative lifestyle habits.

Sex Ratio, Genetic Predisposition

There seems to be a slight male preponderance in GERD in infants and children, but it is much less than the male preponderance in Barrett's esophagus (11).

Increasing anecdotal evidence points to a familial tendency to manifest GERD. Mirroring the familial predisposition recently noted for Barrett's esopha-

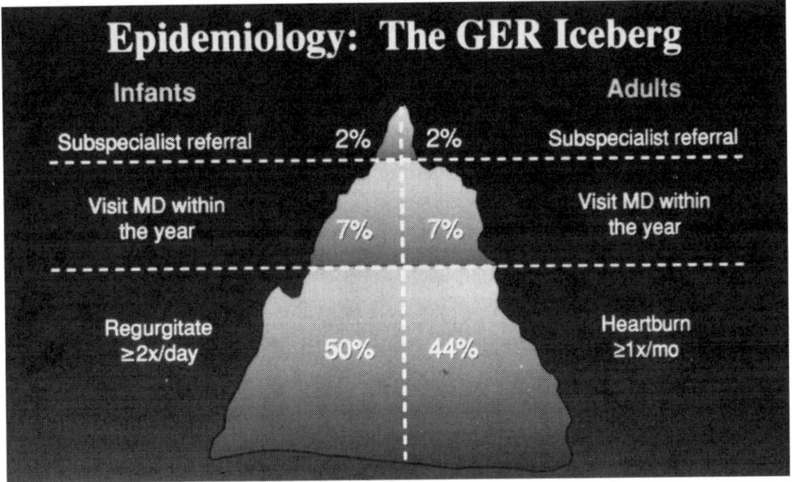

Figure 3 Reflux symptoms range from mild, common ones to less frequent, but more severe ones, both in infants and in adults. Although the incidence of symptoms of varying severities are impressively similar in infants and adults, the primary symptoms, regurgitation and heartburn, are distinctive. (Figure from American Pseudo-obstruction and Hirschsprung's Disease Society Inc., Di Lorenzo C, Flores A, Hyman P, Orenstein S. Pediatric Gastroesophageal Reflux: A Guide for Primary Care Physicians. Slide set 1996; Slide #3. Reproduced by permission. Data from Castell DO. Introduction to pathophysiology of gastroesophageal reflux. In: Castell D, Wu W, Ott D, eds. Gastroesophageal Reflux Disease: Pathogenesis, Diagnosis, Therapy. Mount Kisco, NY: Futura Publishing Company, Inc., 1985:3–9. Gallup Organization. Heartburn Across America. 1988. Kibel MA. In: Report of the 76th Ross Conference on Pediatric Research. 1979.39–42. Orenstein SR. Gastroesophageal reflux. In: Hyman P, Di Lorenzo C, eds. Pediatric Gastrointestinal Motility Disorders. New York: Academy Professional Information Services, Inc. 1994:62–63. Locke GR, Talley NJ, Fett SL, Zinsmeister AR, Melton III LJ. The prevalence and impact of gastroesophageal reflux disease in the United States: A population-based study. Gastroenterology 1994:106(4):A15.

gus in adults, a few reports of clustering of pediatric GERD within families have been reported. If a familial tendency for this very common problem is shown, it will still be necessary to define whether a common environmental factor or a genetic factor is responsible.

Increased in Special Populations

Children with chronic respiratory disease, chronic neurodevelopmental disorders, obesity, and a number of less common disorders manifest increased prevalence of GERD.

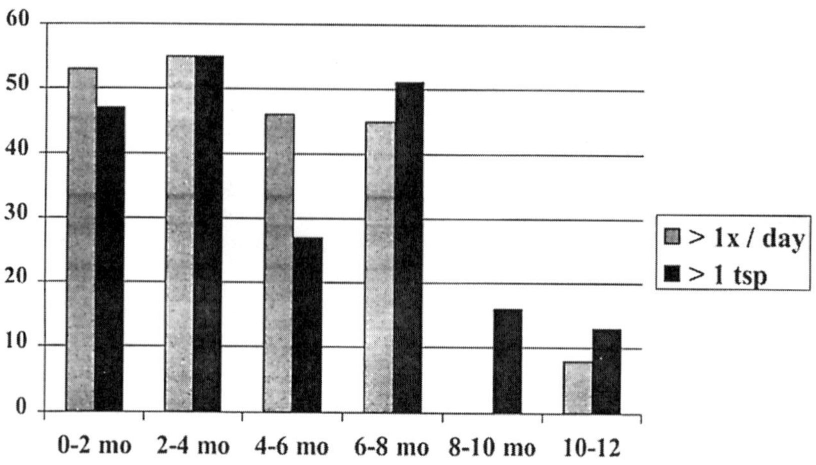

Figure 4 Epidemiology: normal range of observed regurgitant reflux during development. Percent of normal infants exhibiting regurgitation more frequently than once a day (>1×/day) and of an estimated volume more than a teaspoonful (>1 tsp) by parental report. (Unpublished data from the study described in Orenstein SR, Shalaby TM, Cohn J. Reflux symptoms in 100 normal infants: diagnostic validity of the Infant Gastroesophageal Reflux Questionnaire. Clin Pediatr 1996; 35:607–614.)

Chronic Respiratory Disease

Several chronic respiratory diseases of childhood interact with GERD to produce vicious cycles and to worsen GERD in the process (12). Taken all together, they affect more than 10% of children, and form an important arena for attention to GERD.

Asthma affects about 10% of children. Asthma and GERD interact pathophysiologically in complex ways. Both expiration against resistance and coughing increase abdominal pressure and thereby provoke reflux. Some of the medications utilized to treat asthma reduce the lower esophageal sphincter pressure and may also increase reflux. Evidence indicates that the resulting reflux may in turn worsen asthma, by inducing esophagitis, which generates reflexive bronchospasm, or even by promoting microaspiration and subsequent bronchospasm. The actual proportion of children with asthma who also manifest GERD is incompletely defined, but increased over the prevalence of GERD in the general population, and may reach 50%.

Bronchopulmonary disease (BPD), the chronic lung disease that ensues after severe hyaline membrane disease (respiratory distress syndrome) of the surfactant-deficient prematurely born infant, interacts with GERD similarly to asthma. GERD is reported to occur in 10% of premature infants regardless of the presence of BPD, and the pathophysiology of reflux in premature infants has been characterized (13). BPD, occurring in ~1/300 infants, superimposes the pathophysiology of chronic respiratory disease on the developmental predisposition to reflux, thereby exacerbating the reflux of the healthy premature baby. Often incorporating reactive airway disease as well as intrinsic lung damage, BPD is particularly challenging, because it occurs in the smallest infants, with the greatest growth requirements and the greatest caloric requirements for work of breathing. These exaggerated caloric needs challenge the gastric capacity and make supraesophageal migration of refluxate more likely (see Pathophysiology, below). Many of these infants have required tracheostomies for chronic mechanical ventilation. The frequent access of refluxed gastric contents to the pharynx combines with the dysfunctional airway protection engendered by tracheostomy to permit aspiration of refluxate. Chronic supine positioning for mechanical ventilation also facilitates reflux. Infants with bronchopulmonary dysplasia are particularly apt to benefit from fundoplication, which, when combined with gastrostomy feedings, promotes lung growth and healing.

Cystic fibrosis (CF) is a relatively common inherited disease (~1/2000 live births). It often produces reactive airways, so that a pathophysiology similar to asthma facilitates reflux (14). In addition, the increased gastric acid secretion intrinsic to CF makes the refluxate more damaging than in non-CF individuals, and frequent chest physiotherapy provokes reflux on a gravitational basis (15). As medical care for these children with CF improves, more of them reach adulthood; the median survival is now 31 years. Increased survival has unmasked the severity of GERD in these children, and has indicated their increased risk for Barrett's esophagus (16).

Esophageal atresia, with or without tracheoesophageal fistula, is a fourth setting in which chronic lung disease presenting in childhood is associated with increased GERD. This congenital malformation occurs in 1 of 3000 live births, and takes five forms, with the incidence of each indicated in Figure 5. Esophageal atresia does not escape recognition, but delayed diagnosis of the isolated ''H-type fistula'' may be a cause for chronic confusing respiratory symptoms. Reflux is promoted in these infants by a congenital dysfunction of the distal esophageal segment and by the common need for the gastroesophageal junction to be pulled cephalad to the diaphragm (and thus to be unsupported by the diaphragm during straining) when the proximal and distal esophageal segments are anastomosed. It is not uncommon for this increased reflux to engender stricturing at the anastomosis, worsening the dysphagia frequently present in these children (17). They may thus have aspiration during swallowing, as well as during reflux. This aspira-

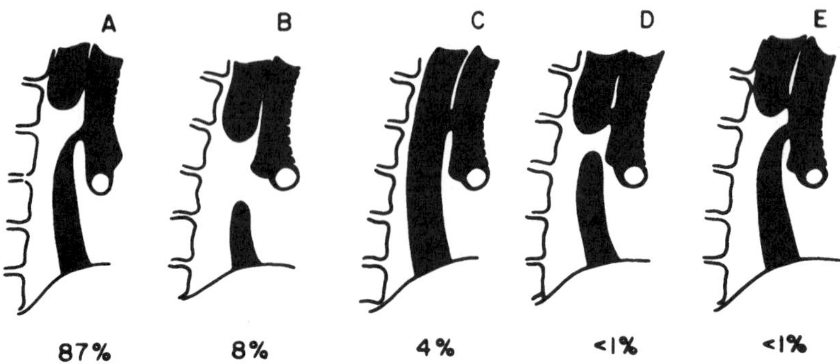

Figure 5 Tracheoesophageal fistula and esophageal atresia. The five forms of this congenital anomaly are diagrammed, and their relative frequencies are indicated. Type C, the "H-type" fistula without esophageal atresia, is the only form that may remain an undiagnosed cause for recurrent aspiration beyond the newborn period, but the other types are associated with increased frequency of reflux disease even after surgical repair. (From Herbst JJ. Esophagus. In: Behrman RE, Kliegman RM, eds. The Digestive System. Nelson Textbook of Pediatrics, 14th ed. Philadelphia: WB Saunders, 1992. Reproduced by permission.)

tion induces lung damage, which combines with GERD-induced reactive airway effects to promote chronic lung disease in these children. Effective therapy of their GERD often improves the lung disease considerably, but the most effective therapy, fundoplication, is made more difficult by the effects of the anastomotic traction on the gastric capacity.

Chronic Neurodevelopmental Disorders

Children with congenital or birth-related severe neurological disease are a second group with increased severity and prevalence of GERD (18). Several aspects of their pathophysiology contribute to the GERD. Spasticity of "cerebral palsy" increases the intra-abdominal pressure, thereby increasing reflux and even promoting hiatal herniation. Similar effects occur during seizures. Severely affected children are often chronically supine, allowing refluxate access to the gastroesophageal junction. Gastrostomy tube feedings, administered to the children whose deficits preclude oral feeding, are frequently administered more rapidly than ordinary meals, challenging gastric receptive relaxation (19).

Obesity

The obese child, like the obese adult, has increased intra-abdominal pressure (as well as increased meal size in many instances) provoking GERD. I have cared for a number of infants whose reflux definitely became more symptomatic as their weight percentiles crossed growth percentiles, ameliorating as their weight returned toward normal for age, without any actual weight reduction.

Miscellaneous

A variety of pediatric syndromes seem to be associated with increased reflux. Familial dysautonomia, trisomy 21, heart-lung transplantation, and chronic renal failure all fall into this category. Clarity about the true incidence of GERD in these disorders, as well as about the pathophysiology for any increased incidence, is limited currently.

CLINICAL PRESENTATIONS, SYMPTOMS, SIGNS

General

It is useful to conceptualize the clinical presentations of pediatric GERD as grouped in clusters, depending on the migration of the refluxate. Refluxate that remains in the esophagus causes inflammation, engendering pain, bleeding (and subsequent anemia), and worsening inflammation resulting in stricturing and Barrett's esophagus. Refluxate that escapes the esophagus into the mouth may be expelled from the mouth, producing malnutrition, or may be reswallowed, possibly producing dental etching by the acid if it remains in the mouth for a time. Refluxate that escapes the esophagus but is allowed into the nasopharynx by dysfunctional soft palate closure may be regurgitated nasally, or may contribute to chronic otitis or sinusitis by inducing inflammation at the eustachian tubes or entry to the sinuses. Upper-airway effects of reflux occur either when the refluxate reaches the pharynx and is not prevented from laryngeal penetration, or when pharyngeal reflux stimulates reflexes affecting laryngeal function. Similarly, lower-airway effects of reflux may be induced by aspirated pharyngeal reflux or by esophagopulmonary reflexes when the refluxate remains in the esophagus. All of these nonesophageal effects of GERD have received increasing attention from diverse subspecialties, and have been termed, ''supraesophageal'' GERD (20). I will discuss the pediatric manifestations of each of these symptomatic groups below. Because these diverse symptomatic presentations have distinct and dissimilar pathophysiologies, diagnostic strategies, and differential diagnoses, I will subsequently detail those aspects for each of the groups separately.

Esophagitis

Pain

Even in adults, verbal descriptions of subjective pain may be misleading; children naturally give less precise descriptions, and infants simply cry to represent a wide variety of negative sensations, from boredom to hunger to pain. The symptom of ''colic'' in infancy is a colloquial term indicating frequent crying, and has been attributed to a variety of causations, including family problems, carbohydrate malabsorption, and protein allergy (21). It occurs, however, at the time that GERD is most prevalent in infants. Several studies have shown GERD to manifest with colicky crying (22), including a pH probe and treatment study that found that 16 of 26 infants with ''colic'' had abnormal pH-metry, and responded to therapy with cisapride and cimetidine (23). However, crying is not sensitive or specific enough for diagnosis of esophagitis (24). The pain of esophagitis in infants may also contribute to any malnutrition due to regurgitation of calories, because the odynophagia leads to refusal to suck and swallow, despite evident hunger (25).

Bleeding

Esophagitis severe enough to cause bleeding from erosions or ulceration occurs in children, as in adults. The mildest chronic bleeding may manifest simply as iron-deficiency anemia. The bleeding may also present as hemoccult positivity in stool samples. More severe bleeding, with hematemesis or even melena, also occurs, but it is rarely the first manifestation of GERD in the neurologically intact child, who can complain of the pain of esophagitis prior to severe bleeding. While rare in infancy, such bleeding has even been reported to occur prenatally, staining the amniotic fluid (26).

Stricture

Esophageal peptic strictures affect pediatric patients as well as adults. An older study, which may have included congenital stenoses along with peptic strictures, identified an unexpected age distribution: 50% of the children presented younger than 2 years of age, 25% between 2 and 5 years, and the other 25% between 5 and 15 years (27). Strictures are less common today than in the past, presumably because of greater recognition and earlier and better therapy of GERD in young children (28). Peptic strictures are generally found in the middle and distal esophagus, and range in length from discrete localized narrowing to several centimeters; a recent study reported nearly half of the children to have strictures longer than 3 cm (28). Recognition of strictures may be delayed during infancy, because the diet contains no solid food. Half of all children with Barrett's esophagus manifest strictures; it is wise to repeat endoscopy after aggressive antireflux therapy to identify Barrett's epithelium in children with strictures.

Barrett's Esophagus

An important pathological study of Barrett's esophagus contrasted pediatric and adult patients (Table 1), finding a lower male preponderance and a lower preva-

Table 1 Barrett's Epithelium (Glandular Intestinal Epithelium)

Child (n = 28; age = 12 y [1–23 y])	Adult (n = 38; age = 56 y [29–80 y])
Male:Female = 2:1 Goblet prevalence = 50% Prevalence and density increase with age Neurological disability = 43% Nissen decr. inflammation but NOT Goblet density	Male:Female = 9:1 Goblet prevalence = 84% Prevalence and density do NOT increase with age >41 y

Source: Ref. 29.

lence of goblet cells in the children's "glandular intestinal epithelium" (29). This study indicated that the prevalence and density of goblet cells increase with age during childhood, both between and within patients, but not after age 41 (29).

Another study, which examined pediatric and adult patients, but only those who already manifested goblet cells, found the prevalence of Barrett's esophagus to be 0.02% of all children undergoing endoscopy between the ages of 8 and 17 years (contrasted with 0.93% of all adults in their ninth decade undergoing endoscopies, and 12% of all adults biopsied during endoscopy, and up to 44% of all adults with strictures) (30).

Provocative factors for Barrett's esophagus in children include chronic neurological disability and chronic respiratory disease, both known to provoke GERD, and the former associated with limited ability to complain of symptoms (29–32). Gastric tube reconstructions of the esophagus also predispose to cervical Barrett's esophagus, for obvious reasons.

While aggressive antireflux therapy, usually incorporating fundoplication, is utilized in these children to prevent adenocarcinoma, there is not much evidence that such therapy induces regression of the abnormal epithelium (29).

Adenocarcinoma subsequent to Barrett's esophagus has been reported in only 10 patients younger than 25 years of age, ranging from 11 to 25 years, with a median of 16 years (31). All but one were male, and at least three had severe neurological disability. All but one presented as a mass or stricture (in the mid- or distal esophagus), and all but one had extraesophageal spread at the time of diagnosis.

Dysmotility due to Esophagitis

Children with severe esophagitis, defined as endoscopic mucosal breaks and inflammatory cells (polymorphonuclear or eosinophilic leukocytes), have decreased amplitude of peristaltic waves, and a more frequent occurrence of simultaneous, broad-based, double-peaked waves (33). In contrast, children with chest pain and mild to moderate esophagitis, but without heartburn or regurgitation and without endoscopic ulceration, had no spontaneous dysmotility (34). A subsequent study by the same group indicated, however, that a subgroup of such children do manifest ''conversion'' of previously normal motility patterns to abnormal ones during esophageal acid perfusion, but that it only occurred in less than half of the children who complained of chest pain during infusion. The findings in these three children included increased duration and amplitude of contractions during wet swallows (35). The disparities among these studies await clarification.

Regurgitation

Malnutrition

Regurgitation, even expelled with enough force to be considered projectile vomiting, is common in infantile GERD. This loss of ingested calories is exacerbated by a refusal to consume adequate calories, due, it seems, to odynophagia caused by esophagitis (25). Marked malnutrition, termed ''failure to thrive'' and most sensitively detected by consecutive plotting of weights and lengths on pediatric growth curves, is thus a fairly common presentation of infantile GERD. As with other causes of inadequate caloric retention, weight percentiles drop prior to length percentiles, and concern should be raised by a decrease in weight percentile, prior to the weight actually becoming ''abnormal'' (less than fifth percentile).

Dental Etching

Lingual surface dental enamel etching produced by regurgitated gastric acid that remains in the mouth has been described (36). It can be distinguished from dental caries by the location on the teeth.

Contrasted with Rumination

Infantile reflux may have more in common with rumination than previously recognized (37). In fact, reflux in infants tends to become regurgitant when propelled by abdominal wall muscle contractions, quite similar to the pathophysiology of rumination (38). The ''psychobehavioral cause'' for the activity may be different—the infant may not be regurgitating intentionally, and the activity may not represent psychopathology. The cause for the frequency of regurgitation in infants is discussed below. I have also observed infants who stuck their fists back into their throat, and were believed to be ''ruminating'' because of some psychosocial deficits, but whose odd behavior ceased when their esophagitis was treated pharmacologically.

Nasopharyngeal

Nasal regurgitation, otalgia, sinusitis, and sneezing have all been associated with gastroesophageal reflux in children recently (39,40). All of them require that the refluxate escapes the esophagus, and, further, that it makes its way between the soft palate and the posterior pharyngeal surface, to access the nasopharynx.

Infants not uncommonly manifest regurgitation as nasal regurgitation, which we have attributed to a developmental immaturity of velopalatal function, which resolves with maturation. Nasopharyngeal pH monitoring has shown more pH below 6 in children with chronic rhinopharyngitis than in control children.

Early reports also suggest a similar role for reflux in sinusitis, indicated by resolution of chronic sinusitis after therapy for GERD (39). An increased frequency of sneezing (a nasopharyngeal protective mechanism parallel to cough for the lower airway) at onset of reflux episodes in infants, demonstrated by linked pH probe and video monitoring, also suggests an access of refluxate into the nasopharynx (40).

Upper Airway

Laryngeal effects of gastroesophageal reflux may result from gastroesophagopharyngeal reflux, which then has access to the larynx, or might even be mediated by esophagolaryngeal reflexes. More data support actual contact of refluxate with upper airway structures, producing symptomatic effects based either on reflexive laryngeal closure or on laryngeal inflammation (39,41,42).

Laryngitis, Hoarseness

Laryngitis and its symptomatic representation, hoarseness, may be caused by acid damage to the laryngeal structures. Frequently, multiple etiologies are operational: reflux laryngitis, ''voice abuse,'' chronic throat clearing, and cigarette smoke exposure may play concurrent roles. Frequently, most efficient identification of reflux as a factor utilizes aggressive empirical antireflux therapy as a diagnostic test (43).

Subglottic Stenosis

Recent otolaryngological literature recognizes GERD, in addition to trauma or infection, as a cause for subglottic stenosis (39). Trauma (from chronic intubation, for example) may interact with reflux-induced injury to potentiate subglottic stenosis and impede its healing. The ability of reflux to induce subglottic stenosis without inducing any reflux esophagitis may be understood as a function of the greater susceptibility of the ciliated columnar epithelium of the airway (in comparison to the squamous epithelium of the esophagus) to acid damage, of the more limited acid clearance functions of the airway (i.e., no peristalsis), and of the lack of bicarbonate-rich salivary washdown in the airway. Indeed, animal models have indicated that relatively brief exposure of the subglottis to gastric contents can have quite profound effects.

Apnea

Obstructive apnea in infants has been clearly shown in some cases to be due to reflux episodes (44). These episodes generally occur within an hour or so following a feeding, while the baby is in the supine or seated position, and produce initial plethoric coloring often followed by cyanosis. Gastric contents may appear at the mouth or nose. These events occur fairly commonly: several such infants may be admitted to a large pediatric hospital for evaluation each week, and significant numbers of others likely do not present to the hospital. Uncommonly, these events may be lethal. Because such ''arrests'' in infants are usually respiratory, in contrast to the predominance of cardiac arrests in adults, they are usually reversible if ventilation is reestablished promptly, and they are often spontaneously reversed if the infant is positioned to clear his or her own pharynx of refluxate.

Concurrent pH probe with polysomnography has convincingly demonstrated temporal relationships between spontaneous reflux and obstructive apnea (Fig. 6), and the same phenomenon produced by experimental acid infusion into the esophagus has confirmed causation (45). A huge series of about 1400 very carefully studied infants with a history of apnea (''apparent life-threatening event,'' ALTE, or ''near-miss sudden infant death syndrome,'' SIDS) found GERD responsible in half (46).

Stridor, Spasmodic Croup

Analogous to infantile apnea, intermittent stridor may be induced by laryngeal closure, which may be seen as a protective reflex. It seems that this phenomenon is more common in infants than in adults, perhaps because, even when unstimulated, the more limited cross-section of their upper airway provides more increased resistance than the lower airway, and perhaps because infants are more susceptible to airway protective reflexes, whose immaturity may inhibit reopening. It is possible that the afferents are located in the esophagus, but studies have not clearly differentiated this scenario from one involving laryngeal afferents (47).

Frightening episodes of spasmodic croup are occasionally due to reflux; the children who manifest this phenomenon are often somewhat older than the infants presenting with infantile apnea, and seem to outgrow the problem as they age. Even adults, however, have demonstrated this manifestation of GERD. Liq-

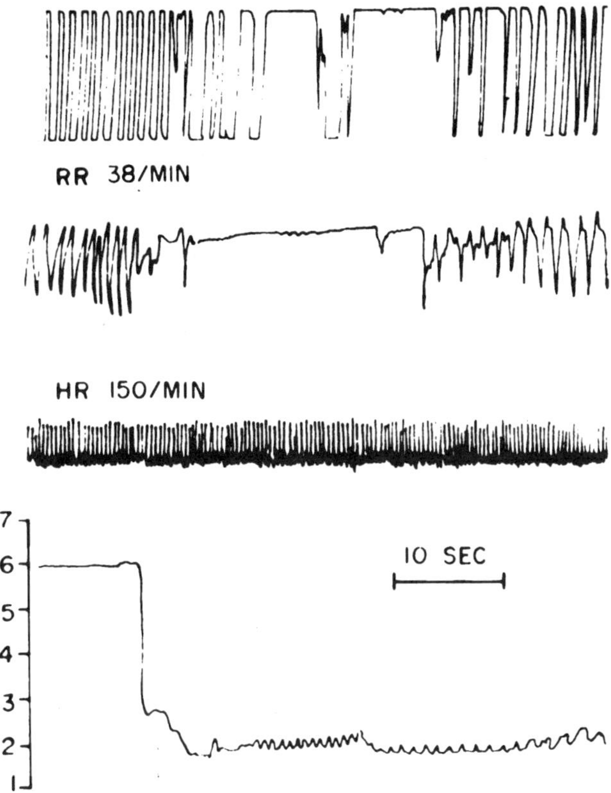

Figure 6 Esophageal acidification causing obstructive apnea in an infant. Spontaneous reflux (distal esophageal pH—bottom channel) is followed immediately by obstructive apnea, documented by cessation of air movement at the nostrils (nasal thermistor—second channel) while respiratory efforts and chest wall movement initially continued (impedance pneumotachogram—top channel); clinically the infant appeared to have laryngospasm. (From Herbst JJ, Minton SD, Book LS. Gastroesophageal reflux causing respiratory distress and apnea in newborn infants. J Pediatr 1979; 95:763–768. Reproduced by permission.)

uid refluxate may not even be required: a report in two adults postulated aerosolized refluxate as provocative of severe acute laryngospasm (48).

Lower Airway

Aspiration Pneumonia, Chronic Bronchitis

Macroaspiration of refluxate causing aspiration pneumonia occurs most frequently in pediatric patients with chronic severe neurological disability. These children, in addition to being chronically supine, which promotes reflux, may have impaired airway protective mechanisms, facilitating actual entry of refluxate into the lower airway. Such aspiration is more often suspected than proven. Chronic bronchitis caused by recurrently aspirated refluxate was one of the earliest suspected reflux-associated respiratory conditions; currently it is not as frequently diagnosed as many of the others (49).

Asthma

Asthma provoked by reflux is likely even more prevalent in children than in adults. Perhaps 10% of children have GERD and perhaps 10% have asthma, but about 50% of pediatric asthmatics have GERD, indicating an association (50). Therapeutic and experimental studies have indicated the likelihood that reflux worsens asthma, but it is also clear that the pathophysiology of asthma can make reflux worse. Chest pain is a marker for esophagitis in asthmatic children whose asthma may improve with pharmacotherapy for GERD (51).

Miscellaneous Symptoms

Sandifer's Syndrome

An odd, uncommon symptom of GERD, Sandifer's syndrome involves contorted posturing, particularly of the neck, in response to reflux. The exact mechanisms are unclear, but one study suggested that peristalsis was improved in one child during these manuevers (52).

Hiccups, Cough, Sneeze

Hiccups have sometimes been identified with reflux, particularly with reflux esophagitis, in children as well as adults (40). Cough represents an upper- and lower-airway response to an irritant; sneeze is a similar reflex designed to clear the nasopharynx (40). A pediatric study of chronic (>1 month) cough in children with normal chest radiographs identified GERD as the cause in 15%, the third most common cause, following asthma and sinusitis (53).

Hypertrophic Osteoarthropathy

Very unusual manifestations attributed to GERD are hypertrophic osteoarthropathy and digital clubbing (54,55). These are extremely infrequent manifestations, and the mechanisms remain obscure.

PATHOPHYSIOLOGY, RISK FACTORS

The pathophysiology of reflux disease in children has many similarities with that in adults, but several areas in which the mechanisms are quite different. In contrast to earlier hypotheses, lower-esophageal-sphincter (LES) tone is adequately established, even in premature infants, and the gastric secretions are adequately noxious to induce esophagitis in infants. However, clearance of refluxate is somewhat impaired in young infants, particularly prematures, both by posture and by some decrements in peristaltic function. Gastric compliance seems to be reduced in infants, provoking reflux. Furthermore, a major difference between infants and adults, is dietary—the meal volume, frequency, and components. Immature respiratory reflexes comprise a final important difference.

For Increased Frequency of Reflux Episodes

Pediatric mechanisms for reflux have been comprehensively reviewed recently (56,57).

Lower Esophageal Sphincter

The LES is the primary barrier to reflux, and is bolstered by the perisphincteric crural diaphragm, in children as in adults.

Tonic Pressure. Although the LES tone was formerly presumed to be inadequate in young children with GERD, improved methods for evaluating it have shown that most children with GERD have adequate LES tone to prevent reflux episodes, and that impaired LES pressure may be a sequel to GERD esophagitis, rather than the primary cause of it.

Phasic Relaxations. In adults, transient LES relaxations (TLESRs) are now understood to be the major mechanism for the occurrence of reflux episodes. Multiple studies have found TLESRs to be the most important event allowing reflux to occur (56,57). These relaxations are probably mediated by nitric oxide (and perhaps vasoactive intestinal peptide), as in adults. A pediatric study found increased levels of nitric oxide and prostaglandins in the esophageal mucosa of children with reflux esophagitis (58).

Perisphincteric Factors (Crural Diaphragm, Hiatal Hernia). The crural diaphragm supports the LES, and the intricate reflexive linkage of the LES and crura assures their working in tandem to allow belching and emesis but to resist strain-induced reflux. Hiatal hernia prevents the bolstering function of the crura from being applied to the LES, and thus facilitates strain-induced reflux. Similar to current understanding in adults, hiatal hernia has also been found to delay esophageal clearance in infants (59). However, in contrast to early writings on the subject (60), hiatal hernia (''partial thoracic stomach'') is relatively uncommon in childhood GERD, and is seen most often in conjunction with severe neurological disability or repaired esophageal atresia.

Location of Gastric Contents Relative to the LES. The stomach generally contains both air and liquid (or semiliquid) material. When air is adjacent to the LES, only belches result from LES relaxation; when liquid is adjacent to the LES, reflux results. This fact is responsible for the beneficial effects of elevation of the head of the bed (in supine individuals, at least) and of prone position in infants (because of the posterior location of the gastroesophageal junction) (61) (Fig. 9). It is also responsible for the detrimental effect of supine and (semisupine) seated position in infants (62).

Gastric Pressure/Volume Relationships

Gastric pressure/volume relationships are crucial differences between infant and adult reflux, and underlie the prevalence of regurgitant reflux in infants.

Gastric Tone and Compliance. Preliminary but exciting work indicates that the young infant has a ''stiffer'' stomach, which relaxes less effectively during mealtime filling (Fig. 7) (63,64). This decreased compliance means in-

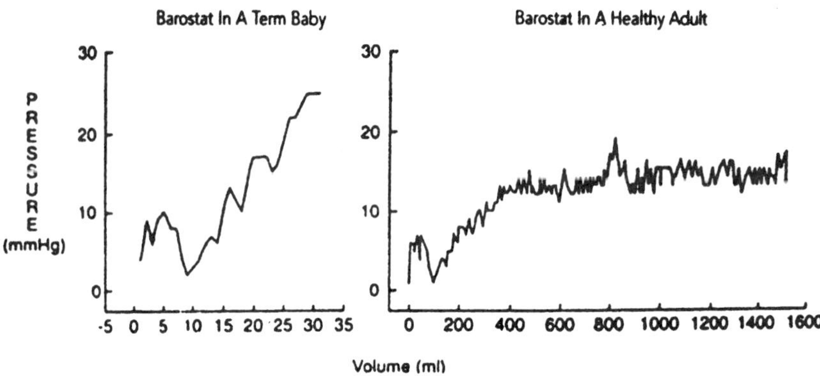

Figure 7 Gastric compliance in a neonate compared to an adult. The pressure-volume relationship in response to intragastric balloon inflation measured by means of an electronic barostat demonstrates less compliance and decreased receptive relaxation in a term baby (left) compared with an adult (right). (From Orenstein SR, Izadnia F, Khan S. Gastroesophageal reflux disease in children. In: Katz P, ed. Gastroesophageal Reflux Disease. Gastroenterology Clinics of North America 1999 28(4). Philadelphia: Saunders, 1999. Courtesy of Carlo Di Lorenzo, MD, Pittsburgh, PA. Reproduced by permission.)

creased pressure at a given volume, and promotes volumetric reflux and regurgitation.

Phasic Gastric Pressure Increases. Superimposed on the increased tonic gastric pressure are phasic increases in gastric pressure produced by straining, via squirming and crying in babies. Sleep reflux seems to occur only during movement (65), and regurgitant reflux (in contrast to reflux, which remains intraesophageal) is associated with phasic increases in gastric pressure induced by contraction of abdominal wall somatic musculature (Fig. 8) (38).

External Contributions to Gastric Pressure (Obesity, Clothing, Slouching). There has not been much evaluation of the role of obesity and tight clothing in children; it is assumed that these factors may play a role similar to that in adults. However, it has been shown that slouching posture of the seated infant induces markedly increased reflux (Fig. 9) (62), likely due both to the positioning of the posterior gastroesophageal junction below the air-fluid interface in the stomach and to the increased gastric pressure allowed by gravity's action on the limited torso tone of the infant.

Meal Volume vs. Gastric Volume. Inadequately appreciated has been the extreme differences between infants and adults with regard to meal-to-gastric-volume relationships. The tripling of weight that occurs in infants during their first year of life mandates a tremendous caloric intake, several times that of the adult on a per-kilogram basis. Even feeding infants up to twice as often as adults eat does not eliminate the necessity for relatively large-volume feeding to the infants (66).

Gastric Emptying. Gastric emptying may be slower in infants than adults, with gastric electrical dysrhythmias possibly playing a role in some children (67,68).

For Esophagitis

Refluxate Components

Hydrochloric acid, secreted by the stomach, is the primary noxious agent inducing esophagitis. Contrary to earlier beliefs that gastric acid secretion was more limited in infants than adults, such secretion reaches levels comparable to those of adults within a month or two after birth (6). (It is true, however, that infants' gastric contents are buffered by their milk formula feedings for much of the day—up to 2 h after each of about six meals. That infant and adult daily esophageal acid exposures are similar—see Fig. 1—implies that infants experience much greater total reflux, in light of this buffering of the infants' gastric acid.)

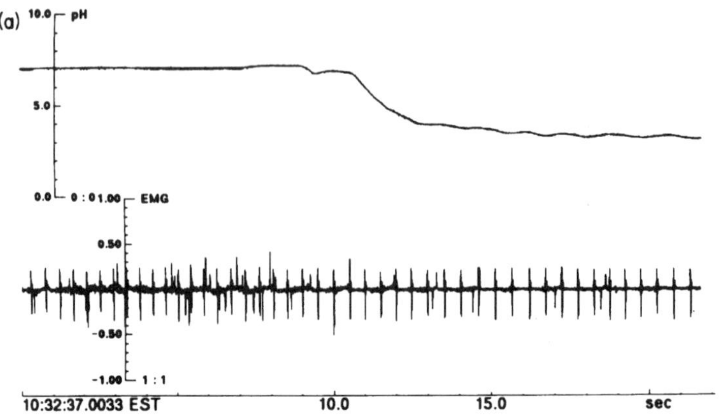

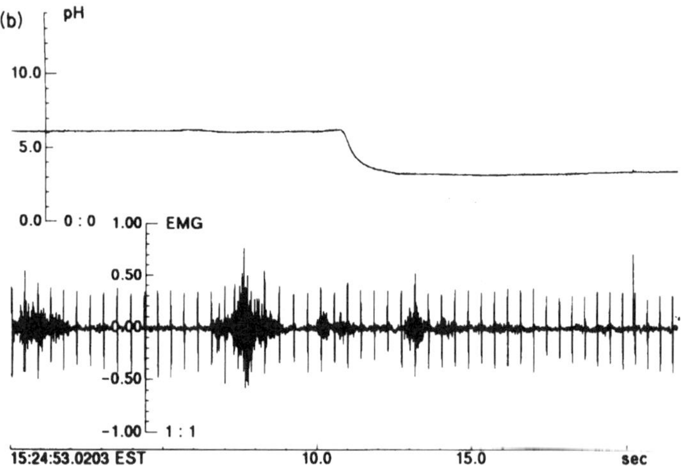

Figure 8 Rectus abdominis contraction is associated with regurgitant reflux. Examples of nonregurgitant (a) and regurgitant (b) reflux. The distal esophageal pH is represented in the top tracing in each panel. The rectus abdominis electromyographic (EMG) activity (with background electrocardiographic signal) is represented in the bottom tracing; the EMG scale units are mV. It can be seen that there is no rectus abdominis activity associated with the nonregurgitant episode, but a burst of rectus abdominis activity a few seconds prior to the esophageal pH drop accompanying regurgitation. (There is also a bit of electromyographic activity following this reflux episode, which probably represents activity that is a response to the regurgitation.) (From Orenstein SR, Dent J, Deneault LG, Lutz JW, Wessel HB, Kelsey SF, Shalaby TM. Regurgitant reflux, vs. non-regurgitant reflux, is preceded by rectus abdominis contraction in infants. Neurogastroenterol Motil 1994; 6(4): 271–277. Reproduced by permission.)

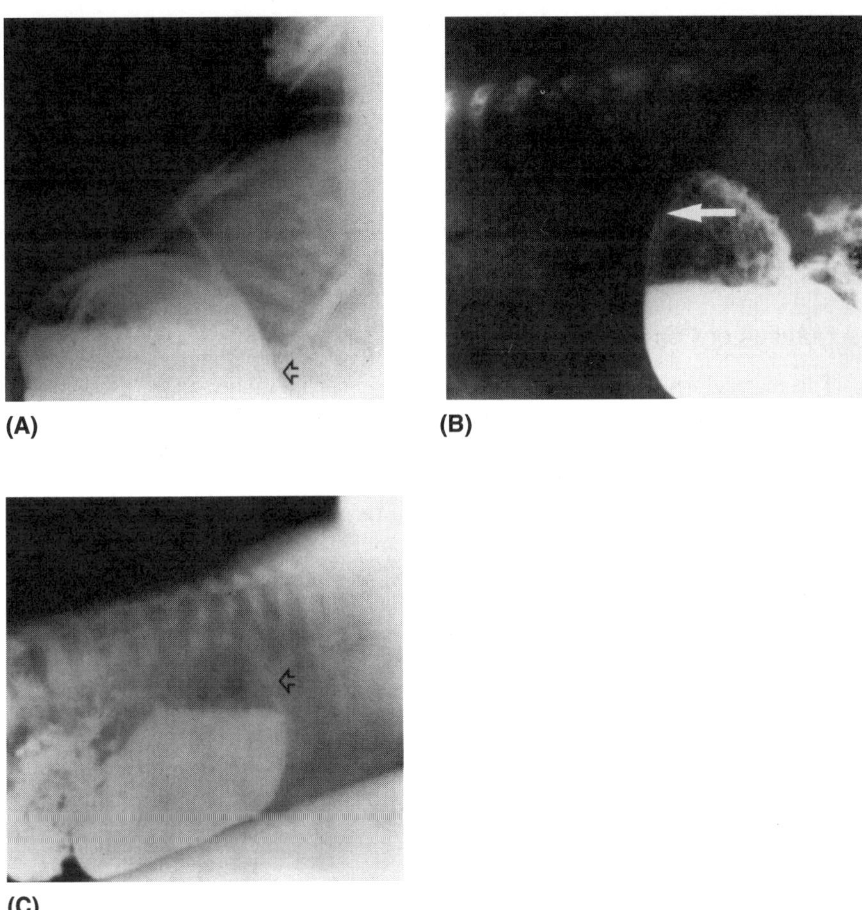

Figure 9 Radiographic demonstration of the relative positions of the gastric air bubble and the gastroesophageal junction in an infant positioned seated (A), prone (B), and prone with head elevated (C). The arrows indicate the locations of the gastroesophageal junction, which is submerged when the child is seated, but not when he is in either prone position. Note the spontaneous reflux of barium occurring while the infant is seated. (From Orenstein SR, Whitington PF, Orenstein DM. The infant seat as treatment for gastroesophageal reflux. N Engl J Med 1983; 309(13):760–763, and from Orenstein SR, Whitington PF. Positioning for prevention of infant gastroesophageal reflux. J Pediatr 1983; 103(4): 534–537. Reproduced by permission.)

Pepsin production requires acid to liberate it from pepsinogen, so that reduction of gastric acidity also decreases the peptic component of injury. Pepsin production reaches 50% of adult levels by 4 months of age, and 100% by about 2 years (6).

Alkaline reflux, predicated on duodenogastric reflux preceding gastroesophageal reflux, occurs in young children as well as in adults. Infants do not secrete bile salts at adult levels until about 1 year of age, but trypsin secretion is at adult levels from birth (6). The importance of alkaline reflux is debated at both ends of the age spectrum (69).

Duration of Contact with Esophagus

The morphometric parameters indicative of esophagitis increase as daily acid exposure increases, in infancy as in adulthood (Fig. 10) (70). This fact highlights the pathogenic importance of esophageal clearance mechanisms: gravity clearance, peristalsis, and salivary washdown.

Gravity clearance is impaired by the recumbency necessitated by the lack of torso tone in infants. Although it was previously believed that supporting infants in a seated position would rectify this problem, experimental investigation indicated that seating actually markedly worsens both reflux frequency and esophageal clearance (Fig. 11) (62).

Peristalsis is adequate for clearance in newborns, but its velocity is slower than in adults (71).

Salivary washdown has not received much attention in infants, but it is likely that improvements in GERD seen with bethanechol therapy in the past had more to do with its increase of salivation than with its increase of tonic LES pressure (72).

Mucosal Protection

The role of mucosal protection in infants is relatively unexamined.

Helicobacter pylori

A study in children suggested that clinical improvement of those with both *H. pylori* infection and esophagitis required antibiotic therapy in addition to acid suppression (73). Because children have more limited chronicity of *H. pylori* infection, as well as less prevalent infection, the induction of esophagitis by eradication of the bacteria may not be as prominent an issue in pediatrics.

For Extraesophageal GERD

General Requirements

Volume, ''height,'' and propulsion of refluxate in the esophagus are interrelated aspects that allow it to have access to extraesophageal sites. The gastric pressure/

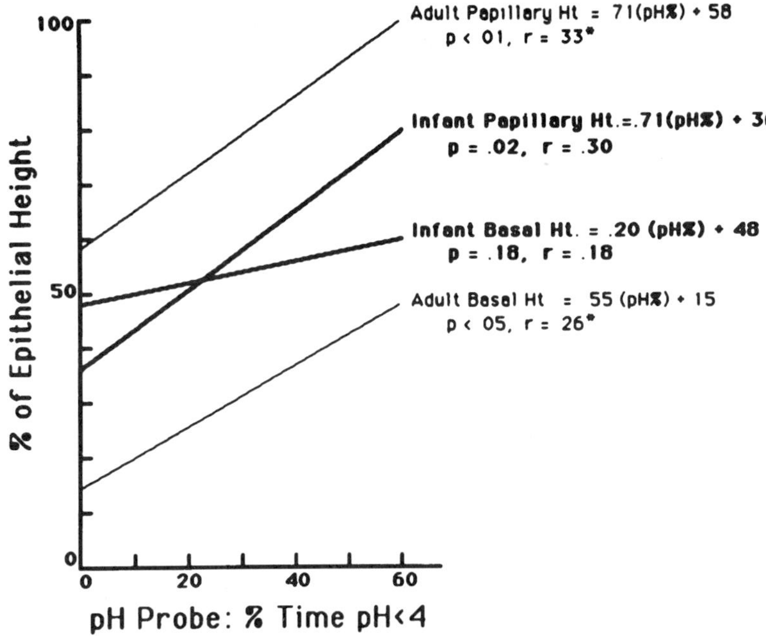

Figure 10 Comparison of the relationship between daily esophageal acid exposure and morphometric measures of esophagitis in infants and adults. Shown is the relationship between daily esophageal acid exposure (pH probe: % time pH < 4) and both papillary height and basal layer thickness in infants and in adults. In infants, papillary height correlates better with the percent time the esophageal pH is less than 4 than does the basal layer thickness, both expressed as a percentage of the total epithelial thickness (% of epithelial height). The slope and correlation coefficient for papillary height versus acid exposure are remarkably similar in infants and adults, but 24-h acid exposure predicts only about 10% of the variability of papillary height for both infants and adults. (Infant data from Orenstein SR, Becich MB, Putnam PE, Shalaby TM, DiGiorgio CJ, Kelsey SF. Correlations between morphometric parameters of esophagitis and pH probe data in infants. Gastroenterology 1994; 106(4,Pt2):A152. Adult data from Johnson L, DeMeester, Haggitt R. Esophageal epithelial response to gastroesophageal reflux: A quantitative study. Dig Dis Sci 1978; 23:498.)

volume relationships discussed above permit this to occur in young children much more frequently than in adults. Regurgitation itself is an ''extraesophageal'' manifestation of reflux, and it occurs daily in the majority of young infants.

Upper-esophageal sphincter (UES) function has received attention in children (74). The UES pressure increases during abdominal straining and during reflux events, but UES relaxations are superimposed on this increased tone, allowing refluxate access to the pharynx while protecting the esophagus from hazardous increases in pressure.

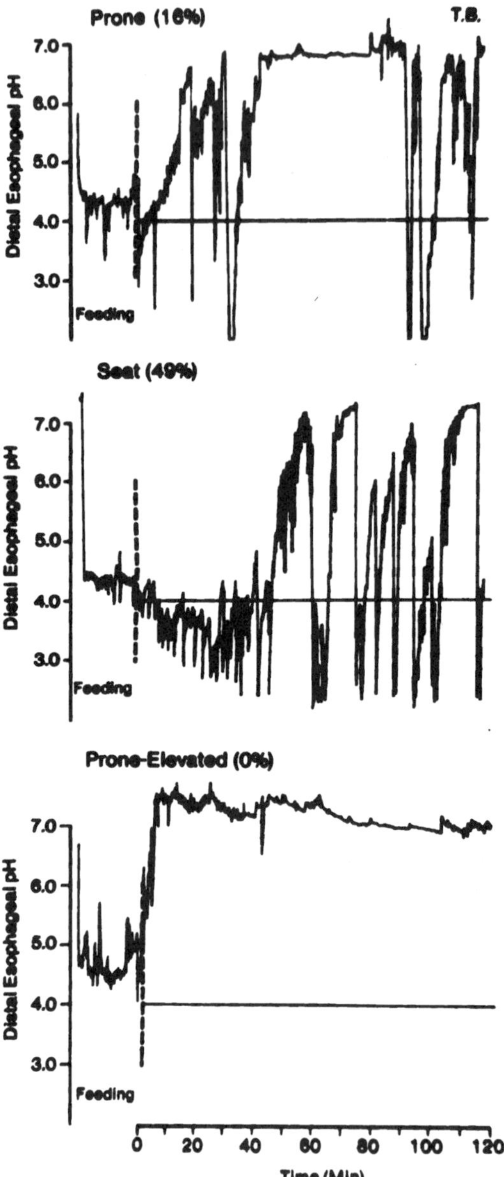

Figure 11 Effect of position on reflux quantity. An infant monitored in three different positions during three otherwise identical postprandial periods for the study reported in Orenstein SR, Whitington PF, Orenstein DM. The infant seat as treatment for gastroesophageal reflux. N Engl J Med 1983; 309(13):760–763. In the prone position the percent of time the esophageal pH was below 4 was 16%, whereas in the seated position it was 49%, and in the prone-elevated position it was 0%. Figure 9 illustrates an explanation for some of this effect of position on reflux quantity.

Failure of normal protections when refluxate achieves access to the pharynx allows it to migrate into the nasopharynx, larynx and lower airway, or mouth. The chief protection is reswallowing via a primary swallow for material that has reached the mouth or a pharyngeal swallow for material that has not. These protections have largely been explored in adults.

Esophagoairway reflexes must be invoked to explain extraesophageal manifestations of GERD when refluxate propulsion and UES relaxation do not occur to allow the actual migration of refluxate above the UES. These reflexes, demonstrated by esophageal acid infusion, have been suggested to cause asthma, stridor, and apnea in children (75–77). It is likely that the apnea, and perhaps stridor, are developmental phenomena, and the reflexes disappear with maturation (78). It has been difficult in these investigations to be certain that there was no extraesophageal migration of acid infused into the esophagus, but it is likely that these reflexes do play a role in some pediatric extraesophageal GERD. It would be illuminating to perform similar studies with a pH probe proximal to the esophageal infusion site, or to perform the studies in duplicate after inhibition of the esophageal sensitivity to the acid (79).

Oral Sites and Emesis

A ''ruminant'' form of regurgitant reflux, which reaches the mouth but is reswallowed, may engender dental disease if it is slowly cleared from the mouth. The ''propelled'' reflux of infants often resembles vomiting, and may even be described as ''projectile'' for reasons noted above.

Nasopharyngeal Sites

Velopalatal closure protects the nasopharynx from refluxate. Some infants seem to display an immaturity of this protective function, manifesting nasopharyngeal reflux and regurgitation through the nose, which disappear with maturation (80).

Laryngeal Sites

The intricate reflexive protections of the upper airway by the epiglottis, aryepiglottic folds, and vocal cord closure have been characterized in detail in adults recently (81,82). Pediatric, and particularly infantile, correlates of these reflexes may be excessively active, producing obstructive apnea as a manifestation of reflux (83,84).

Lower-Airway Sites

Similarly, the lower airway may be involved with pathological reflexes, engendering bronchoconstriction and asthma. Potential mechanisms for lower-airway reactivity are intricate. They include afferent sites in the esophagus or airway;

mediators that may be neural or chemical; and resulting obstruction from aspirated material, secreted material, airway edema, or bronchoconstriction (85).

DIFFERENTIAL DIAGNOSIS

Children differ from adults in the range of differential diagnostic considerations for the varied manifestations of GERD, because of the diversity of congenital and developmental disorders that must be contemplated. Most of the symptomatic presentations of GERD may also be presentations for congenital anatomical abnormalities, genetic metabolic disorders, or acquired infectious diseases in the immunologically naïve young child. Following are some of these differential diagnoses, organized by symptomatic presentation.

For Regurgitation

For Vomiting

The differential diagnosis of emesis in children is broad (Table 2) and varies by age, such that congenital partial gastrointestinal obstructions, metabolic disorders, and formula allergy must be considered in young infants and inflammatory conditions and pregnancy must be considered in adolescents. Because infantile regurgitation resembles rumination pathophysiologically, it may be useful to consider both organic and behavioral antecedents for the symptom in babies.

For Dental Findings

Acid dental etching is differentiated from common dental caries by the lingual location and smoother etched appearance (36).

For Esophagitis

For Pain

The diagnostic considerations for epigastric and substernal pain in older children are quite similar to those in adults (except for the infrequency of cardiac ischemia), including peptic ulceration of the stomach or esophagus, pill esophagitis (86), or spastic esophageal dysmotility (87). Infant crying, or ''colic,'' however, prompts a much broader differential diagnosis (Table 3) (21). While infants may respond to family stress by intractable crying, and the crying induces further stress and contributes to a vicious cycle, it is wise to remain open to the concept of an organic cause for the crying (88). The most common causes, other than reflux esophagitis or familial stress, include formula protein allergy or carbohy-

Table 2 Differential Diagnosis of Vomiting by Anatomic Locus of Stimulus

I. Stimulation of supramedullary receptors:
  - A. Psychogenic vomiting
  - B. Increased intracerebral pressure (subdural effusion or hematoma, cerebral edema or tumor, hydrocephalus, meningoencephalitis, Reye's syndrome)
  - C. Vascular (migraine, severe hypertension)
  - D. Seizures
  - E. Vestibular disease, "motion sickness"

II. Stimulation of chemoceptive trigger zone:
  - A. Drugs: opiates, ipecac, digoxin, anticonvulsants
  - B. Toxins
  - C. Metabolic products (acidemia, ketonemia, hyperammonemia, uremia, etc.):
    - Acidemia, ketonemia (diabetic ketoacidosis, lactic acidosis, phenylketonuria, renal tubular acidosis)
    - Aminoacidemia (tyrosinemia, hypervalinemia, hyperglycinemia, lysinuria, maple syrup urine disease)
    - Organic acidemia (methylmalonic acidemia, proprionic acidemia, isovaleric acidemia)
    - Hyperammonemia (Reye's syndrome, urea cycle defects)
    - Uremia (renal failure)
    - Other (hereditary fructose intolerance, galactosemia, fatty acid oxidation disorders, diabetes insipidus, adrenal insufficiency, hypercalcemia, hypervitaminosis A)

III. Stimulation of peripheral receptors and/or obstruction of the gastrointestinal tract:
  - A. Pharyngeal: gag reflex (sinusitis secretions, post-tussive, self-induced, rumination)
  - B. Esophageal:
    - Functional: reflux, achalasia, other esophageal dysmotility
    - Structural: stricture, ring, atresia, etc.
  - C. Gastric:
    - Peptic ulcer disease (incl. Zollinger-Ellison syndrome), infection, dysmotility/gastroparesis
    - Obstruction (e.g., bezoar, pyloric stenosis, web, chronic granulomatous disease, eosinophilic gastroenteritis)
  - D. Intestinal:
    - Infection, enteritis, enterotoxin, appendicitis
    - Dysmotility (e.g., metabolic or diabetic neuropathy; intestinal pseudo-obstruction)
    - Nutrient intolerance (e.g., cow's milk, soy, gluten, eosinophilic enteropathy)
    - Obstruction (e.g., atresia, web, stenosis, adhesions, bands, volvulus, intussusception, superior mesenteric artery syndrome, duplication, meconium plug, meconium ileus, Hirschsprung's disease, distal intestinal obstruction syndrome in cystic fibrosis)
  - E. Hepatobiliary, pancreatic: hepatitis, cholecystitis, pancreatitis, cholelithiasis
  - F. Cardiac: intestinal ischemia
  - G. Renal: pyelonephritis, hydronephrosis, renal calculi, glomerulonephritis
  - H. Respiratory: pneumonia, otitis, pharyngitis, sinusitis, common cold
  - I. Miscellaneous: peritonitis, sepsis, pregnancy; improper feeding techniques

Source: Modified from Orenstein SR. Vomiting and regurgitation. In: Kleigman RM, ed. *Practical Strategies in Pediatric Diagnosis and Therapy.* Philadelphia: WB Saunders Company, 1996:301–331.

Table 3 Differential Diagnosis of Irritability and Pain from Esophagitis

Infants: Nonspecific irritability	Older children: Chest or epigastric pain or dysphagia
"Colic"	Cardiac pain
Parent-infant dysfunction	Pulmonary, mediastinal, chest well pain (e.g., costochondritis)
Nutrient intolerance	Nonesophagitis upper gastrointestinal inflammation
Otitis	Peptic ulcer disease
Urinary tract infection	Pancreatitis
Miscellaneous other causes	Hepatitis, cholangitis, cholecystitis, cholelithiasis
	Nonesophagitis dysphagia
	Functional, malingering

drate intolerance (both diagnosed and treated by a formula change) and tobacco smoke exposure.

For Stricture

Esophageal stenotic lesions in childhood may be congenital (and only recognized when the older child begins to ingest solid food), eosinophilic, or due to reflux disease (27,28). The clinical situation will identify other strictures as due to caustic ingestions, epidermolysis bullosa dystrophica, or anastomotic stricturing after repair of esophageal atresia, but reflux can also impede the healing of caustic or anastomotic strictures, and must be kept in mind even if GERD is not the primary cause of a stricture (17). Primary reflux strictures tend to be in the distal to mid-esophagus, may range in length from web-like to several centimeters, and often have an irregular and eroded surface radiographically. The histology of the epithelium just distal to the stricture usually reveals reflux changes (see below), but distinguishing nonreflux eosinophilic strictures may be a challenge (89).

For Barrett's Esophagus

Barrett's esophagus is an endoscopic and histological diagnosis, requiring goblet cell metaplasia in the esophagus. Previously, when gastric cardiac epithelium was also encompassed by the diagnosis, distinguishing Barrett's esophagus from hiatal hernia could be difficult.

For Nasopharyngeal Symptoms

Otitis, otalgia, sinusitis, rhinitis, and chronic sore throat have only recently been considered possibly to be related to GERD; the infectious, allergic, anatomical, and irritant causes previously assumed responsible for these symptoms definitely remain in the differential diagnoses (39). Multiple causes may be responsible in a single child.

For Upper-Airway Symptoms

For Laryngitis, Hoarseness

Trauma due to ''voice abuse,'' exposures to irritants like tobacco smoke, infections, and allergic causes for laryngitis may also contribute to these laryngeal symptoms (39).

For Subglottic Stenosis

Trauma and infection are other causes of subglottic stenosis (39).

For Infantile Apnea (Bradycardia, SIDS, ALTE)

Infantile apnea includes *central* apnea, in which respiratory efforts cease, and *obstructive* apnea, in which respiratory efforts continue but are ineffectual in moving air because of airway obstruction, often at the level of the larynx. Monitored premature infants display central ''apnea of prematurity,'' which usually responds to therapy with theophylline or caffeine, both of which treatments theoretically worsen GERD. Older prematures and full-term infants, however, may manifest obstructive apnea as a presentation of GERD. Infants monitored for cardiac rhythm and chest wall movement, but not for nasal air flow, may reveal GERD-associated obstructive apnea only by bradycardia, which results from the hypoxemia caused by the airway obstruction. This bradycardia must be distinguished from physiological bradycardia occurring in association with the presumed increased vagal tone at mealtime, as well as from more pathological variants due to primary cardiac or brainstem disease (90). It is unclear whether GERD is ever manifested as central apnea (91).

Older infants at home may manifest GERD as an ALTE or SIDS—although GERD is responsible for about one-fifth of these, the differential diagnosis is large and challenging to establish in retrospect, after a single episode witnessed by anxious parents (Table 4) (46,92). It includes sepsis, respiratory infections such as pertussis, anatomical lesions such as laryngeal cysts, and metabolic disease. I have found a careful clinical history to be crucial in distinguishing among the possible causes. It is likely that restriction of breathing contributes to the apnea in those babies who become apneic in the ''scrunched'' seated position, which also favors reflux (62).

The differences between GERD-associated infant apnea and SIDS have been highlighted by the current recommendations for normal infants to sleep supine (93–95). SIDS is a syndrome with multiple etiologies, the most common

Table 4 Infants with an ALTE (January 1983 to 1990; $n = 3799$)

Diagnosis	N	%
1. Known Cause		
Digestive	1107	47
Gastroesophageal reflux	770	
Infection	152	
Aspiration	105	
Malformations	75	
Dumping syndrome	5	
Neurological	683	29
Vasovagal syndrome	376	
Epilepsy	150	
Infection	150	
Subdural hematoma	5	
Malformation	2	
Respiratory	353	15
Infection	275	
Airway abnormality	74	
Alveolar hypoventilation	4	
Cardiovascular	82	3.5
Infection	35	
Cardiomyopathy	18	
Arrhythmia	18	
Congenital malformation	11	
Metabolic and Endocrine	59	2.5
Hypoglycemia	23	
Hypocalcemia	12	
Food intolerance	10	
Reye	6	
Hypothyroidism	2	
NEFA metabolism deficiency	2	
Leigh syndrome	1	
Carnitine	1	
Menkes syndrome	1	
Fructosemia	1	
Miscellaneous	71	3
Accidents	39	
Sepsis	11	
Munchausen by proxy	8	
Nutritional error	7	
Drug effect	6	
Total	2355	62
2. Cause Unknown		
Apparently minor incident	874	23
Apparently severe incident (idiopathic ALTE)	570	15
Total	1444	38

of which is probably rebreathing of CO_2 or suffocation, due to lying face down in puffy bedding (96–98). Some infants may have inadequate muscular ability to lift and turn the head from this dangerous position, and others may have congenital or developmental deficits in their ability to sense the need to do so. These factors make the interaction between prone position and puffy bedding potentially hazardous for infants.

Supine position, while evading the risk of suffocation even when hazardous bedding is present, markedly increases reflux episodes, by positioning the gastroesophageal junction below the air-fluid interface in the stomach. The American Academy of Pediatrics' recommendations in favor of supine position for normal infants (''back to sleep'') was promulgated as a simpler public health message than ''avoid puffy material in the baby's bed.'' Infants with GERD, however, deserve the marked benefits that prone sleeping provides, and physicians can take the extra time to clarify that the prone position's safety is comparable to that of the supine position if a firm mattress with a tight sheet is used and puffy materials are excluded from the crib. (Elimination of all tobacco smoke from the environment has marked benefits for both SIDS and GERD, a fact to stress to parents anxious to avoid the dangers of both.)

Spasmodic Croup, Episodic Stridor

Infectious epiglottitis (causing acute airway obstruction by an inflamed and enlarged epiglottis), allergic laryngeal inflammation, infectious croup (causing subglottic inflammation and narrowing), psychologically induced laryngospasm, and developmental laryngotracheomalacea may all present with stridor or apnea resembling GERD induced laryngeal disease. Several causes may coexist: 17% of children with laryngomalacea have a second airway lesion synchronously (39).

For Lower-Airway Symptoms

Recurrent Pneumonia

Cystic fibrosis, immunodeficiency, tracheoesophageal fistula, immotile cilia syndrome, and aspiration during swallowing must be considered in the differential diagnosis of the child presenting with recurrent pneumonia.

Cough

Chronic cough comprehensively studied in 72 children with symptoms persisting longer than 1 month and normal chest radiography was due to cough-variant asthma (32%), sinusitis (23%), GERD (15%), tracheal compression from aberrant innominate artery (12%), and psychogenic cough tic (10%) (53).

Bronchospasm

Wheezing or cough may be the symptomatic presentation of asthma. While foreign body aspiration and anatomical abnormalities must be considered in the young child, allergic and infectious provocations must be considered in children at all ages.

Differentiating Eosinophilic Esophagitis from GERD

Eosinophilic esophagitis is an entity that is just beginning to be identified as distinct from GERD (99). It may present with similar symptoms of pain or vomiting, and occasionally manifests as esophageal stricture. Because eosinophilic infiltration of the esophageal epithelium was identified as a marker for GERD (100), this entity was previously subsumed under GERD esophagitis, but it has become clear that it should be distinguished from it (89). It has a strong male preponderance, is associated with food allergy in up to half of patients, and manifests a furrowed or ringed endoscopic appearance rather than mucosal breaks. Many of the patients have eosinophilic infiltration elsewhere in the gastrointestinal tract, and the density of eosinophilic infiltration in the esophagus is greater than it is in reflux esophagitis. While acid suppression may improve the symptoms of eosinophilic esophagitis, it generally does not give complete relief. Identification and differentiation of this entity from GERD requires histological sampling from esophagus, stomach, and duodenum in individuals endoscoped for GERD symptoms.

DIAGNOSIS, TESTING

For Vomiting

Trial of Dietary Therapy

Normalizing meal volumes in infants receiving abnormally large amounts and thickening feedings to reduce the meal volume further and to minimize regurgitant reflux (101) are useful therapeutic maneuvers prior to formal investigation in infants suspected to have GERD. A trial of an elemental formula for 2 weeks also identifies those infants with allergic emesis (102).

Barium Fluoroscopy (Upper-Gastrointestinal Radiography, UGI)

Any child with GERD manifesting as vomiting should have UGI prior to pharmacotherapy. This precaution is not to confirm the diagnosis of GERD, but to eliminate congenital anatomical (and potentially lethal) malformations such as malrotation from consideration (103). It may also disclose the occasional hiatal hernia or unsuspected esophageal stricture. A paper in the radiological literature has proposed double-contrast esophageal radiography combined with nonendoscopic biopsy for the diagnosis of GERD (104).

Ultrasonography for Pyloric Stenosis

If pyloric stenosis is the primary consideration in the differential diagnosis, ultrasonography may confirm it, but it does not eliminate malrotation or other anatomical abnormalities from consideration, and it does not distinguish pyloric stenosis requiring pyloromyotomy from that due to eosinophilic gastroenteritis, which may respond to diet manipulation alone (105). In the vomiting infant, I therefore prefer fluoroscopy to ultrasonography, and frequently also utilize a dietary trial.

For Esophagitis

Considerable debate has taken place about the relative merits of endoscopic visualization versus histological assessment in the diagnosis of esophagitis. This debate is particularly relevant to pediatric patients.

Endoscopic Evaluation

Endoscopic visualization is useful for identifying lesions in the differential diagnosis of esophagitis, particularly gastroduodenal lesions and *Helicobacter pylori*. It is also useful when endoscopic therapy, of bleeding lesions or stenotic lesions, may be needed. Finally, adequate sampling to identify Barrett's esophagus is best achieved endoscopically.

In children, the differential diagnosis of reflux esophagitis is recognized to encompass eosinophilic esophagitis (89) and eosinophilic gastroenteritis, conditions diagnosed most accurately by histology. Thus most pediatric gastroenterologists obtain histological sampling of every child endoscoped for diagnosis of esophagitis, even when no mucosal breaks are present (106,107).

Furthermore, most infantile GERD lacks endoscopic erosions despite a high prevalence, roughly 65%, of histological changes in infants with GERD (108,109), and few endoscopically diagnosable lesions are in the differential diagnosis of infantile GERD. In addition, the aim of achieving adequate sedation for good visualization, without compromising the patient's safety, is more difficult to achieve in infants than in older children (110). These considerations have prompted some pediatric gastroenterologists to forgo endoscopic visualization in young infants because of the simplicity of obtaining biopsies nonendoscopically (111–113).

Histology

The histological parameters of reflux ''esophagopathy'' in children include the morphometric parameters of papillary lengthening and basal layer thickening, and the inflammatory cell indicators including "squiggle" lymphocytes and eosinophils. Normal infants and young children have papillary heights <53% of the total epithelial thickness, and basal layer thickness <25% of the total epithelial thickness (114), values similar to normals in adults. Papillary lengthening correlates with pH probe data, particularly the total daily esophageal acid exposure, with a nearly identical slope to that found in adults, although the pH probe data predicts only ~10% of the variability of papillary height in both infants and adults (Fig. 10) (70). These morphometric measures lend themselves especially well to objective and quantitative assessment, particularly on well-oriented, non-endoscopic, suction biopsies (115).

The inflammatory cell markers, while the focus of histological analysis in adults because of their accessibility on poorly oriented endoscopic grasp biopsies, are less sensitive markers for reflux disease in children than the morphometric parameters. Eosinophils, previously considered as a sensitive and specific marker for reflux disease, are not very sensitive compared to morphometric parameters, and are not specific enough to distinguish reflux disease from primary eosinophilic esophagitis (89), though they are increased in babies who are older and who have greater papillary height (116).

Whether dilated intercellular spaces, newly identified as a marker for reflux esophagitis (117), will be so in children as well awaits investigation.

A summary proposal for diagnosis and management of pediatric esophagitis has been developed by a European pediatric gastroenterology group (118).

For Nasopharyngeal and Upper- and Lower-Airway Symptoms

Extraesophageal (airway) symptoms of GERD require testing tailored to the symptom.

Modified Barium Swallow

The "cookie swallow" or modified barium esophagogram allows the clinician to examine various aspects of food ingestion if airway penetration during swallowing, rather than during reflux, is suspected (119). Velopalatal insufficiency and laryngeal penetration can be observed. The study is often performed jointly by a speech pathologist and a radiologist, and swallowing function is evaluated with different textures and under different conditions.

Scintigraphy

Nuclear medicine evaluation of children suspected to have GERD has developed from a simple scintigraphic study in which occasional images were obtained after a radiolabeled meal to a variety of tailored studies examining various aspects of upper-digestive-tract function. Its ability to detect postprandial reflux, prior to acidification of the gastric contents, makes it particularly relevant to children. However, the requirement to remain still during the imaging makes it particularly challenging for them.

Reflux scintigraphy currently monitors a child for several hours following a (usually liquid) meal labeled with technetium 99m. Because the half-life of this radioisotope is about 6 h, the study cannot examine an entire day, as the pH probe can do, but continuous monitoring for a somewhat briefer time is feasible. Formatting the resulting images at varying durations (from a few seconds to a number of minutes, for example) changes the sensitivity of the study for reflux episodes of varying durations. The study is particularly sensitive for nonacid and larger-volume reflux episodes (120,121).

Overnight reflux scintigraphy may be more sensitive for reflux with aspiration in children suspected to have nocturnal supine reflux and inadequate pulmonary protective function. It does not have wide utilization at present.

Radionuclide salivagram is particularly useful in identifying aspiration during swallowing (122).

Gastric emptying may be assessed during reflux scintigraphy, to determine whether delayed emptying is part of the pathophysiology of GERD in a particular child. It is frequently performed prior to fundoplication, to assess the need for concurrent pyloroplasty (123). A dual-labeled meal, in which solid and liquid components are differentially labeled, can distinguish the slower solid-phase emptying, often combined with faster liquid emptying, characteristic of vagal dysfunction or inadvertent vagotomy during fundoplication.

Laryngobronchoscopy

Visualization of laryngeal changes associated with GERD suggests reflux as pathogenetic and also eliminates other laryngeal abnormalities in the differential diagnosis. The GERD-associated changes include posterior erythema involving the arytenoids and posterior commissure, pachydermia involving the same area, vocal cord nodules (although these are probably more often due to ''voice abuse'' in children), contact ulcers and granulomas on the vocal process of the arytenoids, and laryngeal stenosis. Most of these findings, however, have several potential pathogenic factors, of which GERD is one. Utilization of a small flexible fiberoptic scope in young children allows observation of the dynamic functions of the larynx during spontaneous respiration, and facilitates diagnosis of laryngomalacia.

Bronchoscopy allows similar assessment of the lower airway and sampling of secretions, which can be evaluated for lipid-laden macrophages or lactose, which imply aspiration (124–126).

pH Probe

Quantification and characterization of the 24-h esophageal acid exposure seems somewhat less useful than previously, although it still provides helpful information and is fairly widely used (127). Various scoring systems have been advocated as a means to distinguish children whose GERD is responsible for their respiratory disease (Table 5). Pediatric gastroenterologists identified a score using the number of reflux episodes and the number of episodes longer than 5 min as selecting children with GERD pathogenic for pulmonary disease or apnea (128). A pediatric surgical group has proposed the ''ZMD,'' or ''mean duration of reflux episodes during sleep,'' as a diagnostic criterion to distinguish those infants whose apneic episodes are due to reflux from those with other causes (129). Similar to work in adult patients, advocates of dual probes identify increased upper-esophageal-acid exposure as an important marker for extraesophageal GERD, and even pharyngeal and tracheal monitoring have been proposed, although concern about technical aspects remains.

Bernstein Test

A modification of the original Bernstein test, using experimental esophageal infusion of acid to generate the proposed GERD-associated symptom, has been used for asthma and for stridor (51,76).

Table 5 pH Probe Scoring Systems: Respiratory Symptoms Due to GERD

RI (reflux index, i.e., percent of total time with pH < 4)
Score $> \sim 10\%$
AUC (area ''under'' the curve of pH 4)[a]
Score > 20 (pH units) (min)/h
No. episodes/day + 4 (No. episodes > 5 min/day)[b]
Score > 50
ZMD (mean duration of reflux during sleep)[c]
Score $> \sim 4$ min

[a] Vandenplas Y, Franckx GA, Pipeleers MM, Derde MP, Sacre SL. Area under pH 4: advantages of a new parameter in the interpretation of esophageal pH monitoring data in infants. J Pediatr Gastroenterol Nutr 1989; 9: 34–39.

[b] Euler AR, Byrne WJ. Twenty-four-hour esophageal intraluminal pH probe testing: a comparative analysis. Gastroenterology 1981; 80:957–961.

[c] Johnson DG, Jolley SG, Herbst JJ, Cordell LJ. Surgical selection of infants with gastroesophageal reflux. J Pediatr Surg 1981; 16:587–594.

Flexible Endoscopic Evaluation of Swallowing with Sensory Testing (FEESST)

This exquisite testing protocol evaluates the pathogenesis of defective airway protection, using puffs of air applied to the arytenoids to quantify deficits in reflexive airway closure (81,119). Developed in adults, it is being applied to children in an exploratory way currently (JE Aviv, personal communication, 1998). Like the modified esophagogram and the radionuclide salivagram, it characterizes defective airway protection rather than reflux, thus indicating patients who may be aspirating during swallowing as well as during reflux.

For Apnea

Pneumocardiogram (±pH Probe)

Polysomnography, in which cardiac impulses, chest wall movement, and pulse oximetry are combined (see Fig. 6), is used to identify apneic episodes in infants, and to distinguish them from other causes of cyanotic or other ''spells'' (130). To differentiate between obstructive and central apnea, a measure of airflow at the nares is also required, and obtained by nasal thermistor or nasal measurement of end-tidal CO_2. Infants who have had several apneic events may benefit from further characterization by such polysomnography, particularly if the events have been at a frequency to make them likely to occur during a 24-h testing period (46,131). When GERD is in the differential diagnosis, such testing is frequently combined with pH probe testing, to facilitate correlation of apneic events and reflux events (132).

Such testing is frequently frustrating, and less definitive than hoped. The normal infant diet of milk formula every 3 or 4 h buffers the gastric contents for much of the day, particularly postprandially, when reflux-associated apnea is likely to occur. Pediatric gastroenterologists have adapted the pH probe study to this challenge by feeding apple juice (pH 3.5–4.0), either for all the meals or for alternate meals; this markedly increases reflux detection, and probably also increases reflux frequency itself. The acid apple juice feedings themselves make some young prematures apneic! It is questionable in many cases whether the somewhat invasive pH probe evaluation provides more helpful diagnostic information than a very careful history combined with a willingness to use empirical therapy.

Bernstein Test

The modified Bernstein test has been proposed as a useful tool for evaluation of infants with apnea (133).

Role of pH Probe

Much has been written recently regarding the role of the pH probe in pediatric GERD (134). Several professional societies have published guidelines for its use in children (135,136).

Infant Feeding Type

The issue of milk versus acid feedings identified above has prompted the development of an acidified, but noncurdled, milk formula, but it is not widely used (137). The differing amount of reflux promoted by breast versus milk formula feedings has also been identified (138).

Distal Esophageal Probe Placement

Optimal placement of distal esophageal pH probes is more challenging in children because of the huge variability of size, and several regression equations have been developed to relate pH probe length to patient height or to crown-rump length (Fig. 12) (139).

Other Probe Placement—Proximal Esophageal, Pharyngeal, Tracheal

As noted above, alternative placements have been suggested when the focus is on extraesophageal manifestations of GERD (140).

Scoring

Several scoring methods have been contrasted, with no clear optimal method (134). The ''area under the curve'' (AUC), aimed at quantifying both the duration of acid exposure and the intensity of the exposure, has conceptual merit, but requires computerized quantification, and definitive validation as a useful measure (141).

"Drifting Onsets"

pH drops with drifting onsets were previously considered to be artifacts, but they likely represent a distinct mechanism of slow, seeping reflux (142).

Alkaline Reflux

As in adults, the importance of duodenogastroesophageal reflux, characterized as alkaline reflux, has been debated (143). Some have proposed the relative rigor of identifying bilirubin-containing reflux in place of alkaline reflux, which may

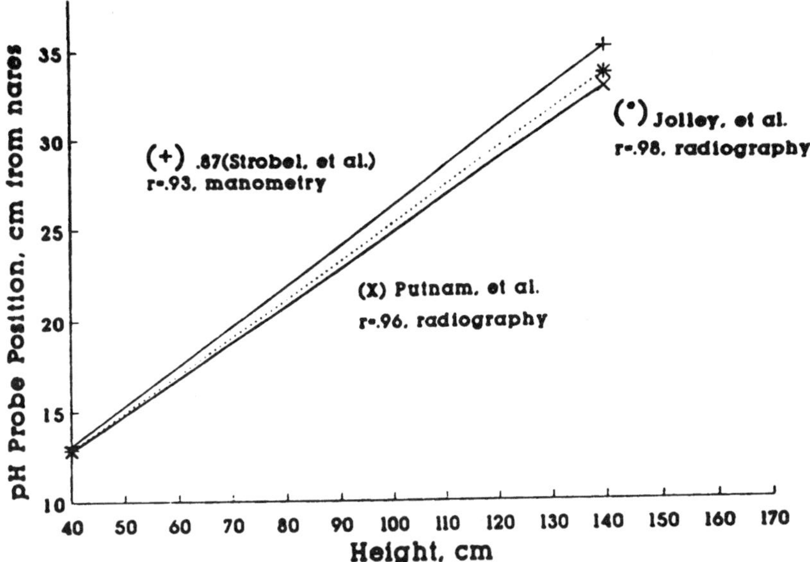

Figure 12 Regression equations associating esophageal length to height in children of various sizes. Three separate studies have confirmed a fairly constant ratio between a child's height (''Height, cm'') and the esophageal length, which is proportionate to the optimal location for pH probe position (''pH Probe Position, cm from nares''). Each line designates a linear regression found in a published study; the method for determining the esophageal length is indicated on the graph following each regression coefficient (*r*). (From Putnam PE, Orenstein SR. Crown-rump length and pH probe length: author's reply. J Pediatr Gastroenterol Nutr 1992; 15:222–223. Reproduced with permission.)

be artifactually increased by swallowed saliva and artifactually decreased by mixing with gastric acid.

New Modalities

Ultrasonography

Proposed as a method to identify reflux noninvasively and without radiation exposure, this method awaits validation (144). Ultrasound has also been utilized to quantify gastric emptying, so it could have a dual function similar to scintigraphy, but without radiation exposure, which is particularly important for young children (145).

Intraluminal Impedance and Electrical Impedance Tomography

These novel techniques are in very early stages of validation but are intriguing (146,147).

Role of Symptom Questionnaires and Empirical Therapy

Symptom questionnaires have just begun to be evaluated for their diagnostic validity in children, particularly in the infant age group (148). The noninvasive nature of questionnaires is particularly appealing for these vulnerable patients.

Empirical therapy as a diagnostic test for reflux disease causing a particular symptom has been examined in adults, but not in children. However, it is clinically used in children, following the adult models. Its optimal role also awaits definition.

Testing Prior to Surgical Therapy

Children referred for fundoplication require upper-gastrointestinal radiography to define anatomy. Many surgeons like to evaluate pediatric patients with gastric-emptying scans to assess the need for pyloroplasty, and some also utilize manometry to identify children for whom a tight wrap might produce dysphagia.

TREATMENT

Conservative, Life-Style

General Feeding Practices

Because the volumes of infant meals are so close to the limits of their gastric capacity, any feeding practices that increase those volumes (such as less frequent meals) provoke reflux. Infants and older children should avoid acidic beverages, which include most drinks other than milk or water (149). Breast feeding seems to improve clearance of reflux episodes, but it is unlikely that the choice to breast-feed an individual infant will be modulated by considerations of reflux treatment (138). The type of infant formula, including whether it contains medium chain triglycerides, may affect gastric emptying, but no clear benefit in minimizing reflux has been proven (150,151).

Because of the similarity of symptoms of GERD to those of formula protein intolerance (allergy), a 2-week trial of hypoallergenic formula is a useful diagnostic test (102). Alimentum and Pregestamil are two comparable casein hydralysate formulas that are hypoallergenic because of their oligopeptides; Neocate, containing amino acids as the protein source, is even more hypoallergenic, and even more expensive. Because a large proportion of babies sensitive to cow's milk will demonstrate sensitivity to soy protein, a time-consuming 2-week trial of soy formula is inefficient in management of the baby with significant symptoms.

Thickening

Adding dry rice cereal to milk formula for infants produces tremendous benefits for the infant with regurgitant reflux, particularly if caloric loss is generating weight deficits. The simple dietary adjustment of adding 1 tablespoon (15 mL) per ounce (30 mL) of milk formula reduces emesis (to about one-third of prethickened frequency and daily volume), increases the caloric density of the meal (from 20 cal/oz to 30 cal/oz), and decreases caloric expenditure in crying (101). The use of rice cereal in this way makes babies fatter and can induce constipation, and has no effect on nonregurgitant reflux.

Recently, commercial production of prethickened formulas provides similar benefits, while retaining the ideal caloric distribution of breast milk. As formulated, these prethickened milk formulas do not provide increased caloric density, however.

Positioning

In contrast to formula thickening, positioning may not change regurgitation, but has marked effects on nonregurgitant reflux. The flat supine position and the semisupine seated position markedly increase reflux frequency and duration in infants, and should be avoided in babies with reflux (see Fig. 9) (62). The seated position may induce oxygen desaturation in term infants, an effect even more pronounced in prematures, who have much more limited torso tone. I have evaluated multiple infants who became apneic in car seats, some to the point of requiring resuscitation. The commercial availability of nonseated car restraints may save these babies from succumbing to GERD while being protected from injury in an automobile (152).

Contrary to expectations, elevation of the head of the bed for infants positioned prone provides no significant additional benefit (61). Rather obviously, the head-down positions utilized for chest physiotherapy worsen reflux.

The issues of positioning in the era of ‘‘back to sleep’’ to minimize SIDS have been discussed above.

Elimination of Tobacco Smoke Exposure

As in adults, exposure to tobacco smoke worsens reflux in infants, and has been shown to be a risk factor for pediatric esophagitis (153). Even prenatal exposure to cigarettes is associated with obstructive sleep apnea (154); the role of reflux as a potential intermediary is unknown. Tobacco smoke exposure has multiple other risks for infants and children, including increasing risks of SIDS, asthma, pneumonia, and eventual lung cancer, so its strong proscription when an infant presents with symptoms of GERD has many potential benefits (155).

Pharmacotherapy

Pharmacotherapy (Table 6) is utilized for children with GERD that does not respond adequately to conservative measures. Because pediatric GERD is more a disorder of motility and less a disorder of acid, compared to adult GERD, prokinetic pharmacotherapy has precedence, particularly in the young child and the child with regurgitation predominating over pain. Pediatric studies have not adequately addressed the relative benefits of prokinetic, acid-suppressive, or combination therapy for children.

A great challenge facing practitioners prescribing pharmacotherapy for pediatric GERD is the very limited data available to rationalize such prescription, in terms of efficacy, safety, and dosing. This data gap was partially caused by concerns about the liability for studying these most vulnerable patients, but left pediatricians with the greater danger of prescribing unstudied drugs for young children who needed therapy. The recent Federal Drug Administration Modernization Act rewards pharmaceutical manufacturers for rectifying this dearth of data. The importance of this type of investigation is highlighted by recent work suggesting that young children often need much higher dosing on a per-kilogram-of-body-weight basis than adults (156,157).

The requirement for liquid dosing of these medications, both for dose titration and to compensate for inability to swallow pills, makes the other components of liquid medications important. The tremendous amount of alcohol and sorbitol in some of these medications is of interest: a 6-kg infant treated with both cimetidine and cisapride may receive about 6.5 g sorbitol per day, for example (158).

Prokinetic

Prokinetic agents have been reviewed recently with special attention to pediatric issues (159). Prokinetic pharmacotherapy is often the foundation of antireflux pharmacotherapy in young children.

Cisapride has become the most frequently prescribed prokinetic agent because of its apparent efficacy and safety (160,161). Its efficacy may relate to effects on esophageal motility, LES tone, and gastric emptying, mediated by its enhancement of cholinergic tone (162,163).

Concern was raised in the last few years about cardiac toxicity leading to prolonged QT when cisapride is used in higher-than-recommended doses and in conjunction with drugs that impair its normal metabolism (164,165). These concerns must be put in the context of the huge number of patients treated without serious events and the preventability of most events related to toxicity. A review

Table 6 Therapy for Reflux

I. Conservative
  A. Position: prone or completely upright (avoid supine, semi-seated)
  B. Thicken infant feedings: 1 Tbsp dry rice cereal/oz formula (= 30 cal/oz, if original formula is 20 cal/oz)
  C. Fast before bedtime
  D. Avoid large meals, obesity, light clothing
  E. Avoid foods and medications that lower LES tone or increase gastric acidity:
    Fatty foods, citrus, tomato, carbonated or acid beverages, coffee, alcohol, smoke exposure
    Anticholinergics, adrenergics, xanthines (theophylline, caffeine), calcium channel blockers, prostaglandins

II. Pharmacologic*
  A. Prokinetic:
    Metoclopromide (0.1 mg/kg/dose qid: AC, HS)
      [restlessness, drowsiness, dystonic reactions—antidote: diphenhydramine]
      [(gastrointestinal obstruction, perforation, hemorrhage; pheochromocytoma; extrapyramidal risk)]
    Bethanechol (0.1–0.3 mg/kg/dose tid or qid: AC, HS)
      [cholinergic: hypotension, flushing, headache, bronchospasm, salivation, abdominal cramping]
      [(urinary or gastrointestinal obstruction, perforation, hemorrhage, recent surgery, peritonitis, hypotension, bradycardia, epilepsy, asthma, hyperthyroidism, peptic ulcer)]
    Cisopride (0.2 mg/kg/dose qid AC, HS)
      [cramping, arrhythmias]
      [(concurrent use of macrolide or antifungal antibiotics: ketoconazole, itraconazole, miconazole, troleandomycin, erythromycin, clarithromycin)]
  B. Anti-Acid:
    Cimetidine (5–10 mg/kg/dose qid AC, HS) [headache, confusion, pancytopenia, gynecomastia, cholestasis]
    Ranitidine (4–5 mg/kg/day divided bid to tid) [similar to cimetidine, less gynecomastia, more hepatitis]
    Famotidine (0.5 mg/kg/dose bid or tid; adult 40 mg HS)
    Omeprazole (0.7–3.3 mg/kg/dose qd or divide bid; adult 20 mg HS or bid)
    Antacids (0.5–1 mL/kg/dose, 3–8 times a day: 1–2 hr PC, HS) [diarrhea, constipation, rickets, aluminum or magnesium toxicity]
  C. Barrier or miscellaneous mechanism
    Sucralfate slurry (1 g in 5 to 15-mL solution, qid PC, HS)—protects against bile salts, trypsin, acid [constipation, gastric concretions, potential binding of other medications]
    Alginate-antacid (0.2–0.5 mL/kg/dose 3–8 times a day PC)

III. Surgical
    Fundoplication (complete vs. loose wrap; ± gastrostomy, ± pyloroplasty)

* Usual course is 8 weeks.
( ) = Common doses.
[ ] = Partial list of side effects.
[( )] = Partial list of contraindications.

of 22,960 patients treated with cisapride found five arrythmias, and noted that this calculates to 0.4 arrhythmias/1000 patients treated, a lower risk than 33 other drugs (166). Several other studies have emphasized the relative safety of cisapride if it is used carefully: only prescribed for pathological GERD, using established doses, and avoiding medications that impair its metabolism (167,168). It is useful to provide a handout listing the medications to be avoided concurrently.

Bethanechol is a cholinergic medication that is occasionally used. Its efficacy is unclear, and it should be avoided in asthmatics (72).

Metoclopramide is a reasonable alternative to cisapride, with a dopaminergic mechanism of action. It increases LES pressure and facilitates gastric emptying. It has a narrow therapeutic dosing range, producing central nervous system effects at doses close to the therapeutic range. Although children are more resistant to the most ominous of these effects, chronic tardive dyskinesia, it has been seen in a child given high doses chronically (169).

Domperidone is unavailable in the United States, although it has been found useful for pediatric GERD (170).

Erythromycin markedly improves gastric emptying, but has not proved very useful in GERD. It is one of the medications whose use is contraindicated in conjunction with cisapride.

Antacid

Antacids are useful for their immediate relief of acid-induced pain, and can thus be used as a diagnostic test for infant crying due to esophagitis (21). Magnesium-containing antacids may cause diarrhea, which may be useful for the infant who is constipated intrinsically or due to rice cereal used to thicken formula. Aluminum-containing antacids have the opposite effect. There is concern about toxicity of these medications (171–173) if they are used in the doses required for efficacy comparable to the H_2-receptor antagonists (174).

H_2-Receptor Antagonists (H_2RAs)

The moderate acid suppression available from this class of agent is useful for many children with GERD (175). Two-thirds or more of infants with GERD have esophagitis, prompting the addition of an H_2RA. For young children, in most of whom a four-times-daily prokinetic agent is usually used, the addition of acid inhibition in the form of a four-times-daily H_2RA simplifies administration. Currently, cimetidine also allows more rational dosing at the higher levels supported by clinical investigation (157).

Optimal pediatric dosing of ranitidine will likely require higher doses given more frequently than is currently the case (176,177).

A European study of nizatidine (178) and an American study of intravenous famotidine (179) are beginning to facilitate the use of these other H_2RAs.

Proton Pump Inhibitors (PPIs)

The frequency with which PPIs will be indicated in pediatrics is yet to be determined. It is likely that they will be particularly useful in those populations susceptible to the most severe GERD—those with chronic respiratory and neurological disability. Omeprazole is the most frequently studied PPI in children, and has shown the ability to heal esophagitis refractory to H_2RAs (180–182).

Omeprazole must be given before a meal to obtain optimal inhibition of the proton pump by activating the pump first. When one daily dose of omeprazole is used, it should be given before breakfast; when a second dose is used, it should be given before dinner. If adequate nocturnal acid suppression is not obtained by twice-daily dosing, the addition of an H_2RA may be useful, as in adults (183).

Administration of omeprazole to children unable to take a capsule or to those requiring administration of the intact granules via gastrostomy tube has been somewhat challenging, but can be done (184).

Other

Several other medications use physical properties to augment their effects. Sucralfate binds to mucosal breaks, and is thus particularly useful in erosive disease, used as a slurry. Gaviscon has a theoretical benefit of establishing a floating "barrier" on top of the gastric contents (161).

Surgical Fundoplication or Tube Feedings

Fundoplication

A recent review of nearly 7500 children treated with fundoplication provides an excellent summary of the operation (185).

Complications of the surgery include disturbances of esophageal function producing dysphagia (186) and of antroduodenal function producing dumping, gas/bloat, gastric stasis, and retching (187,188). Because of the prevalence of postfundoplication stasis, many surgeons recommend anteroplasty or pyloroplasty prophylactically (189,190).

The challenges and complications of the surgery are particularly pronounced in exactly those children who most stand to benefit from it—those with chronic neurological and respiratory disease. This fact, combined with the increasing efficacy of pharmacotherapy for GERD, have led some to favor medical over surgical therapy even for severe GERD (191). The large majority of children with GERD do not require surgery.

Preoperative evaluation is important when surgery is contemplated, because of failure to control GERD or to avoid prolonged pharmacotherapy. In addition to radiographic evaluation to assess the anatomy, various combinations of pH probe studies, esophageal manometric evaluation (192), and gastric emptying quantification have been recommended. Whether the ZMD, or ''mean duration of reflux during sleep,'' is a useful pH probe measure, whether an abbreviated pH probe study is adequate, and whether surgery should ever be done in the context of a normal pH probe study are debated (193,194). It has been suggested that one should never attempt to apply surgery to a problem that was not manageable with the powerful pharmacotherapy now available. Certainly, endoscopic evaluation for eosinophilic esophagitis is worthwhile in intractable GERD prior to fundoplication (195).

Surgery for special groups has been addressed recently. Children with severe neurological disability have received the most attention, as they are most likely to require fundoplication and most likely to suffer complications and side effects from it (196–198). Many of them will have had feeding gastrostomy tubes placed; superimposing a fundoplication later is possible for children who require it (199). Children with familial dysautonomia are also among those with particular benefit but increased morbidity from fundoplication, and methods to limit the morbidity have been summarized (200).

Premature babies have more provocative ratios between their meal volumes and their gastric volumes; many also suffer from chronic lung disease—bronchopulmonary dysplasia. Fundoplication may be particularly useful in this group also. Many of them, like the neurologically disabled, can benefit from feeding via a gastrostomy placed at the time of fundoplication for venting and for feeding (201). Esophageal atresia is also associated with chronic lung disease and may warrent fundoplication. Fundoplication in these children is often particularly challenging because of the tension already applied to the stomach to close the atretic gap (202).

Fundoplication is generally recommended for Barrett's esophagus, to provide optimal safeguards against the development of adenocarcinoma (203).

Laparoscopic fundoplication has been performed successfully even in very small children (204). Long-term efficacy of this procedure remains to be assessed; the issue of long-term function is particularly relevant for young children.

Tube Feedings

Continuous intragastric feedings have been used (infused via a gastrostomy or via a nasogastric tube) to treat reflux in children. Their efficacy is based on the elimination of the volumetric issues provoking reflux in young children. However, children treated in this way generally require pharmacotherapy in addition to the continuous tube feedings, and this therapy provides short-term benefit. Augmented protection of the esophagus from reflux of tube feedings is provided by continuous feedings into the small intestine, via a tube introduced through the nose or through a gastrostomy, and passed radiographically, endoscopically, or by gravity past the pylorus. This type of therapy for reflux has compared favorably with fundoplication, but does not allow normal oral feedings, and replacement of tubes that have migrated orad is frequently necessary (205). In contrast, a ''gastrostomy with antireflux properties'' has been described (206).

Therapy of Esophageal Strictures

Esophageal strictures due to GERD require particularly aggressive therapy. Fundoplication is usually necessary to induce long-term remission, and dilation of the stricture with balloons or bougies, under endoscopic or fluoroscopic control, is required (207–210). Even strictures from other causes, such as corrosive injury or anastomotic in esophageal atresia, often persist because of continuing acid damage due to reflux, and benefit from aggressive antireflux therapy (211). Sometimes injection of steroid into the stricture will help to heal a stricture refractory to a program of dilations (212). Some strictures are so severe that only surgical repair, using stricturoplasty, resection, or esophageal replacement, is sufficient (213).

Special Considerations for Supraesophageal GERD

Although asthma was appreciated as a complication of GERD in pediatric patients perhaps sooner than in adults, understanding of the required aggressiveness of therapy of GERD needed to reverse the asthma has progressed more rapidly in adults than in children. This has been due in part to reluctance to investigate such aggressive therapy rigorously in children who cannot as readily give informed consent. Currently pediatric therapy must be extrapolated from adult therapy, but hopefully studies will eventually allow pediatric management to be as evidence-based as that in adults. It is likely that therapy must include a PPI or fundoplication, and be carried out for months, to achieve adequate efficacy for many of the supraesophageal complications of GERD, including asthma.

Gastroesophageal reflux disease in children is prevalent and often severe, and has the potential for lifelong morbidity. Optimal recognition and treatment of GERD in this group has the greatest potential for improvement in long-term quality of life.

REFERENCES

1. Orenstein S. Infantile reflux: different from adult reflux. Am J Med 1997; 103: 114S–119S.
2. Jeffery J, Page M. Developmental maturation of gastro-oesophageal reflux in preterm infants. Acta Paediatr 1995; 84:245–250.

3. Isolauri J, Luostarinen M, Isolauri E, Reinikainen P, Viljakka M, Keyrilainen O. Natural course of gastroesophageal reflux disease: 17–22 year follow-up of 60 patients. Am J Gastroenterol 1997; 92:37–41.
4. Carre IJ. The natural history of the partial thoracic stomach (hiatus hernia) in children. Arch Dis Child 1959; 34:344–353.
5. Carre I, Astley R. The fate of the partial thoracic stomach (''hiatus hernia'') in children. Arch Dis Child 1960; 35:484–486.
6. Orenstein SR. Gastroesophageal reflux. In: Stockman J, Winter R, eds. Current Problems in Pediatrics. Chicago: Mosby Year Book Medical Publishers, 1991:193–241.
7. Booth IW. Silent gastro-oesophageal reflux: how much do we miss? Arch Dis Child 1992; 67:1325–1327.
8. Orenstein S. What are the boundaries between physiologic and pathologic reflux in relation to age in infancy? In: Giuli R, Tytgat G, DeMeester T, Galmiche J-P, eds. The Esophageal Mucosa: 300 Questions . . . 300 Answers. Amsterdam: Elsevier Science, 1994:741–745.
9. Orenstein S, Shalaby T, Cohn J. Reflux symptoms in 100 normal infants: diagnostic validity of the infant Gastroesophageal Reflux Questionnaire. Clin Pediatr 1996; 35:607–614.
10. Treem W, Davis P, Hyams J. Gastroesophageal reflux in the older child: presentation, response to treatment and long-term follow-up. Clin Pediatr 1991; 30:435–440.
11. Peeters S, Vandenplas Y. Sex ratio of gastroesophageal reflux in infancy. J Pediatr Gastroenterol Nutr 1991; 13:314.
12. Simpson H, Hampton F. Gastro-oesophageal reflux and the lung. Arch Dis Child 1991; 66:277–283.
13. Omari T, Barnett C, Snel A, Goldsworthy W, Haslam R, Davidson G, Kirubakaran C, Bakewell M, Fraser R, Dent J. Mechanisms of gastroesophageal reflux in healthy premature infants. J Pediatr 1998; 133:650–654.
14. Cucchiara S, Santamaria F, Andreotti MR, Minella R, Ercolini P, Oggero V, de Ritis G. Mechanisms of gastro-oesophageal reflux in cystic fibrosis. Arch Dis Child 1991; 66:617–622.
15. Button B, Heine R, Catto-Smith A, Phelan P, Olinsky A. Postural drainage and gastro-oesophageal reflux in infants with cystic fibrosis. Arch Dis Child 1997; 76:148–150.
16. Hassall E, Israel D, Davidson A, Wong L. Barrett's esophagus in children with cystic fibrosis: not a coincidental association. Am J Gastroenterol 1993; 88:1934–1938.
17. Chittmittrapap S, Spitz L, Kiely EM, Brereton RJ. Anastomotic stricture following repair of esophageal atresia. J Pediatr Surg 1990; 25:508–511.
18. Ravelli A, Milla P. Vomiting and gastroesophageal motor activity in children with disorders of the central nervous system. J Pediatr Gastroenterol Nutr 1998; 26:56–63.
19. Launay V, Gottrand F, Turck D, Michaud L, Ategbo S, Farriaux J. Percutaneous endoscopic gastrostomy in children: influence on gastroesophageal reflux. Pediatrics 1996; 97:726–728.

20. American Journal of Medicine (supp). (In press). Proceedings of the Second Multi-Disciplinary International Symposium on Supraesophageal Complication of Reflux Disease, Aug 6–8, 1998; Seattle.
21. Treem W. Infant colic. Pediatric Clin North Am 1994; 41:1121–1138.
22. Vandenplas Y, de Pont S, Devreker T, Peeters S, Hauser B, Goossens A. Gastroesophageal reflux (GER) as a cause for excessive crying in infants. J Pediatr Gastroenterol Nutr 1995; 21:333.
23. Berkowitz D, Naveh Y, Berant M. ''Infantile colic'' as the sole manifestation of gastroesophageal reflux. J Pediatr Gastroenterol Nutr 1997; 24:231–233.
24. Orenstein S, Putnam P, Shalaby T, Becich M, DiGiorgio C, Kelsey S. Symptoms of infantile reflux esophagitis, using validated techniques for symptoms and histopathology. Gastroenterology 1994; 106:A153.
25. Dellert S, Hyams J, Treem W, Geertsma M. Feeding resistance and gastroesophageal reflux in infancy. J Pediatr Gastroenterol Nutr 1993; 17:66–71.
26. Bedu A, Faure C, Sibony O, Vuillard E, Mougenot J, Aujard Y. Prenatal gastrointestinal bleeding caused by esophagitis and gastritis. J Pediatr 1994; 125:465–467.
27. Nihoul-Fekete C, Mitrofanoff P, Lortat-Jacob S. Les stenoses peptiques de L'oesophage chez l'enfant. Ann Pediatr 1979; 26:692–698.
28. Rode H, Millar AJW, Brown RA, Cywes S. Reflux strictures of the esophagus in children. J Pediatr Surg 1992; 27:462–465.
29. Qualman S, Murray R, McClung J, Lucas J. Intestinal metaplasia is age related in Barrett's esophagus. Arch Pathol Lab Med 1990; 114:1236–1240.
30. Hassall E. Barrett's esophagus: new definitions and approaches in children (invited review). J Pediatr Gastroenterol Nutr 1993; 16:345–364.
31. Hassall E, Dimmick JE, Magee JF. Adenocarcinoma in childhood Barrett's: case documentation and the need for surveillance in children. Am J Gastroenterol 1993; 88:282–288.
32. Hassall E. Co-morbidities in childhood Barrett's esophagus (invited review). J Pediatr Gastroenterol Nutr 1997; 25:255–260.
33. Cucchiara S, Staiano A, DiLorenzo C, et al. Esophageal motor abnormalities in children with gastroesophageal reflux and peptic esophagitis. J Pediatr 1986; 108: 907–910.
34. Berezin S, Halata MS, Newman LJ, Glassman MS, Medow MS. Esophageal manometry in children with esophagitis. Am J Gastroenterol 1993; 88:680–682.
35. Ganatra J, Medow M, Berezin S, Newman L, Glassman M, Bostwick H, Halata M, Schwarz S. Esophageal dysmotility elicited by acid perfusion in children with esophagitis. Am J Gastroenterol 1995; 90:1080–1083.
36. Aine L, Baer M, Maki M. Dental erosions caused by gastroesophageal reflux disease in children. J Dent Child 1993; 210–214.
37. Amarnath RP, Perrault JF. Rumination in normal children: diagnosis and clinical considerations (abstr). Gastroenterology 1991; 100:A25.
38. Orenstein S, Dent J, Deneault L, Lutz J, Wessel H, Kelsey S, Shalaby T. Regurgitant reflux, vs. non-regurgitant reflux, is preceded by rectus abdominis contraction in infants. Neurogastroenterol Motil 1994; 6:271–277.
39. Yellon R. The spectrum of reflux-associated otolaryngologic problems in infants and children. Am J Med 1997; 103:125S–129S.

40. Feranchak A, Orenstein S, Cohn J. Behaviors associated with onset of gastroesophageal reflux episodes in infants: prospective study using split-screen video and pH probe. Clin Pediatr 1994; 33:654–662.
41. Bauman N, Sandler A, Smith R. Respiratory manifestations of gastroesophageal reflux disease in pediatric patients. Ann Otol Rhinol Laryngol 1996; 105:23–32.
42. Burton DM, Pransky SM, Katz RM, Kearns DB, Seid AB. Pediatric airway manifestations of gastroesophageal reflux. Ann Otol Rhinol Laryngol 1992; 101:742–749.
43. Gumpert L, Kalach N, Dupont C, Contencin P. Hoarseness and gastroesophageal reflux in children. J Laryngol Otol 1998; 112:49–54.
44. de Ajuriaguerra M, Radvanyi-Bouvet M-F, Huon C, Moriette G. Gastroesophageal reflux and apnea in prematurely born infants during wakefulness and sleep. Am J Dis Child 1991; 145:1132–1136.
45. Herbst JJ, Book LS, Bray PF. Gastroesophageal reflux in the ''near miss'' sudden infant death syndrome. J Pediatr 1978; 92:73–75.
46. Kahn A, Rebuffat E, Franco P, N'Duwimana M, Blum D. Apparent life-threatening events and apnea of infancy. In: Beckerman R, Brouilette R, Hunt C, eds. Respiratory Control Disorders in Infants and Children. Baltimore: Williams & Wilkins, 1992:178–189.
47. Nielson DW, Heldt GP, Tooley WH. Stridor and gastroesophageal reflux in infants. Pediatrics 1990; 85:1034–1039.
48. Curtis D, Crain M. Aerosol regurgitation as a laryngeal-sensitizing event explaining acute laryngospasm. Dysphagia 1987; 2:93–96.
49. Chen P-H, Chang M-H, Hsu S-C. Gastroesophageal reflux in children with chronic recurrent bronchopulmonary infection. J Pediatr Gastroenterol Nutr 1991; 13:16–22.
50. Vandenplas Y. Asthma and gastroesophageal reflux (invited review). J Pediatr Gastroenterol Nutr 1997; 24:89–99.
51. Berezin S, Medow MS, Glassman MS, Newman LJ. Esophageal chest pain in children with asthma. J Pediatr Gastroenterol Nutr 1991; 12:52–55.
52. Puntis J, Smith H, Buick R, Booth I. Effect of dystonic movements on oesophageal peristalsis in Sandifer's syndrome. Arch Dis Child 1989; 64:1311–1313.
53. Holinger L, Sanders A. Chronic cough in infants and children: an update. Laryngoscope 1991; 101:596–605.
54. Greenwald M, Couper R, Laxer R, Durie P, Silverman E. Gastroesophageal reflux and esophagitis-associated hypertrophic osteoarthropathy. J Pediatr Gastroenterol Nutr 1996; 23:178–181.
55. Herbst JJ, Johnson DG, Oliveros MA. Gastroesophageal reflux with protein-losing enteropathy and finger clubbing. Am J Dis Child 1976; 130:1256–1258.
56. Cucchiara S, Bartolotti M, Minella R, et al. Fasting and postprandial mechanisms of gastroesophageal reflux in children with gastroesophageal reflux disease. Dig Dis Sci 1993; 38:86–92.
57. Kawahara H, Dent J, Davidson G. Mechanisms responsible for gastroesophageal reflux in children. Gastroenterology 1997; 113:399–408.
58. Zicari A, Corrado G, Cavaliere M, Frandina G, Rea P, Pontieri G, Cardi E, Cucchi-

ara S. Increased levels of prostaglandins and nitric oxide in esophageal mucosa of children with reflux esophagitis. J Pediatr Gastroenterol Nutr 1998; 26:194–199.
59. Stewart R, Johnston B, Boston V, Dodge J. Role of hiatal hernia in delaying acid clearance. Arch Dis Child 1993; 68:662–664.
60. Carre IJ. The natural history of the partial thoracic stomach (hiatus hernia) in children. Arch Dis Child 1959; 34:344–353.
61. Orenstein SP. Prone positioning in infant gastroesophageal reflux: is elevation of the head worth the trouble? J Pediatr 1990; 117:184–187.
62. Orenstein SR, Whitington PF, Orenstein DM. The infant seat as treatment for gastroesophageal reflux. N Engl J Med 1983; 309:760–763.
63. DiLorenzo C, Mertz H, Alvarez S, Mori C, Mayer E, Hyman P. Gastric receptive relaxation is absent in newborn infants. Gastroenterology 1993; 104:A498.
64. DiLorenzo C, Mertz H, Rehm D, Meyer E, Hyman P. Postnatal maturation of gastric response to distension in newborn infants. Gastroenterology 1994; 107:1222.
65. Jeffery H, Heacock H. Impact of sleep and movement on gastro-oesophageal reflux in healthy, newborn infants. Arch Dis Child 1991; 66:1136–1139.
66. Orenstein SR, Izadnia F, Khan S. Gastroesophageal reflux disease in children and adolescents. Gastroenterol Clin North Am 1999; 28(4):947–969.
67. Cucchiara S, Salvia G, Borrelli O, Ciccimarra E, Az-zeqeh N, Rapagiolo S, Minella R, Campanozzi A, Riezzo G. Gastric electrical dysrhythmias and delayed gastric emptying in gastroesophageal reflux disease. Am J Gastroenterol 1997; 92:1103–1108.
68. Cucchiara S, Bortolotti M, Minella R, Pagano A. Study of antro-duodeno-jejunal (A-D-J) motility in children with refractory gastro-oesophageal reflux (GOR) disease. J Pediatr Gastroenterol Nutr 1991; 13:325.
69. Vandenplas Y, Loeb H. Alkaline gastroesophageal reflux in infancy. J Pediatr Gastroenterol Nutr 1991; 12:448–452.
70. Orenstein S, Becich M, Putnam P, Shalaby T, DiGiorgio C, Kelsey S. Correlations between morphometric parameters of esophagitis and pH probe data in infants. Gastroenterology 1994; 106:A152.
71. Hosokawa M, Kosuge N, Tsukada K, Umezu R, Murata M. The evaluation of the esophageal function in newborn infants. Pediatr Res 1992; 31:108A.
72. Orenstein SR, Lofton SW, Orenstein DM. Bethanechol for pediatric gastroesophageal reflux: a prospective, blind, controlled study. J Pediatr Gastroenterol Nutr 1986; 5:549–555.
73. Rosioru C, Glassman MS, Halata MS, Schwarz SM. Esophagitis and *Helicobacter pylori* in children: incidence and therapeutic implications. Am J Gastroenterol 1993; 88:510–513.
74. Willing J, Furukawa Y, Davidson G, Dent J. Strain induced augmentation of upper oesophaeal sphincter pressure in children. Gut 1994; 35:159–164.
75. Davis RS, Larsen GL, Grunstein MM. Respiratory response to intraesophageal acid infusion in asthmatic children during sleep. J Allergy Clin Immunol 1983; 72:393–398.
76. Orenstein SR, Kocoshis SA, Orenstein DM, Proujansky R. Stridor and gastroesophageal reflux: diagnostic use of intraluminal esophageal acid perfusion (Bernstein test). Pediatr Pulmonol 1987; 3:420–424.

77. Ramet J, Egreteau L, Curzi-Dascalova L, Escourrou P, Dehan M, Gaultier C. Cardiac, respiratory, and arousal responses to an esophageal acid infusion test in near-term infants during active sleep. J Pediatr Gastroenterol Nutr 1992; 15:135–140.
78. Bauman N, Sandler A, Schmidt C, Maher J, Smith P. Reflex laryngospasm induced by stimulation of distal esophageal afferents. Laryngoscope 1994; 104:209–214.
79. Becker K, Enck P, Kuhlbusch R, Lubke H, Frieling T. Topical anesthesia selectively inhibits esophageal sensitivity without affecting tone or motility. Dysphagia 1994; 9:262.
80. Plaxico D, Loughlin G. Nasopharyngeal reflux and neonatal apnea. Am J Dis Child 1981; 135:793–794.
81. Aviv J. Sensory discrimination in the larynx and hypopharynx. Otolaryngol Head Neck Surg 1997; 116:331–334.
82. Shaker R. Airway protective mechanisms: current concepts. Dysphagia 1995; 10: 216–227.
83. Menon AP, Schefft GL, Thach BT. Airway protective and abdominal expulsive mechanisms in infantile regurgitation. J Appl Physiol 1985; 59:716–721.
84. Pickens DL, Schefft G, Thach BT. Prolonged apnea associated with upper airway protective reflexes in apnea of prematurity. Am Rev Respir Dis 1988; 137:113–118.
85. Putnam PE, Ricker DH, Orenstein SR. Gastroesophageal reflux. In: Beckerman R, Brouilette R, Hunt C, eds. Respiratory Control Disorders in Infants and Children. Baltimore: Williams & Wilkins, 1992;322–341.
86. Biller JA, Flores A, Buie T, Mazor S, Katz AJ. Tetracycline-induced esophagitis in adolescent patients. J Pediatr 1992; 120:144–145.
87. Glassman MS, Medow MS, Berezin S, Newman LJ. Spectrum of esophageal disorders in children with chest pain. Dig Dis Sci 1992; 37:663–666.
88. Poole S. The infant with acute, unexplained, excessive crying. Pediatrics 1991; 88: 450–455.
89. Orenstein S, Mousa H, Di Lorenzo C, Kocoshis S, Putnam P, del Rosario J, Sigurdsson L, Shalaby T. The spectrum of eosinophilic esophagitis in children. Gastroenterology 1998; 114:A248.
90. Suys B, De Wolf D, Hauser B, Blecker U, Vandenplas Y. Bradycardia and gastroesophageal reflux in term and preterm infants: is there any relation? J Pediatr Gastroenterol Nutr 1994; 19:187–190.
91. Beyaert C, Marchal F, Dousset B, Serres M-A, Monin P. Gastroesophageal reflux and acute life-threatening episodes: role of a central respiratory depression. Biol Neonate 1995; 68:87–90.
92. Arens R, Gozal D, Williams J, Davidson Ward S, Keens T. Recurrent apparent life-threatening events during infancy: a manifestation of inborn errors of metabolism. J Pediatr 1993; 123:415–418.
93. AAP Task Force on Infant Positioning and SIDS. Positioning and SIDS. Pediatrics 1992; 89:1120–1126.
94. Orenstein SP. Throwing out the baby with the bedding: a commentary on the A.A.P. statement on positioning and SIDS (editorial). Clin Pediatr 1992; 31:546–548.
95. Orenstein SR, Mitchell AA, Davidson Ward S. Concerning the American Academy

of Pediatrics Recommendation on Sleep Position for Infants. Pediatrics 1993; 91: 497–499.

96. Bolton D, Taylor B, Campbell A, Galland B, Cresswell C. Rebreathing expired gases from bedding: a cause of cot death? Arch Dis Child 1993; 69:187–190.
97. Gilbert-Barness E, Hegstrand L, Chandra S, et al. Hazards of mattresses, beds, and bedding in deaths of infants. Am J Forens Med Pathol 1991; 12:27–32.
98. Kemp J, Livne M, White D, Arfken C. Softness and potential to cause rebreathing: differences in bedding used by infants at high and low risk for sudden infant death syndrome. J Pediatr 1998; 132:234–239.
99. Liacouris CA, Markowitz JE. Eosinophilic esophagitis: a subset of eosinophilic gastroenteritis. Curr Gastroenterol Reports. JE Richter, ed. Pediatric Gastroenterol 1999; 1(3):253–258.
100. Winter H, Madara J, Stafford R, Grand R, Quinlan J-E, Goldman H. Intraepithelial eosinophils: a new diagnostic criterion for reflux esophagitis. Gastroenterology 1982; 83:818–823.
101. Orenstein SR, Magill HL, Brooks P. Thickening of infant feedings for therapy of gastroesophageal reflux. J Pediatr 1987; 110:181–186.
102. Forget P, Arends JW. Cow's milk protein allergy and gastro-oesophageal reflux. Eur J Pediatr 1985; 144:298–300.
103. Bissett GI, Miller C, Frush D. Pediatric imaging perspective: the vomiting infant. J Pediatr 1998; 132:306–307.
104. Bender G, Makuch R. Double-contrast barium examination of the upper gastrointestinal tract with nonendoscopic biopsy: findings in 100 patients. Radiology 1997; 202:355–359.
105. Khan S, Orenstein S. Eosinophilic gastroenteritis masquerading as pyloric stenosis. Am J Gastroenterol 1998; 93:1724.
106. Hassall E. Macroscopic versus microscopic diagnosis of reflux esophagitis: erosions or eosinophils? J Pediatr Gastroenterol Nutr 1996; 22:321–325.
107. Vandenplas Y. Reflux esophagitis: biopsy or not? J Pediatr Gastroenterol Nutr 1996; 22:326–327.
108. Shub MD, Ulshen MH, Hargrove CB, Siegal GP, Groben PA, Askin FB. Esophagitis: a frequent consequence of gastroesophageal reflux in infancy. J Pediatr 1985; 107:881–884.
109. Hyams JS, Ricci AJ, Leichtner AM. Clinical and laboratory correlates of esophagitis in young children. J Pediatr Gastroenterol Nutr 1988; 7:52–56.
110. Casteel HB, Fledorek SC, Kiel EA. Arterial blood oxygen desaturation in infants and children during upper gastrointestinal endoscopy. Gastrointest Endosc 1990; 36:489–493.
111. Putnam PE, Orenstein SR. Blind esophageal suction biopsy in children less than 2 years of age. Gastroenterology 1992; 102:A149.
112. Bern E, Mobassaleh M. Cost-effectiveness analysis of diagnostic procedures to detect esophagitis in infancy. J Pediatr Gastroenterol Nutr 1995; 21:334.
113. Friesen C, Zwick D, Streed C, Zalles C, Roberts C. Grasp biopsy, suction biopsy, and clinical history in the evaluation of esophagitis in infants 0–6 months of age. J Pediatric Gastroenterol Nutr 1995; 20:300–304.
114. Black DD, Haggitt RC, Orenstein SR, Whitington PF. Esophagitis in infants: mor-

phometric histologic diagnosis and correlation with measures of gastroesophageal reflux. Gastroenterology 1990; 98:1408–1414.
115. DiGiorgio C, Orenstein S, Shalaby T, Mahoney T, Wisniewski S, Becich M. Quantitative computer-assisted image analysis of suction biopsy in pediatric gastroesophageal reflux. Pediatr Pathol 1994; 14:653–664.
116. Orenstein S, Becich M, Putnam P, Shalaby T, DiGiorgio C, Kelsey S. Infants with esophageal epithelial eosinophils are older and have greater papillary height and basal layer thickness than those without eosinophils. Gastroenterology 1994; 106: A153.
117. Tobey N, Carlson J, Alkiek R, Orlando R. Dilated intercellular spaces: a morphological feature of acid reflux-damaged human esophageal epithelium. Gastroenterology 1996; 111:1200–1205.
118. Vandenplas Y. Reflux esophagitis in infants and children: a report from the Working Group on Gastro-oesophageal Reflux Disease of the European Society of Paediatric Gastroenterology and Nutrition. J Pediatr Gastroenterol Nutr 1994; 18:413–422.
119. Aviv J, Sacco R, Mohr J, Thompson J, Levin B, Sunshine S, Thomson J, Close L. Laryngopharyngeal sensory testing with modified barium swallow as predictors of aspiration pneumonia after stroke. Laryngoscope 1997; 107:1254–1260.
120. Orenstein SR, Klein HA, Rosenthal MS. Scintigraphic images for quantifying pediatric gastroesophageal reflux: a study of simultaneous scintigraphy and pH probe using multiplexed data and acid feedings. J Nucl Med 1993; 34:1228–1234.
121. Tolia V, Kuhns L, Kauffman RE. Comparison of simultaneous esophageal pH monitoring and scintigraphy in infants with gastroesophageal reflux. Am J Gastroenterol 1993; 88:661–664.
122. Bar-Sever Z, Connolly L, Treves S. The radionuclide salivagram in children with pulmonary disease and a high risk of aspiration. Pediatr Radiol 1995; 25:S180–S183.
123. Cannon R, Stadalnik R. Postprandial gastric motility in infants with gastroesophageal reflux and delayed gastric emptying. J Nucl Med 1993; 34:2120–2123.
124. Nussbaum E, Maggi JC, Mathis R, Galant SP. Association of lipid-laden alveolar macrophages and gastroesophageal reflux in children. J Pediatr 1987; 110:190–194.
125. Colombo J, Hallberg T. Recurrent aspiration in children: lipid-laden alveolar macrophage quantitation. Pediatr Pulmonol 1987; 3:86–89.
126. Moran JR, Block SM, Lyerly AD, Brooks LE, Dillard RG. Lipid-laden alveolar macrophage and lactose assay as markers of aspiration in neonates with lung disease. J Pediatr 1988; 112:643–645.
127. Andze GO, Brandt ML, St. Vil D, Bensoussan AL, Blanchard H. Diagnosis and treatment of gastroesophageal reflux in 500 children with respiratory symptoms: the value of pH monitoring. J Pediatr Surg 1991; 26:295–300.
128. Euler AR, Byrne WJ. Twenty-four-hour esophageal intraluminal pH probe testing: a comparative analysis. Gastroenterology 1981; 80:957–961.
129. Jolley S, Halpern L, Tunnell W, Johnson D, Sterling C. The risk of sudden infant death from gastroesophageal reflux. J Pediatr Surg 1991; 26:691–696.
130. Spitzer A, Newbold M, Alicea-Alvarez N, Gibson E, Fox W. Pseudoreflux syn-

drome: Increased periodic breathing during the neonatal period presenting as feeding-related difficulties. Clinical Pediatrics 1991; 30:531–537.

131. Poets C, Samuels M, Noyes J, Hewertson J, Hartmann H, Holder A, Southall D. Home event recordings of oxygenation, breathing movements, and heart rate and rhythm in infants with recurrent life-threatening events. J Pediatr 1993; 123:693–701.
132. Kahn A, Rebuffat E, Sottiaux M, Blum D, Yasik EA. Sleep apneas and acid esophageal reflux in control infants and in infants with an apparent life-threatening event. Biol Neonate 1990; 57:144–149.
133. Friesen C, Streed C, Carney L, Zwick D, Roberts C. Esophagitis and modified Bernstein tests in infants with apparent life-threatening events. Pediatrics 1994; 94: 541–544.
134. Friesen CA, Hayes R, Hodge C, Roberts CC. Comparison of methods of assessing 24-hour intraesophageal pH recordings in children. J Pediatr Gastroenterol Nutr 1992; 14:252–255.
135. Colletti R, Christie D, Orenstein S. Indications for pediatric esophageal pH monitoring: statement of the North American Society for Pediatric Gastroenterology and Nutrition (NASPGN). J Pediatr Gastroenterol Nutr 1995; 21:253–262.
136. Working Group of the European Society of Pediatric Gastroenterology and Nutrition. A standardized protocol for the methodology of esophageal pH monitoring and interpretation of the data for the diagnosis of gastroesophageal reflux. J Pediatr Gastroenterol Nutr 1992; 14:467–471.
137. Sutphen J, Dillard V. pH-adjusted formula and gastroesophageal reflux. J Pediatr Gastroenterol Nutr 1991; 12:48–51.
138. Heacock HJ, Jeffery HE, Baker JL, Page M. Influence of breast versus formula milk on physiological gastroesophageal reflux in healthy, newborn infants. J Pediatr Gastroenterol Nutr 1992; 14:41–46.
139. Putnam PE, Orenstein SR. Crown-rump length and pH probe length (author's reply). J Pediatr Gastroenterol Nutr 1992; 15:222–223.
140. Cucchiara S, Santamaria F, Minella R, Alfieri E, Scoppa A, Calabrese F, Franco M, Reea B, Salvia G. Simultaneous prolonged recordings of proximal and distal intraesophageal pH in children with gastroesophageal reflux disease and respiratory symptoms. Am J Gastroenterol 1995; 90:1791–1796.
141. Tovar J, Eizaguirre I. Automatic measurement of the "area under the curve" in the diagnosis of gastroesophageal reflux. J Pediatr Gastroenterol Nutr 1993; 17: 345–346.
142. Sondheimer J, Hoddes E. Gastroesophageal reflux with drifting onset in infants: a phenomenon unique to sleep. J Pediatr Gastroenterol Nutr 1992; 15:418–425.
143. Tovar J, Wang W, Eizaguirre I. Simultaneous gastroesophageal pH monitoring and the diagnosis of alkaline reflux. J Pediatr Surg 1993; 28:1386–1392.
144. Westra S, Derkx H, Taminiau J. Symptomatic gastroesophageal reflux: diagnosis with ultrasound. J Pediatr Gastroenterol Nutr 1994; 19:58–64.
145. LiVoti G, Tulone V, Bruno R, Cataliotti F, Iacono G, Cavataio F, Balsamo V. Ultrasonography and gastric emptying: Evaluation in infants with gastroesophageal reflux. J Pediatr Gastroenterol Nutr 1992; 14:397–399.
146. Skopnik H, Silny J, Heiber O, Schulz J, Rau G, Heimann G. Gastroesophageal

reflux in infants: evaluation of a new intraluminal impedance technique. J Pediatr Gastroenterol Nutr 1996; 23:591–598.
147. Ravelli A, Milla P. Detection of gastroesophageal reflux by electrical impedance tomography. J Pediatr Gastroenterol Nutr 1994; 18:205–213.
148. Orenstein SR, Cohn JF, Shalaby TM, Kartan R. Reliability and validity of an infant gastroesophageal reflux questionnaire. Clin Pediatr 1993; 32:472–484.
149. Feldman M, Barnett C. Relationships between the acidity and osmolality of popular beverages and reported heartburn. Gastroenterology 1995; 108:125–131.
150. Tolia V, Lin C-H, Kuhns L. Gastric emptying using three different formulas in infants with gastroesophageal reflux. J Pediatr Gastroenterol Nutr 1992; 15:297–301.
151. Sutphen J, Dillard V. Medium chain triglyceride in the therapy of gastroesophageal reflux. J Pediatr Gastroenterol Nutr 1992; 14:38–40.
152. Bull M, Weber K, Stroup K. Automotive restraint systems for premature infants. J Pediatr 1988; 112:385–388.
153. Shabib S, Cutz E, Sherman P. Passive smoking is a risk factor for esophagitis in children. J Pediatr 1995; 127:435–437.
154. Kahn A, Groswasser J, Sottiaux M, Kelmanson I, Rebuffat E, Franco P, Dramaix M, Wayenberg J. Prenatal exposure to cigarettes in infants with obstructive sleep apneas. Pediatrics 1994; 93:778–783.
155. American Academy of Pediatrics Committee on Environmental Health. Environmental tobacco smoke: a hazard to children. Pediatrics 1997; 99:639–642.
156. Hassall E, Israel D, Shepherd R, Radke M, Dalvag A, Junghard O, Lundborg P, The International Pediatric Omeprazole Study Group. Omeprazole for chronic erosive esophagitis in children: a multicenter study of dose requirements for healing. Gastroenterology 1997; 112:A143.
157. Lambert J, Mobassaleh M, Grand R. Efficacy of cimetidine for gastric acid suppression in pediatric patients. J Pediatr 1992; 120:474–478.
158. Feldstein T. Carbohydrate and alcohol content of 200 oral liquid medications for use in patients receiving ketogenic diets. Pediatrics 1996; 97:506–511.
159. Horn J. Use of prokinetic agents in special populations. Am J Health-Syst Pharm 1996; 53:S27–S29.
160. Cucchiara S. Cisapride therapy for gastrointestinal disease. J Pediatr Gastroenterol Nutr 1996; 22:259–269.
161. Greally P, Hampton FJ, MacFadyen UM, Simpson H. Gaviscon and Carobel compared with cisapride in gastro-oesophageal reflux. Arch Dis Child 1992; 67:618–621.
162. Cucchiara S, Staiano A, Boccleri A, De SM, Capozzi C, Manzi G, Camerlingo F, Paone F. Effects of cisapride on parameters of oesophageal motility and on the prolonged intraoesophageal pH test in infants with gastro-oesophageal reflux disease. Gut 1990; 31:21–25.
163. Vandenplas Y, deRoy C, Sacre L. Cisapride decreases prolonged episodes of reflux in infants. J Pediatr Gastroenterol Nutr 1991; 12:44–47.
164. Hill S, Evangelista J, Pizzi A, Mobassaleh M, Fulton D, Berul C. Proarrhythmia associated with cisapride in children. Pediatrics 1998; 101:1053–1056.
165. Shulman P. Report from the NASPGN Therapeutics Subcommittee (Medical Posi-

tion Paper): clsapride and the attack of the P-450s. J Pediatr Gastroenterol Nutr 1996; 23:395–397.

166. Wager E, Tooley P, Pearce G, Wilton L, Mann R. A comparison of two cohort studies evaluating the safety of cisapride: prescription-event monitoring and a large phase IV study. Eur J Clin Pharmacol 1997; 52:87–94.
167. Janssens G, Melis K, Vaerenberg M. Long-term use of cisapride (Prepulsid) in premature neonates of <34 weeks gestational age. J Pediatr Gastroenterol Nutr 1990; 11:420–422.
168. Ward R, Lemons J, Moltoni R. Cisapride: A survey of the frequency of use and adverse events in premature newborns. Pediatrics 1999; 103:469–472.
169. Putnam PE, Orenstein SR, Wessel HB, Stowe RM. Tardive dyskinesia associated with metoclopramide use in a child. J Pediatr 1992; 121:983–985.
170. Bines JE, Quinlan J-E, Treves S, Kleinman RE, Winter HS. Efficacy of domperidone in infants and children with gastroesophageal reflux. J Pediatr Gastroenterol Nutr 1992; 14:400–405.
171. Brand JM, Greer FR. Hypermagnesemia and intestinal perforation following antacid administration in a premature infant. Pediatrics 1990; 85:121–124.
172. Pivnick E, Kerr N, Kaufman R, Jones D, Chesney R. Rickets secondary to phosphate depletion: a sequela of antacid use in infancy. Clin Pediatr 1995; (February): 73–78.
173. Tsou V, Young R, Hart M, Vanderhoof J. Elevated plasma aluminum levels in normal infants receiving antacids containing aluminum. Pediatrics 1991; 87:148–151.
174. Cucchiara S, Staiano A, Romaniello G, Capobianco S, Auricchio S. Antacids and cimetidine treatment for gastro-oesophageal reflux and peptic oesophagitis. Arch Dis Child 1984; 59:842–847.
175. Kelly D. Do H2 receptor antagonists have a therapeutic role in childhood? J Pediatr Gastroenterol Nutr 1994; 19:270–276.
176. Orenstein S, Blumer J, Li B, Lavine J, Grunow J, Treem W, Czinn S, Pappa K, Williams B, Kellerman D, Ciociola A. Pediatric gastric pH data following ranitidine 75mg (abstr). Gastroenterology 1999; 116(4,Pt2):4273.
177. Fontana M, Tornaghi R, Petrillo M, Lora E, Porro GB, Principi N. Ranitidine treatment in newborn infants: effects on gastric acidity and serum prolactin levels. J Pediatr Gastroenterol Nutr 1993; 16:406–411.
178. Simeone D, Caria M, Miele E, Staiano A. Treatment of childhood peptic esophagitis: a double-blind placebo-controlled trial of nizatidine. J Pediatr Gastroenterol Nutr 1997; 25:51–55.
179. Treem W, Davis P, Hyams J. Suppression of gastric acid secretion by intravenous administration of famotidine in children. J Pediatr 1991; 118:812–816.
180. Alliet P, Raes M, Bruneel E, Gillis P. Omeprazole in infants with cimetidine-resistant peptic esophagitis. J Pediatr 1998; 132:352–354.
181. Gunasekaran T, Hassall E. Efficacy and safety of omeprazole for severe gastroesophageal reflux in children. J Pediatr 1993; 123:148–154.
182. Israel D, Hassall E. Omeprazole and other proton pump inhibitors: pharmacology, efficacy, and safety, with special reference to use in children. J Pediatr Gastroenterol Nutr 1998; 27:568–579.

183. Peghini P, Katz P, Castell D. Ranitidine controls nocturnal gastric acid breakthrough on omeprazole: a controlled study in normal subjects. Gastroenterology 1999; 115:1335–1339.
184. Sharma V, Heinzelmann E, Steinberg E, Vasudeva R, Howden C. Nonencapsulated, intact omeprazole granules effectively suppress intragastric acidity when administered via a gastrostomy. Am J Gastroenterol 1997; 92:848–851.
185. Fonkalsrud E, Ashcraft K, Coran A, Ellis D, Grosfeld J, Tunell W, Weber T. Surgical treatment of gastroesophageal reflux in children: a combined hospital study of 7467 patients. Pediatrics 1998; 101:419–422.
186. Mattox HI, Albertson D, Castell D, Richter J. Dysphagia following fundoplication: ''slipped'' fundoplication versus achalasia complicated by fundoplication. Am J Gastroenterol 1990; 85:1468–1472.
187. DiLorenzo C, Flores A, Hyman PE. Intestinal motility in symptomatic children with fundoplication. J Pediatr Gastroenterol Nutr 1991; 12:169–173.
188. Samuk I, Afriat R, Horne T, Bistritzer T, Barr J, Vinograd I. Dumping syndrome following Nissen fundoplication, diagnosis, and treatment. J Pediatr Gastroenterol Nutr 1996; 23:235–240.
189. Dunn J, Lai E, Webber M, Ament M, Fonkalsrud E. Long-term quantitative results following fundoplication and antroplasty for gastroesophageal reflux and delayed gastric emptying in children. Am J Surg 1998; 175:27–29.
190. Brown R, Wynchank S, Rode H, Millar A, Mann M. Is a gastric drainage procedure necessary at the time of antireflux surgery? J Pediatr Gastroenterol Nutr 1997; 25: 377–380.
191. Hassall E. Antireflux surgery in children: time for a harder look. Pediatrics 1998; 101:467–468.
192. Cullu F, Gottrand F, Lamblin M, Turck D, Bonnevalle M, Farriaux J. Prognostic value of esophageal manometry in antireflux surgery in childhood. J Pediatr Gastroenterol Nutr 1994; 18:311–315.
193. Eizaguirre I, Tovar JA. Predicting preoperatively the outcome of respiratory symptoms of gastroesophageal reflux. J Pediatr Surg 1992; 27:848–851.
194. Tovar JA, Angulo JA, Gorostiaga L, Arana J. Surgery for gastroesophageal reflux in children with normal pH studies. J Pediatr Surg 1991; 26:541–545.
195. Liacouras C. Failed Nissen fundoplication in two patients who had persistent vomiting and eosinophilic esophagitis. J Pediatr Surg 1997; 32:1504–1506.
196. Rice H, Seashore J, Touloukian R. Evaluation of Nissen fundoplication in neurologically impaired children. J Pediatr Surg 1991; 26:697–701.
197. Smith C, Blemann Otherson HJ, Gogan N, Walker J. Nissen fundoplication in children with profound neurological disability: high risks and unmet goals. Ann Surg 1992; 215:654–659.
198. Pearl R, Robie D, Ein S, Shandling B, Wesson D, Superina R, Mctaggart K, Garcia V, O'Connor J, Filler R. Complications of gastroesophageal antireflux surgery in neurologically impaired versus neurologically normal children. J Pediatr Surg 1990; 25:1169–1173.
199. Sulaeman E, Udall J, Brown R, Mannick E, Loe W, Hill C, Schmidt-Sommerfeld E. Gastroesophageal reflux and Nissen fundoplication following percutaneous endoscopic gastrostomy in children. J Pediatr Gastroenterol Nutr 1998; 26:269–273.

200. Udassin R, Seror D, Vinograd I, Zamir O, Godfrey S, Nissan S. Nissen fundoplication in the treatment of children with familial dysautonomia. Am J Surg 1992; 164: 332–336.
201. Jolley SG, Halpern CT, Sterling CE, Feldman BH. The relationship of respiratory complications from gastroesophageal reflux to prematurity in infants. J Pediatr Surg 1990; 25:755–757.
202. Wheatley MJ, Coran AG, Wesley JR. Efficacy of the Nissen fundoplication in the management of gastroesophageal reflux following esophageal atresia repair. J Pediatr Surg 1993; 28:53–55.
203. Hassall E, Weinstein WM. Partial regression of childhood Barrett's esophagus after fundoplication. Am J Gastroenterol 1992; 87:1506–1512.
204. Rothenberg S. Experience with 220 consecutive laparoscopic Nissen fundoplications in infants and children. J Pediatr Surg 1998; 33:274–278.
205. Albanese C, Towbin R, Ulman I, Lewis J, Smith S. Percutaneous gastrojejunostomy versus Nissen fundoplication for enteral feeding of the neurologically impaired child with gastroesophageal reflux. J Pediatr 1993; 123:371–375.
206. Stringel G. Gastrostomy with antireflux properties. J Pediatr Surg 1990; 25:1019–1021.
207. Allmendinger N, Hallisey M, Markowitz S, Hight D, Weiss R, McGowan G. Balloon dilation of esophageal strictures in children. J Pediatr Surg 1996; 31:334–336.
208. Dalzell AM, Shepherd RW, Cleghorn GJ, Patrick MK. Esophageal stricture in children: fiber-optic endoscopy and dilation under fluoroscopic control. J Pediatr Gastroenterol Nutr 1992; 15:426–430.
209. Shah MD, Berman WF. Endoscopic balloon dilation of esophageal strictures in children. Gastrointest Endosc 1993; 39:153–156.
210. Gandhi R, Barlow B. Successful management of esophageal strictures without resection or replacement. J Pediatr Surg 1994; 24:745–750.
211. Capella M, Goldberg P, Quaresma E, Araujo E, Pereima M. Persistence of corrosive esophageal stricture due to gastroesophageal reflux in children. Pediatr Surg Int 1992; 7:180–182.
212. Berenson G, Wyllie R, Caulfield M, Steffen P. Intralesional steroids in the treatment of refractory esophageal strictures. J Pediatr Gastroenterol Nutr 1994; 18:250–252.
213. Ohhama Y, Tsunoda A, Nishi T, Yamada R, Yamamoto H. Surgical treatment of reflux stricture of the esophagus. J Pediatr Surg 1990; 25:758–761.

Index